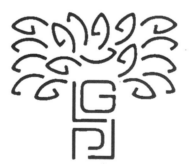

BODY CONFIDENCE

BODY CONFIDENCE

VENICE NUTRITION'S 3-STEP SYSTEM
THAT UNLOCKS YOUR BODY'S FULL POTENTIAL

MARK MACDONALD

HarperOne
An Imprint of HarperCollinsPublishers

HarperOne

Chelsea Handler Photo: Russell James for Shape *magazine. Used courtesy of* Shape *magazine.*
Mark Macdonald's After Photo: Martin Ryter
Tally Sanders's After Photo: David Robinet
Megan Hall's After Photo: Keiko Guest
All other Success Story After Photos: Chris Calhan
Graphics: Vaughan Risher
Recipes: Venice Nutrition's Chef, Valerie Cogswell

FIRST EDITION

Library of Congress Cataloging-in-Publication Data
    Macdonald, Mark (Mark Michael).
    Body Confidence : Venice Nutrition's 3-Step System That Unlocks Your Body's
Full Potential / by Mark Macdonald. — First Edition.
        p.   cm. Includes index.
    ISBN 978–0–06–199727–3
        1. Nutrition.   2. Blood sugar.   3. Food habits.   I. Title.
    RA784.M275   2011
    613.2—dc22   2010048679

11   12   13   14   15   RRD (H)   10   9   8   7   6   5   4   3   2   1

I dedicate this book to my foundation—my wife, Abbi;

and to my greatest teacher—our son, Hunter.

You both are my everything.

CONTENTS

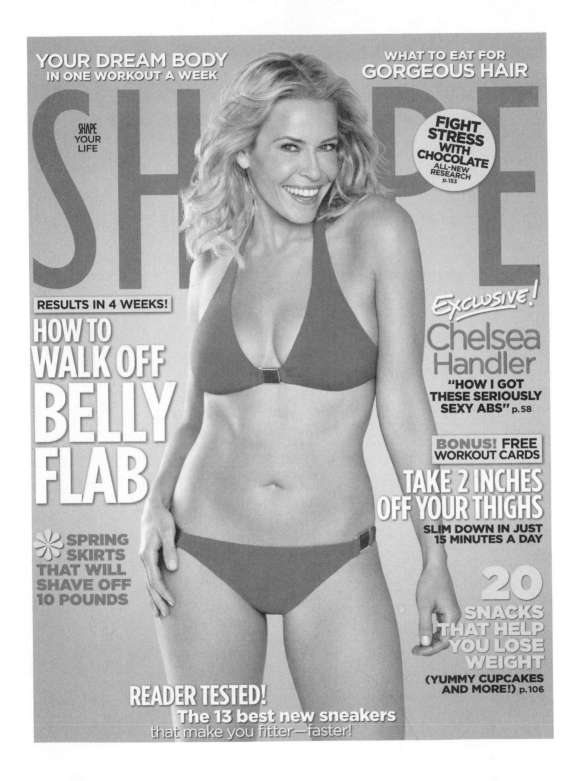

YOUR DREAM BODY
IN ONE WORKOUT A WEEK

WHAT TO EAT FOR
GORGEOUS HAIR

SHAPE

SHAPE
YOUR
LIFE

FIGHT
STRESS
WITH
CHOCOLATE
ALL-NEW
RESEARCH
p. 153

RESULTS IN 4 WEEKS!

HOW TO
WALK OFF
BELLY
FLAB

EXCLUSIVE!
Chelsea
Handler
"HOW I GOT
THESE SERIOUSLY
SEXY ABS" p. 58

BONUS! FREE
WORKOUT CARDS

TAKE 2 INCHES
OFF YOUR THIGHS
SLIM DOWN IN JUST
15 MINUTES A DAY

SPRING
SKIRTS
THAT WILL
SHAVE OFF
10 POUNDS

20
SNACKS
THAT HELP
YOU LOSE
WEIGHT
(YUMMY CUPCAKES
AND MORE!) p. 106

READER TESTED!
The 13 best new sneakers
that make you fitter—faster!

FOREWORD

I met Mark Macdonald three weeks before my twenty-seventh birthday, and he changed my life forever. I was sick of starving myself and never losing any weight, and not exactly open to the idea of cutting alcohol out of my life. After spending an hour with Mark, I realized how little I knew about food, and how many bad habits had been formed from my childhood in New Jersey.

Growing up in a household where you would find Twix bars in your nightstand, and where a bowl of freshly made macaroni and cheese was considered an after-school snack, it became clear that I had a lot of mental deprogramming to do. I was basically starving my body and weighing myself three to four times a day. I had gotten so delusional about my food that I believed a chicken wing was a more logical snack than an apple because it weighed less.

When Mark explained to me how important it was to feed your body every three to four hours, I was elated. When he told me I had to cut back on alcohol, but not eliminate it completely, I was furious.

Mark gently explained to me how the body works and showed me how much actual fat, protein, and carbohydrate was necessary for me to feel satisfied. I had no idea that a salad drenched in dressing was basically the equivalent of a piece of pizza. He broke down all the components of fueling my body and what ratios would be effective in retraining it to stop storing fat—and finally release a little. It had never occurred to me that by starving my body, it was holding on to fat.

The first time I walked out of Mark's office, I was intent on following all his directions to a tee. Within the first three days, I had more energy than I knew what to do with, I felt satisfied after every meal, and I actually began to crave working out. In the first week, I lost 2 percent body fat—but I gained three pounds. I was beside myself and had a complete breakdown in Mark's office, where he urged me to stay with the program and not worry about the number on the scale. He had warned me that, because of all the years I'd been tricking my body, I would probably gain a few pounds before I lost. But he encouraged me to focus on the fact that I had been successful in losing fat, and he reminded me about my increase in energy and workout stamina.

It was only one more week before I lost another 2 percent body fat and my body started to drop weight due to my muscle/fat ratio. My clothes all fit better than before, and my muffin top started to dissipate. I watched my body lean out everywhere: my arms, stomach, and face. It was the first time anyone in my family could claim to have a set of abs. I was euphoric and so relieved to know that my body wasn't that different from everyone else's and that there was an actual program that would work for me.

I have learned that with a busy lifestyle, it's not always easy to eat right, so it's important to get in the habit of carrying healthy options with you and filling your refrigerator with clean food. I'll prepare grilled chicken, shrimp, and turkey meatballs for the week and eat something different each day. I always have arugula salad with me, and protein powder that I mix with water for a snack at least once a day. My mind-set has changed in that I now know that I am fueling my body, and not snacking because of cravings. The healthier and leaner I am, the fewer cravings I have. I always start with protein and work my way from there. If I'm drinking, I skip heavy starches and know I can fill up on fresh steamed veggies and small amounts of fat. I eat more frequently than I've ever eaten before, and my mind and body are sharper because of it.

Since that time, I have fallen on and off Mark's nutrition plan, but he has always been there for me when I decided I didn't like the dimples forming on the back of my ass. Most recently, I posed for the cover of *Shape* magazine and worked with Mark daily to get myself back on the program and back to healthy, lean eating. It took less than a week for me to see the definition in my stomach and arms. Any cellulite on the back of my legs had completely disappeared, and I have to say, I looked borderline amazing. I did combine the nutrition with Pilates and some cardio, but in the past I'd done an hour of cardio a day without focusing on nutrition, and I didn't have the same results. I now know that the nutritional component is the most important aspect, and I know that If I want to maximize my energy level and feel great about myself in a bikini, I have to be responsible about my food. I get to drink my Belvedere, stay lean, and help my friends when they're serious about getting their bodies in better condition.

—Chelsea Handler

INTRODUCTION

In a world where we are all searching for the right answers, often without results, have you ever given thought to what the right questions are?

—Steven Clarke

I vividly remember watching my mom struggle with her weight year after year. She would start one diet, believing that she had found the solution, and then gain back everything she lost, becoming overwhelmed by feelings of failure and shame. She felt she was destined to struggle with her health and weight forever.

I remember the frustration I felt for years as an athlete when I looked for the information I needed to take my ability to another level and realized that no one had the answers. I remember the desperation I felt after my athletic career ended and how I started on a vicious cycle of weight gain followed by severe dieting alongside calorie and carbohydrate restriction. I remember the pain of living for a fitness model's physique. For years I looked great while I felt horrible. Every day I was scared that one meal or one missed workout would cause me to get fat. I remember the anger I felt when I could not find a solution for my wife, Abbi, when her world was turned upside down by what seemed like a minor injury. Over the time span of one year, Abbi's injury caused her body to deteriorate so severely that she could barely walk more than five minutes at a time without severe muscle spasms and pain. I remember the disappointment, bitterness, and loss of hope that so many people shared with me through the years as they attempted to be healthy every day and yet thought, for some reason, that they lacked the discipline to succeed.

I created Venice Nutrition because there had to be a solution for my mom, myself, my wife, and now *you.*

This book and the program it describes are my life's work. They will provide you with the answers and education you need to help you get on the path to permanently achieving your health goals and taking your Body Confidence to the next level. This is true whatever your goals, gender, or age may be. You might want to lose anywhere from five to one hundred pounds. . . . You might be an athlete or a fitness model who wants to gain weight and improve your performance. . . . You might live a busy lifestyle and frequently travel or eat in restaurants. . . . You might have a medical challenge like high cholesterol, high blood pressure, diabetes, digestive irregularities, hormonal imbalances, or autoimmune issues. . . . You might be looking for more energy. . . . You might want to eliminate your sugar cravings. . . . You might even just want to better understand how food affects your body. . . .

Simply put, this book is for you, *whatever health goal you want to achieve.*

We live in a time of available information, and a new diet or amazing solution for your health seems to appear every day. Some claim that you can achieve the body you want in two weeks through severe calorie restriction, easy ten-minute workouts, or a new magic dietary supplement. Each of these "solutions" keeps the focus on hype and is marketed to appeal to the desperation that so many feel due to their lack of results. People will try anything to overcome the challenges they have with their bodies. Millions of people hunger for information that will lead to results; they just don't know where to find it and who they can trust. I know, because I used to be one of these people, searching for answers year after year. Time and time again I thought I had found the solution, only to end up realizing that the "solution" I found was incomplete. Then I would go right back into the fray, hunting for the missing pieces to the puzzle.

You would think that finding a way to prioritize health as part of your lifestyle would be simple. Unfortunately, the reality is very different. *Until recently, there was a hole in the health industry.*

The answers that so many look for cannot easily be found, causing them to grasp for solutions that are incomplete and incorrect. I discovered this during my own journey from being a student and a college athlete to a fitness model, a personal trainer, a nutritionist, a health club manager, a wellness speaker, and, finally, a business owner. I have personally coached over thirty thousand clients. Our nutrition centers throughout the United States and the world have coached hundreds of thousands of clients. I am a believer in the power of "living the experience," since I think each experience molds an individual's purpose and ignites their passion. As I look back at my journey, it's clear that every part of my life provided me with the education I needed to create Venice Nutrition and fill the hole in the health industry. I have always wanted to know why things work, and I am relentless in my pursuit of the answers. Albert Einstein said it best: "Learn from yesterday, live for today, hope for tomorrow. The important thing is not to stop questioning."

To me, this book is much more than a nutrition and fitness program; it is the possibility for you to change your health and, as a result, change your life. I know that I can provide you with the answers you are looking for, along with the high quality of life that you desire.

To help you see this possibility, I would like to share my story with you, in the hope that you can use it to solidify your belief in the process and reinforce your commitment to your health.

Currently the industry can be seen as having two halves. One half is *medical and educational* and the other is *weight loss and fitness*. Each half has its strengths, and each has its challenges. Unfortunately, neither half represents the complete picture, nor does either half have enough information to fill the hole. Let's begin with the medical and educational half.

The nutrition education system, from the government and medical community to the universities, has been outdated for decades. The industry's current focus on BMI (body mass index), BMR (basal metabolic rate), the food pyramid, and the "calories in versus calories out" philosophy are simply not working. The evidence of this (as of 2010) can clearly be seen in the continual rise over the past thirty years in the percentage of overweight and obese adults and children throughout the United States. Simultaneously, the demand for pharmaceuticals and weight-loss programs is at an all-time high. Each year more people are seeking health advice, and yet as a society, our health continues to regress. Something is obviously broken. The Organization for Economic Cooperation and Development (OECD) released a study in 2010 stating that if the current health trends continue, 75 percent of American adults will be overweight or obese by the year 2020! Not only is this fact shocking; it reinforces Albert Einstein's wise words: "The world we've made, as a result of the level of thinking we have done thus far, creates problems we cannot solve at the same level of thinking." Now, on to the second half: weight loss and fitness. As I shared with you, I watched my mom drop and then regain fifty-plus pounds over and over again. I saw how this cycle created overwhelming sadness and stress. My mom tried many different "solutions," just as I and thousands of my clients have done. She tried every type of diet, a few being appetite suppressants; liquid, prepared food; and carbohydrate/calorie restriction. Each "solution" provided temporary results along with a sense of hope, but the trouble was that this was *false* hope. Several months later she would once again regain all of the weight and fat.

I never truly understood the pain my mom went through until I lived it myself.

In college, I was a star soccer player. My entire focus since I was a young boy had been on playing soccer. I lived and breathed the sport and was fortunate enough to accomplish the goals I set for myself. I always knew that after college I would end my soccer dream and move on to the next chapter of my life. What I did not anticipate was the void I would feel. I was a typical athlete, training four to five hours every day and eating whatever I wanted: pizza, hamburgers, French fries, soda . . . and a whole lot more. My weight challenges began the moment I stopped playing soccer. I went from an abundance of exercise to no exercise at all, and from eating unhealthy to eating extremely unhealthy. As you can guess, this was a bad combination. I felt lost and uncertain about what my next adventure would be. The escape from my fear and anxiety was food. My life became centered on the all-you-can-eat pizza and ice cream buffet. I would wake up feeling excited about eating, go to the lunch buffet and fill up, see an afternoon movie on the days I did not work, then go home for TV and bedtime, looking forward to repeating the same routine the following day. My daily life focus became food because I was addicted. I transferred my obsession with soccer to an obsession with food. I lived this way for six months, and during this time I gained sixty pounds! The scariest thing was that I didn't even realize what was happening until my wife, Abbi, filled me in.

I was standing in front of the mirror with my shirt off, and Abbi walked into the room. I had a typical male mind-set, thinking that the sixty pounds I'd put on was all muscle. (It is comical to think about how many men believe that any weight they gain is all muscle.) I turned to her and said, "Abbi, can you believe I am 250 pounds and still have a six-pack stomach?" Her expression was the same one you see when someone's going to be honest with you even though they know you won't like what they're going to say. Her look caused me some concern, so I immediately followed up with: "Look at my abs, they're right here. Can't you see the definition?" Abbi then continued to hesitate. . . . She still hadn't said anything. I was getting worried. . . . How could she not see my abdominal muscles? Was she blind? So I followed up one last time: "Abbi, come over here so you can see them in the same light." I then took her hand and rubbed it over my stomach. Her look just became more uncomfortable. She then looked at me as if she was going to tell me the worst news I had ever heard and said, "Baby, I just don't see your abs anymore." I was in shock and disbelief, and immediately thought she was kidding. . . . She then followed up with: "What do you expect when you eat pizza and ice cream buffets every single day?" Ouch! At that moment I felt like the world around me crumbled. I felt shattered. . . . How did I miss gaining sixty pounds?

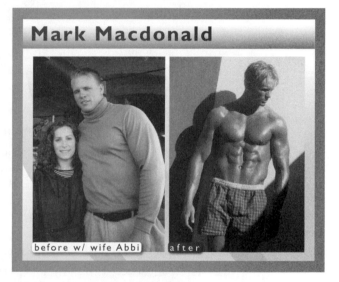

Mark Macdonald

before w/ wife Abbi   after

I reacted like most people do: with a feeling of desperation and a willingness to do anything to get the weight/fat off. I knew that the anatomy and physiology I learned in school would provide only some of the answers I was looking for, so I chose to look deeper into the weight-loss and fitness world. For years I had gravitated to this half of the health industry because the information seemed cutting-edge and more relevant than what I was learning in school. I didn't care how I got the weight off and didn't give any thought to rebounding. I just needed to get it off! After researching every method of losing weight on the market, I decided to start a ketogenic diet (a high-fat, high-protein diet with a very low intake of carbohydrates, designed specifically for fitness models), drastically cut calories (down to fifteen hundred per day), took fat-burner supplements, and exercised six days a week, at least two hours per day. I was determined and on a mission. . . . Within four months, I lost sixty pounds and 20 percent body fat!

For the next four years, my life became focused on what my body looked like and nothing else. I lived as a fitness model, nutritionist, and personal trainer. I lived in misery six days a week (the days when I ate very few carbohydrates), having severe sugar cravings, low energy, and extreme irritability.

All week, the only thing I could think of was making it to my cheat day, when I could eat whatever I wanted. The fear and anxiety I felt when I finished playing soccer were nothing compared with this amped new fear and anxiety. Though I achieved the weight and body fat that I desperately wanted, I was also in a constant state of panic about getting fat again. Every time I walked past a mirror, I would feel an urgent desire to lift up my shirt and make absolutely certain I still had a lean stomach. When I missed a workout I felt that the weight would come right back, and when Abbi wanted to eat out, I *needed* to bring my own food, not trusting myself in a restaurant.

I lived this way because this is exactly what I thought I had to do to shed my excess body fat and weight. At this time (the mid-1990s), most diet books and magazines I read focused on creating deficits through calorie and/or carbohydrate restriction, with some promoting a regimen of supplements. The saying I constantly heard from my buddies was: "If you look like crap, you feel good; if you look good, you feel like crap." All I cared about at the time was looking good, so I *believed* I had to suffer and feel deprived. Then, simultaneously, two life-changing "moments" occurred, one personal and the other professional.

My Personal "Moment"

I was the most unbalanced and the unhappiest I had ever been. I made the transition from soccer being my sole purpose to my "pizza and ice cream" phase to the overwhelming focus on my body. I would always fill my void with another obsession and let it dominate everything else in my life. One day Abbi came to me again and brought her words with her. They woke me up. She told me that my distance, my lack of intimacy, and my vanity were only getting worse. This was not the life she wanted. All I seemed to care about was my body and food. The qualities she loved about me seemed to be fading away, replaced by what she called the "prison" of my body image.

We all have defining moments where one choice alters our future. This was my moment. It was time for me to make a choice: either keep the obsession with my body, or keep Abbi. Abbi has been with me every step of the way, providing the insight and strength I needed to break through my challenges and helping me accomplish things I never thought were possible. She is my foundation. As you've probably already guessed, my choice was easy: I chose Abbi.

My Professional "Moment"

The second moment had to do with my personal training and nutrition clients. Our society typically looks at success in health by gauging a person's appearance. To achieve a health goal, most people hire the person that looks the part. Most don't truly know or care whether the person they hire actually understands how the body works. I was fitness-modeling and looked the part, so clients wanted to work with me. They would share their goals, and I would put them on a nutrition and exercise plan. I encouraged them to eat exactly the way I ate, and each of them got fantastic results and achieved their goals . . . in the beginning. This is when I started to see a trend. Typically about three to four months later, my clients began to gain the weight and fat right back. I was witnessing the same yo-yo effect in them that my mom experienced countless times. The most troubling aspect about this was that I was the one who facilitated it! My clients came to me for solutions and answers, and I ended up causing the same feelings of initial success and long-term failure that my mom suffered for so many years. Once I realized what I was doing, I refused to keep walking that path.

. . .

These two moments made me realize that there had to be a better way and that it was time to learn more. Why couldn't you look good *and* feel good? Why was it one or the other? Why did you have to deprive yourself to get healthier? That concept seemed to be filled with contradictions. When in life is creating a deficit ever a positive thing? How can being obsessed with your body and with food be healthy? There were gaping holes everywhere, and it was time to find the answers that would fill those holes.

I took a step back and looked at my education up to this point. From college I had gained a full understanding of the body's anatomy and physiology. I had uncovered the benefits and problems of low-calorie and low-carbohydrate diets from my research and personal dieting experiences—both my own and those of my clients. From reading books, articles, and case studies, along with completing multiple certification courses, I knew how to optimize and diversify exercise to maximize results. I had all the pieces of the puzzle in front of me; I just needed to fit them together. I began researching the systems in the body more deeply: the nervous system, the endocrine system, the digestive system, the respiratory system, the circulatory system, and the muscular system. I knew I would find the answers to my questions if I could get at the root of how the body creates internal balance.

Then all the answers came together for me. My research led me to the concept of blood-sugar stabilization (explained in chapter 1). You see, blood sugar is essential for the body to function. Blood sugar is what provides the fuel for each of the body's systems to correctly move and function. It fills a role very similar to the one gasoline plays in a car. For the next couple of years I worked alongside some of the most well-respected professionals in the field of blood-sugar stabilization. Their expertise took my skill set to a higher level.

Once I fully understood the concept of blood-sugar stabilization, I began working with clients and teaching them how to consistently stabilize their blood sugar. This is how the foundation of the Venice Nutrition Program was built. (The name "Venice Nutrition" comes from my first nutrition consulting practice, in Venice Beach, California.) I was finally able to coach clients as to how to work nutrition and fitness into their lifestyle on a daily basis to achieve permanent results.

I felt a huge weight lift from my shoulders. My clients began to get results without deprivation, without sugar cravings, and without the fear of rebounding. They were eating foods they liked, and they were enjoying the process. Most important, they were becoming educated about how their body works and thus would have this education for life. I, by the same token, had finally achieved balance with my own food, body, and quality of life. For a moment, everything seemed complete . . . and then I realized there was still more to uncover.

The majority of my clients, about 70 percent, were getting great results. The challenge was that 30 percent were still struggling. I knew that the foundation was the stabilization of blood-sugar levels, but the problem was that the calories per meal and nutrient ratios (protein, fat, and carbohydrates) used to stabilize blood sugar were not working for about 30 percent of my clients. This formula was based on overall body composition and the amount of lean body mass, or LBM (everything in the body minus fat content). Unfortunately, the formula did not take into account the person's lifestyle, metabolism, past and current dietary habits, and existing hormonal and/or digestion challenges. You have probably heard the saying "You are what you eat." The saying should be: "You are what you metabolize." The 30 percent who were struggling seemed to have a difficult time awakening their body's metabolism. It made sense that all factors had to be taken into account to optimally stabilize a person's blood sugar. This is when I started adjusting the calories per meal and nutrient ratios for my clients based on all factors and immediately saw how quickly their metabolism responded.

The new formula began to work for 100 percent of my clients and provided a pathway to success for all those who had challenges with diets.

This breakthrough was a moment of peace for me . . . a brief time where all the questions seemed answered . . . a time when all my clients were succeeding with their weight, lean-muscle mass, and health goals . . . a time when I was confident and content. Of course, as I've learned through the years, at moments like these, life has a way of showing up and testing your strength more than before. Life showed up for me and Abbi in March 2000, and our world was turned upside down.

Around this time, Abbi had a minor-impact injury to her neck and back. . . . This was something we both assumed would heal in only a few weeks. However, what initially seemed minor became the hardest and most frustrating year and a half of our lives. From the moment of injury, Abbi's condition began to deteriorate, to the point where she was wracked with muscle spasms and pain. None of the doctors we went to (a total of thirteen) could provide us with real answers. She was eventually diagnosed with fibromyalgia. The treatment consensus was medication and possibly surgery. Within a year, Abbi was taking medication for sleep, medication for pain, and even medication for stomach and intestinal challenges. She was in a constant state of spasms and discomfort, and my wife, once active and full of life, was now struggling to function. As with many people suffering from fibromyalgia, Abbi used food in an attempt to temporarily escape from her condition. Her lack of exercise combined with a high intake of calories caused her to gain weight and store body fat. She put on twenty pounds over a six-month time span, and for someone five-foot-two with back and soft-tissue pain, that additional weight put a heavy burden on her body.

The frustration and desperation we both felt was unbearable. No one could provide insight into why this was happening. There were millions of others suffering from the same symptoms as Abbi, so why weren't there any answers?

I kept searching, and then one day I was discussing back surgery with a client. He had had two of them, and Abbi and I were in the process of deciding whether she was going to give surgery a go. He recommended that, before she went through with the surgery, I read the book *Mind Body Prescription*, by Dr.

John E. Sarno. I bought it that day, and within a week I began to understand what was happening with Abbi. Fibromyalgia is an autoimmune challenge affecting the body's soft muscle tissue. Her body had ceased being able to heal. A year of desperation immediately shifted into a point of inspiration: the possibility that Abbi would get better was within our grasp.

I realized that stabilizing blood sugar was only part of the equation in creating balance in the body. Other components like sleep, exercise, water, vitamins/minerals, and stress management also play vital roles in optimizing the body's performance. Abbi's injury greatly affected her sleep and stress levels. Without quality sleep her body could not repair her soft tissue, and the lack of sleep only made her stress levels worse. (We all know how quickly stress levels rise with fatigue.) With little quality sleep and with high stress, Abbi's body constantly was in pain, and this directly affected her ability to exercise and to metabolize her food, water, and vitamins/minerals. It became evident that I needed to look beyond her nutrition and begin to focus on balancing all six components—sleep, nutrition, exercise, vitamins/minerals, water, and stress—in Abbi's program. Within four months I created what I called the Body Confidence Plan, to balance these six components. The Body Confidence Plan was the key to Abbi's recovery. The six components of the Plan worked together to create internal balance in her body. This provided the proper environment for it to heal.

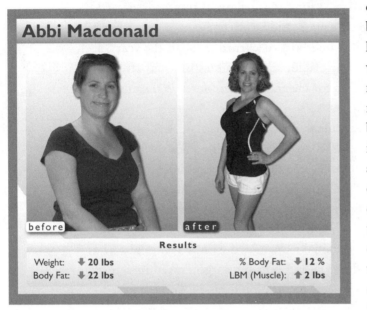

Abbi Macdonald

Results

Weight:	⬇ 20 lbs	% Body Fat:	⬇ 12 %
Body Fat:	⬇ 22 lbs	LBM (Muscle):	⬆ 2 lbs

Each week Abbi's comfortable days grew more frequent and her pain lessened. Within six months she was completely off medication, had lost her extra weight and body fat, and had her life back.

Abbi's recovery unequivocally expanded my mission. If we hadn't kept searching, a negative future for her was absolutely determined. She would have suffered her entire life, and neither of us would have experienced the greatest moment of our lives: the birth of our son, Hunter.

I knew there were people all over the world experiencing the same challenges Abbi had as well as the challenges that my mom, I, and my clients experienced. I knew I had the solution they were searching for, and at that time only our clients in Venice, California, could get coaching. It was time for expansion. The first step was to create our own nutrition certification so that fellow health professionals could teach blood-sugar stabilization and the Venice Nutrition Program. In March 2003, we launched three new additions to Venice Nutrition: our medical board; a complete online nutrition certification course; and a robust licensing system for health-related businesses. The second step was to provide clients a way to engage in the program in addition to working with a Venice Nutrition coach. In May

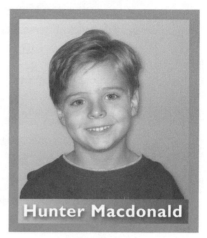

Hunter Macdonald

2006, we launched Venice Nutrition Online, a fully interactive online version of the program. This eliminated all logistical boundaries for the program and provided people the opportunity to take on the program from anywhere in the world. The final step was writing this book—the one source that captures all of the principles that make up the Venice Nutrition Program.

This book is about your possibility of change and how to make your health goals attainable. This book is written for you. We will work together as a team, and I will guide you every step of the way, just as I would if we were doing a ninety-day coaching program together. Through this process I will share real-life tools, inspirational stories, testimonials, and, most important, the science and physiology behind the workings of your body. It's time for a change. There *is* a better way to look good *and* feel good at the same time.

There are many things we cannot control in life;
the one thing we can control is how we
choose to take care of ourselves.

Making your health a priority is not about doing more; rather, it's about becoming better at what you do when you do it. Making your health a priority requires courage, knowledge, desire, and patience. It takes courage to look in depth at all aspects of your life and find a way to open up enough space to take care of your health. It takes knowledge to let go of quick fixes and begin to understand your body. It takes desire to persevere through the necessary lifestyle adjustments. Most of all, it takes patience to stay the course.

I propose that you ask yourself two questions:

Do I feel my best every day?

What quality of life do I want to have?

If your goals are to feel great every day, achieve your internal and external physical goals, and have the highest quality of life possible, this book is for you. Being your best is possible only through great health.

Each chapter is designed to lead you through the entire Venice Nutrition process. I invite you to pace yourself and fully understand the content in each chapter before you move on to the next.

This is a new beginning for you and a new understanding of your body. Now, let's dive in and take your Body Confidence to the next level!

1

WHY DIETS FAIL

If you live in the past, your future is already determined.

—Anonymous

We've all had that one moment in our lives (brief as it may be) when we felt in control of our health. We got there somehow—through exercise, a diet, our genetics, or some other means. For whatever reason, everything just seemed to work; we felt and looked great. Then, for some other reason, everything that was once working seemed to vanish suddenly. Each day we tried to get back to that place and those circumstances, attempting to relive that moment. We spent endless hours focusing on the past, trying to figure out what had changed.

That moment becomes our hope, our future possibility—our ace in the hole (an advantage held in reserve until needed). We believe that at any time we can pull out that ace and get back to where we were during that moment. Of course, we have our justifications for not immediately doing it—like: "Life is too busy" or "Once this project is completed" or "After the holidays" or "When the timing is right." We take on each day feeling just a bit worse, having less energy, getting more stressed, and watching our weight and body fat slowly increase. We tell ourselves that it is not a problem, that we know what we need to do but are just not doing it. We keep tight hold of that ace in the hole, ready to use it at any time.

This thought process could continue for years until eventually we hit a tipping point—a moment when we can't take it anymore. The trigger could be many things: our clothes are too tight, our exercise program isn't working, we're tired all the time, our weight is at its highest point, our wedding is in three months, or maybe we have health complications. . . . This is when we pull out the ace in the hole, feeling that it will get us back to where we were, back to that moment we held on to.

You dive right in, confident in your success as if it were guaranteed. The first day comes and goes, and you briefly think, "It seemed to be easier before. . . ." You might struggle and tell yourself, "I'll start fresh tomorrow." Tomorrow comes. The same challenges arrive, and you just shake it off. You enter the third day, and you still can't get on track. And now the doubts settle in. . . . You begin to think, "I didn't remember it being this hard, so what changed?" This pattern can continue for days, weeks, months, or even years, eventually leading us to the realization that we've lost control of our health and that the ace in the hole we've held on to for so long no longer works. This harsh reality hits like a ton of bricks, and we begin to accept the fact that we don't actually know what to do. . . . *This is when panic sets in.* We spent so much time holding on to that past moment, keeping it as our ace in the hole, that we stopped learning and stopped listening to our body.

This is when diets attack; they are life's quick fixes. People use diets in their moments of frustration and desperation. Diets are the magic spell we are told to believe in, hoping that it really will be *that* easy to solve our problems. We become so overcome by the pain of our current status that we will do practically anything to alleviate it, including believing in smoke and mirrors. Our sense of reason is at its lowest point, and we've become more vulnerable than ever before, so we reach for the magic potion. We go on a calorie- and/ or carbohydrate-restrictive diet, a liquid diet, a doctor-prescribed (medication) appetite-suppression diet, or even a lemon and honey diet. . . . We'll do basically anything out there that's designed to rapidly drop weight through deprivation, even if it lacks common sense, provides little structure, and is devoid of any history of long-term success.

A diet will accomplish the initial goal by temporarily yielding results and relieving some frustration. Unfortunately, once you begin eating normally again, the weight returns as fast as it was lost. What in life can successfully be accomplished by reaching for a quick fix? Can a business succeed without a plan? Can a relationship succeed without continued communication? Can you parent your children successfully without leading by example?

Your health is no different from any of these things. The fact is that anything we do that's worth the effort takes a proper foundation, hard work, and commitment.

Your first step in taking your Body Confidence to the next level is to let go of your old aces in the hole and any attachments you might have to diets. Your hormones, physiology, lifestyle, profession, and environment are all continually changing and evolving. Whatever worked for you in the past is exactly that—your past. It will not work the same for you again. Embracing this fact is the key. The truth is that if your ace in the hole was the right thing for your body, your health would never have regressed.

If you choose to let go of the past now, your health possibilities for the future are endless. Your mind will be open, and you'll be ready to learn how your body truly works *now*.

Let's get into the actual physiological reasons that diets will always fail you. . . .

There are two main philosophies in nutrition: *dieting* and *blood-sugar stabilization*. One is a catalyst that leads to what we call the Yo-Yo Syndrome (weight loss followed by weight gain in repetitive cycles), while the other creates an internal hormonal balance within your body that ignites your metabolism to optimally burn body fat.

The dieting philosophy is centered on caloric and/or carbohydrate restriction and deprivation. It is a philosophy that leads you to create deficits in your nutrition and use restrictions to lose weight. This is the most common nutrition philosophy, most clearly explained by the phrase "calories in versus calories out." The thought process is this: if you are burning two thousand calories per day and you eat fifteen hundred calories a day, you are creating a daily five-hundred-calorie deficit. This deficit will initially assist in weight loss. . . . Unfortunately, because dieting is based on deprivation, your body will always hit an immovable and impenetrable plateau (known as your body's internal *set point*, explained in chapter 2). This calorie deprivation will cause your body to burn fat. However, it will also cause your body to burn muscle. Losing muscle negatively affects the speed of your metabolism, because muscle is the primary place where body fat is burned (less muscle equals less fat burning), and muscle increases the rate at which your body burns calories.

Typically, after you reduce your initial weight and/or reach a plateau on a diet, you'll begin eating the same way you did before you started, only now your body has lost some of its muscle, resulting in a slower metabolism.

Eventually all the weight you lost is regained, but it contains more body fat. What I'm describing is what I earlier called the Yo-Yo Syndrome (in which your weight and body fat go up and down like a yo-yo, and many times your rebound weight is higher than your previous starting weight).

Think about it: eventually every deficit must somehow be paid back. By dieting, you are training your metabolism to slow down, not speed up. The truth is that dieting is based on incorrect physiology.

Anything that causes you to burn muscle is working against you, not for you. Millions of people have gotten caught up in dieting, including thousands of my clients *and* me. It's taught everywhere—at the doctor's, on TV, in magazines, in books, on infomercials, and even at universities. The reality is that dieting is outdated information, and is a billion-dollar industry designed specifically to keep you coming back. Now, the excitement of dieting is that it typically yields fast, temporary results (until you've done enough damage to your metabolism) and that it seems so simple: just eat less. The challenge is that dieting will yield only one outcome: long-term failure. If your goal is to make progress with your health and unlock your body's full potential, it's time to learn a better way.

Somewhere along the way we got so caught up in the quick-fix mentality that we chose to forget about how our body actually works. We abandoned physiological facts and accepted hype and theories. This happened through the years because as time passes, our lives seem only to get busier and more stressful. Instead of wanting to do the work, we choose to take shortcuts with dieting.

In the introduction I described the journey I went on to learn that the nutrition solution was *blood-sugar stabilization*. Debates about different diets become pointless once you truly understand how the body creates and utilizes blood sugar, and balances blood-sugar levels. What elevated my passion and motivated me to further understand the importance of stable blood sugar was living through the experience of Abbi's pregnancy as well as the birth and first year of Hunter's life.

I still have some trouble understanding why most of the health industry lost focus on stable blood-sugar levels. You see, a fetus's core developmental factor is its mother's blood-sugar levels. Keeping them stable is vital for its survival.

During Abbi's pregnancy she was diagnosed with gestational diabetes (the type of diabetes that occurs during pregnancy). The concern with this is that if a fetus is constantly exposed to high levels of glucose (sugar), it is as if the fetus were overeating. A fetus inside a mother who's living with gestational diabetes produces more insulin to absorb the excess glucose (sugar), which results in a gain in fetal size and fetal weight. It's interesting how our adult bodies work the same way a fetus does. A fetus getting too much glucose (sugar) can become too large, leading to birth complications for the fetus and mother. Once Abbi was diagnosed with gestational diabetes, the number-one focus during her pregnancy became keeping her blood-sugar levels stable.

Fortunately, Abbi was already active, healthy, and eating correctly. . . . She had a great foundation. When our doctor diagnosed Abbi with gestational diabetes, he brought one of the hospital's dietitians into the room to provide us with proper nutrition information. Abbi and I were given information that was outdated by a couple of decades. The hospital's dietician was a nice lady, and both she and our doctor had the best intentions . . . they were just out of touch. Just imagine, if you will, Abbi and me, having already trekked along a path filled with years of frustration, sitting in a doctor's office listening to outdated and inaccurate methods for stabilizing her blood sugar for the health of our baby. As you can guess, we thanked the dietician for her time, and I proceeded to design Abbi's nutrition and exercise program throughout her pregnancy, while our doctor monitored her insulin requirements. We monitored her blood-sugar levels very carefully, and Hunter was born at a normal weight and size. He was a healthy seven-pound baby boy.

What was very interesting was what occurred within the first five minutes of Hunter's life, when the nurses tested his blood sugar. His survival depended on his blood sugar being within the normal range. If his blood sugar was too low, we would have had to immediately get food into his little body to stabilize his levels to make sure that his body could function correctly. Fortunately, since Abbi controlled her blood-sugar levels throughout the pregnancy, Hunter was of normal size and his body immediately processed glucose correctly. In the first few hours of his life, the nurses wanted Hunter to drink breast milk or formula (made to match breast milk). Both of these food sources are a combination of protein, fat, and carbohydrates. The nurses also spoke about the importance of meal frequency: Hunter should be breast-feeding every three hours. I knew this meal structure, along with the balance of protein, fat, and carbohydrates in Abbi's breast milk, would naturally keep his blood sugar stable and assist in his body's proper development and growth. To emphasize the importance of this information, the hospital offered a class for new mothers specifically focused on "how to properly feed your baby." This approach to proper nutrition continued through Hunter's first year of life. At every single doctor visit, the number-one topic was Hunter's nutrition, particularly his caloric intake and meal intervals.

During Hunter's first year of life, an industry that I thought was outdated was actually teaching blood-sugar stabilization for babies. This led me to ask a few questions: First, how could most medical professionals be so correct with a baby's nutrition and so off with an adult's nutrition? Our physiology doesn't change, our body's ability to create energy doesn't change, and our need for nutrients doesn't change. If our bodies are meant to be fed a certain way during the first year of life, why should our focus change afterward?

I took a step back, thought about the questions, and realized that the answers are simple. We choose to abandon how the body is supposed to be fed because, after the first year, the business and complicated nature of life get in the way. We are extremely fragile in the first year of life. During that time, we develop at a rapid pace every day. To ensure proper development as well as to survive, we need to be correctly fed. Once we pass that one-year mark, our bodies have stored enough body fat, and we've become strong enough, that our meal intervals and nutrient ratios are capable of change. Now, even though it makes sense for us to continue following the same pattern that we did during the first year of life (the way our bodies are meant to be fed), society, life, and lack of education become roadblocks that shift our focus away from eating correctly. Once Hunter turned one year old, his doctor's appointments shifted focus to height/weight charts and food pyramid recommendations, not blood-sugar stabilization. The reason everything seems to work so well for the first year of a child's life is that meal intervals, calories per meal, and nutrient ratios are based on instinct. Whether with breast milk or formula, a baby must be fed this way. Every study supports these facts. Think about it: doctors never explain why we feed our babies like this . . . it's just what we're supposed to do. Now, the truth is that I already knew why Hunter was supposed to eat like this, but parents without this knowledge do not. Once babies have enough energy stored in reserve (enough weight, body fat, and so on), they begin to be fed like everyone else . . . people in "normal" society. They eat three meals a day and try to be healthy. The three-meal system (breakfast, lunch, and dinner) is how most medical professionals eat. It's how most of society eats. Immediately after our first year of life, this system is ingrained in us by everyone we know. Because of this lack of knowledge, parents teach only what they know to their children. Children grow up, have their own children, and then repeat the pattern. There is a simple solution to end this pattern: we simply continue feeding ourselves according to the same structure we used throughout our first year of life.

Blood Sugar:
Your Body's Fuel Source

Blood sugar is sugar in the form of glucose within the bloodstream. The body must maintain stable blood sugar because glucose fuels our nervous system. Glucose creates the bulk of our body's energy source: ATP (adenosine triphosphate). ATP fuels every movement, every heartbeat, and every breath you take. This is why there is so much attention paid to a baby's first year of life. Their blood-sugar level equals life.

The concentration of glucose in the blood is measured in milligrams of glucose per deciliter of blood (1 deciliter equals 100 milliliters). Simply stated, what you need to know is this: if you keep your blood-sugar levels between 80 and 120 milligrams per deciliter (mg/dl)— the range for stable blood sugar—you will *not* store fat or burn muscle, because your blood-sugar hormones will be in balance.

How Your Body Keeps Your
Blood Sugar Stable

First, it is important to understand that your body's main goal is to maintain a continual state of homeostasis (balance) in all of its systems. You have two choices to help it achieve that balance. Either effectively take care of your body and let your positive actions keep it in balance, or do not and make your body balance itself. Any time the body is taken out of balance in its blood-sugar level, it must take measures to counter the rise or drop in blood sugar in order to regain a steady equilibrium. It does this by releasing hormones into the bloodstream. Hormones are chemical substances produced by your body that control and regulate the activity of certain cells or organs.

Your blood sugar is controlled by the pancreas, a part of the endocrine system. Your endocrine system is a system of glands that produce hormones to regulate your body. A few of these glands are your thyroid gland (your metabolism), your adrenal gland (your energy levels), and your pancreas (your blood-sugar regulator). The two main hormones in the pancreas are *insulin* and *glucagon*. Insulin's purpose is to lower the body's blood sugar, and glucagon's purpose is to raise the body's blood sugar. Your pancreas is continually creating and releasing insulin and glucagon (unless you are a type 1 diabetic), with the sole purpose of keeping your blood-sugar levels in the 80–120 mg/dl range. If your blood sugar drops below 80 mg/dl (low blood sugar), your pancreas overreleases glucagon, which causes the rapid breakdown of stored glucose and amino acids (muscle) to get the blood sugar elevated and in balance. If your blood sugar rises above 120 mg/dl (high blood sugar), your pancreas overreleases insulin, which triggers your body to store all nutrients (a lot of the time they're stored as fat) to get the blood sugar lowered and in balance.

Here's a perfect example of how the pancreas works: Think of a time when you were desperately looking for something to eat because you waited too long to get a meal inside you and you were ravenous, irritable, and shaky . . . Those are the symptoms caused by low blood sugar. While in this state, your body consumes itself in an attempt to regain balance, triggering a severe hunger reaction. This is how and why your body tells you it needs food. When you are in this state and eventually do find food, you tend to dash right for the carbohydrates, since they're what your body craves. You see, carbohydrates are broken down directly into glucose—which your body needs desperately at this moment. Then you begin an eating frenzy, feeling like you cannot get enough. . . . About twenty minutes into the meal, you'll begin to feel very full, uncomfortable, and even a little sleepy. (It takes your brain twenty minutes to realize you've eaten once your blood sugar gets that low.) Now your body's blood sugar is elevated, your pancreas overreleases insulin, and all the excess food you have just eaten is stored by your body—some of it as fat.

This is a prime example of how a large percentage of people eat every day. All the body is attempting to do is keep its blood-sugar levels balanced. So my suggestion is this: rather than have the body trigger these responses to stabilize your blood sugar, learn how your actions beforehand can stabilize your blood sugar, and prevent the scenario I've just described from ever happening again.

Stabilizing Your Blood Sugar: The Three Factors

There are three factors that will keep your blood sugar stable and your body in homeostasis. Your best point of reference when reading these three factors is the baby analogy that I used earlier.

The first factor is *meal intervals*. Your body is a "refuel as it goes" machine. This means that in order for it to work correctly, the body needs to be fed *consistently*. On the Venice Nutrition Program, you'll be eating within the first hour after waking, then again every three to four hours throughout the day, and finally within an hour of going to sleep. Yes, you *can* eat before bed! (I will explain why in chapter 5.)

The second factor is *nutrient ratios*. There are three nutrients that contain calories and are essential for our survival: protein, fat, and carbohydrates. All three combined in the correct ratio (just like breast milk) will provide your body with the proper amount of glucose (carbohydrates), amino acids and nitrogen (protein), and fatty acids (fat), which will slow down the rate of digestion, keep your blood sugar stable, and ensure that your body maintains homeostasis. (You will learn more about your nutrient ratios in chapter 5.)

The third factor is *calories per meal*. Yes, I'm talking about calories per *meal,* not per day. Your body can process only a certain amount of food at once, and that amount is based on many individual factors. The most important thing about the quantity of food per meal is that you should be ready to eat before a meal (never starving), satisfied after a meal (not full), and then ready to eat again approximately three to four hours later. This is a clear indication that your blood sugar is stable and your body is in balance. The most important thing to remember in regards to your calories per meal is how to adjust your food quantity for optimal blood-sugar maintenance. (In chapter 5, I will teach you how to do this.)

These three factors constitute the foundation you must maintain to keep your blood sugar stable. The amount of calories per meal, nutrient ratios, and meal intervals to stabilize your blood sugar will be explained in chapter 5.

Permanently Achieving Your Health Goals Through Blood-Sugar Stabilization

Nutrition should be used to create internal balance. This is what separates maintaining stable blood sugar from dieting.

When nutrition is used to create balance, the body is in homeostasis and will release whatever it does not need, like stored body fat, toxins, and excess sodium. The state of homeostasis also creates an anabolic environment (a positive growth state) in the body, which optimizes cell reproduction, energy, focus, sleep, stress management, and the amount of lean body mass (your muscle).

Diets, on the other hand, create deficits through deprivation and restriction—the opposite of balance. These deficits create unstable blood-sugar levels and trigger low blood-sugar responses. As I shared, low blood sugar shifts your body into a panic state in which it begins consuming amino acids (muscle) and converting it into the glucose (sugar) it needs to supply your body with energy (ATP). The dieting misconception is that your body will use its stored fat for energy in times of deprivation. Physiologically speaking, this is not possible. Stored body fat cannot be converted to glucose (sugar), which means your body must attack its muscle to produce glucose for energy. Deprivation actually causes your body to hold its stored fat and burn muscle. This is why dieting results in an overall slower metabolism.

With stable blood sugar, the result is much different. When the body's blood sugar is stable, it will continually release stored fat (each pound of stored fat has approximately 3,500 calories—a *lot* of fuel), which is then burned primarily within the muscle tissue through daily activity and exercise.

Quite often I have had female clients concerned about increasing their muscle mass through eating more protein and exercising. . . . Trust me: male or female, muscle is your friend; it makes up your metabolism. The fact is that one pound of muscle is approximately three times smaller than one pound of fat. This means that if you build muscle and lose fat, you actually become smaller and more toned. The only time muscle causes bulk is when you are *not* stabilizing your blood sugar. This will prevent your body from releasing fat and cause it to build muscle while keeping your fat. That's what causes the

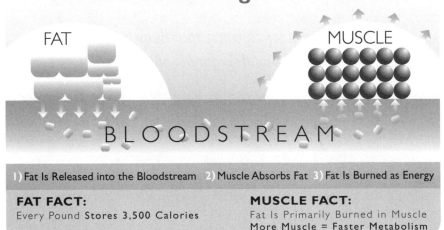

When Blood Sugar Is Stable

FAT   MUSCLE

BLOODSTREAM

1) Fat Is Released into the Bloodstream   2) Muscle Absorbs Fat   3) Fat Is Burned as Energy

FAT FACT:
Every Pound Stores 3,500 Calories

MUSCLE FACT:
Fat Is Primarily Burned in Muscle
More Muscle = Faster Metabolism

"bulky" look. So as long as you keep your blood sugar stable, your body will release its fat and build lean muscle mass at the same time (with an efficient and diverse exercise plan, explained in chapter 6), which will increase your metabolism and improve your overall body composition.

Of course, the leaner you become, the more food you must consume. This is because your body will have less stored fat to use as fuel and will require more calories (possibly even more meals) to keep your blood sugar stable. This is the number-one sign that your metabolism is speeding up. This is similar to what happens when a child grows, since they, too, have a larger appetite. The larger the appetite, the more the child needs to consume. This is truly a positive sign of a healthy metabolism for babies, children, teenagers, and adults.

Eliminating Your Sugar Cravings and Increasing Your Energy

Through all my years of working with clients. I've seen that the majority of them initially have little concern about the quality of their energy. They are so attached to reaching their target weight and seeing their external results that they lose sight of actually feeling good while they go through the process. Many of us think that to get in shape means to feel deprived, eat less, have low energy, be grumpy, and basically feel horrible. The reality is this: it's just not true. . . . What I've described is an outdated way of thinking. The improved way to achieve the same external goals—through blood-sugar stabilization—has the benefit of producing more energy and no sugar cravings. To achieve external results, you must first create internal balance. Your blood-sugar maintenance has a direct effect on both your sugar cravings and your energy.

When your blood-sugar level is low, your body starts panicking because it needs glucose (sugar) to create energy. Your body's way of telling you this is your feeling of hunger and cravings for sugar. Most of the time, people don't realize its sugar they're craving. Many think that sugar is just sweets like candy, regular soda, juice, or anything that has a significant amount of sugar listed on the product's food label. But the reality is that *all* carbohydrates—grains, breads, fruit, vegetables, and such (the exception being fiber)—are broken down by your body's digestive system into glucose (sugar). The only difference between the digestion of different types of carbohydrates is how quickly they get broken down by the body into glucose. (We will cover this topic in detail in chapter 5.)

When our blood sugar is low, we crave sugar. That sugar craving will simply manifest itself in you as a craving for the kind of carbohydrates that *you* like. For example, if you are a candy person, you probably will have a craving for candy. If you love chocolate, you probably will have a craving for chocolate. Each one of us has different cravings for different types of carbohydrates based on our taste buds.

The Two Types of Cravings: Physiological and Psychological

My favorite food is pizza, as you can tell from my storied pizza days. When my blood sugar is low, I crave pizza for two reasons. The first reason is that I love pizza, and the second is that pizza is loaded with carbohydrates. This is both a physiological and psychological craving. Since my blood sugar is low, my body physically needs carbohydrates (a physiological craving), and I choose pizza because I just want it (a psychological craving). Our body's mechanism for basic survival is to create a sense of urgency to consume carbohydrates when our blood sugar is low, causing a physiological craving. A physiological craving is a physical "need" controlled by the feeding drives of your body. Now, when my blood sugar is stable, and the pizza is front of me, of course I still "want" it (because I love it). I just do not physically "need" it. Since my blood sugar is stable, I have control over my eating decisions. Words cannot express the liberation I felt once I understood this. During my dieting years I would spend days beating myself up because I had a cheat meal, thinking I lacked the will power to abstain, not understanding that my body's essential food *needs* will always overpower my *wanting* to not succumb to my sugar cravings. The reality is that if your blood sugar is low, you will crave, and you will eventually give in to those cravings (for whatever carbohydrates you crave). The way to control your psychological cravings is to maintain stable blood-sugar levels that prevent your physiological cravings.

Blood-sugar levels also have a direct correlation to energy. Think about the last time you were starving and you overate. How did you feel? What was your energy like? What was your mood like? How long did it take you to recover? Remember that our energy, ATP, is created by glucose. Any time your blood sugar becomes unstable, your energy levels drop, since your body's fuel source is compromised and your blood-sugar hormones are out of balance. Stable blood sugar, on the other hand, will provide you with consistent energy throughout the day and eliminate any midmorning or midafternoon energy crashes. (Your sleep and stress also play a role in energy—a topic discussed in chapter 4.)

In summary, the food you eat throughout the day can create internal balance, release stored fat, provide an anabolic environment, and optimize the energy within your body. Exercise activates muscle, burns fat, and increases lean body mass (muscle). Blood-sugar stabilization is the key to achieving your health goals and taking your Body Confidence to the next level. By stabilizing your blood sugar, you likewise shift your mind-set. You learn to believe in nutrition and use it as your foundation. This way, when life shows up, you can temporarily shift your body into a maintenance mode. When it calms down, you can shift your body back into progression mode. By viewing nutrition in this light, you guarantee that you will progress with your body year after year—and never regress!

Whether you believe it is possible, or you believe it is not possible, you are right

We all have good days and tough days, moments of calm and moments of chaos, times of frustration and times of peace. Even though each of us lives a different life and has different strengths and challenges, we all share a similar experience: life always shows up (unforeseen circumstances). In those moments, we can push through or we can check out. One thing I know is that the success of others can provide the necessary motivation and inspiration to help push us through to the other side. A perfect example of this is the running feat of Roger Bannister. Roger Bannister was the first person to break the four-minute mile. For nearly a decade the record held at 4:01.4. Runners of amazing ability attempted to beat the record over and over again, always coming up short. It was a number that many thought was impossible to break. That is, they all thought it could not be broken until May 6, 1954. On that day Mr. Bannister ran the mile of his life and made history. His effort showed other runners what was possible, and then an interesting thing happened: one month later, John Landy broke Bannister's record by a full second. The record that had stood for a decade was broken again in only one month. Then runners all over started to break the four-minute mark as if it was something easy. Roger Bannister showed others that if you believe you can, you can. Anything is possible. I believe this with all my heart. You can win. You can succeed. You can gain the Body Confidence you desire if you believe it is possible.

Two of my clients, Shana and Tom, embody this belief.

Shana's story shows the possibility of switching from the mind-set of dieting to the mind-set of blood-sugar stabilization. I remember the first time I met Shana and how she shared her story with me. Her story touched a special place in my heart. Shana started her dieting days as a preteen. She was twelve and felt she was bigger than she should be. Her mom took her to a doctor, and she was immediately put on a low-calorie, low-carbohydrate diet. It was her first encounter with food restriction, and as most kids do, she rebelled when something she loved was taken away. Unfortunately, as you now know, when a caloric deficit is created, your cravings become uncontrollable. Shana spoke about how she would follow her diet throughout the day and then start closet-eating her candy bars come nighttime. As each day passed, her guilt over binge eating continued to build. She initially did drop a few pounds; then, as her binge eating became more frequent, every pound she lost was regained and she became heavier than she was when she started the diet.

Over the next twenty-five years Shana would jump on any new diet on the market and would follow the same pattern—drop initially and then gain all her weight back, plus, as she would put it, "a little extra insurance weight." She was trapped within the classic behavior called the Yo-Yo Syndrome. When all was said and done she was one hundred pounds overweight, her highest weight ever: 228 pounds. In the beginning of this chapter I spoke about a *tipping point*, a moment when we tell ourselves enough is enough. For Shana, reaching 228 pounds was her tipping point. She joined a gym, began eating healthier and exercising four days a week, and slowly and steadily began to lose weight and feel better. She proceeded to drop twenty-eight pounds over a four-month period and was on her way . . . until her old habits came back. Her dieting mind-set caught up to her, and over the next couple of months she gained back all the weight she had lost—once again back at 228 pounds.

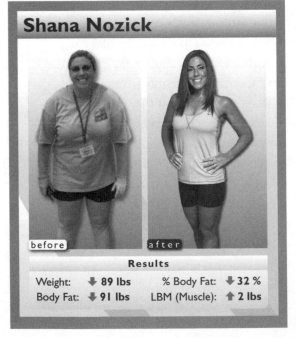

Shana Nozick

before · after

Results

| Weight: | ⬇ 89 lbs | % Body Fat: | ⬇ 32 % |
| Body Fat: | ⬇ 91 lbs | LBM (Muscle): | ⬆ 2 lbs |

At this point, Shana had a choice: continue going down the same path she had followed since the age of twelve; or choose to actually overcome her twenty-five years of dieting frustration. This was the moment when Shana was introduced to Venice Nutrition. As she began to understand the concepts of calories per meal, nutrient ratios, and meal intervals, she realized that she could eat the foods she wanted and still drop weight and body fat. Over the next ten months, Shana worked the program into her lifestyle (while still having her "off plan" meals; she does really love those candy bars!). The thing is that she never felt deprived. Each month, her body progressed and became leaner.

Then, after her ten-month journey, she stepped on the scale and weighed 139 pounds! She was extremely excited. She just stood there looking at the number in disbelief, her face full of pride; she was in shock that she had finally broken the 140-pound mark. What was even more impressive was that she did not lose any muscle through her weight loss; she actually gained two pounds of muscle, increasing her metabolism. For me, the classic moment was when I pulled up her "before" picture on the computer screen and she said, "Who is that girl? There is no way I was ever that big." She had transformed so much she did not even recognize her old self anymore. Now, that is cool! Shana has truly learned how to make her body work for her, inside and outside, and has permanently reprogrammed her body. She took what she thought in the beginning was impossible and made it a reality by the time she stepped onto that scale.

My client Tom Barone is a great example of how to successfully work the program into your world. Tom owns and operates two preschools. The first time I met Tom was when Hunter was four years old and starting prekindergarten. I dropped Hunter off, and Tom and I began to talk. He knew I was a nutritionist, and he wanted to ask me a few questions. I took a seat in Tom's office, and he told me how he'd always been into fitness, loved sports, and especially had a passion for tennis. His spirits were a little low since he had recently developed a minor shoulder injury that put his tennis playing on hold, causing his weight to begin creeping up. He was frustrated and puzzled with his lack of results: he was eating healthy and working out at the gym, yet his weight was only increasing.

I asked him about his health history. Tom said that he had been working in corporate America for over twenty years and that at certain times in his life he had points at which he gained weight. At those points, he would usually step up his exercise routine or jump on a quick diet to get back to where he wanted to be. That would seem to do the trick for a while, only to finally lead back to regressing once again. He wanted to speak with me because he felt like he was missing something; just eating healthy and exercising was not working for him. Tom then clued me in to what he was doing with his nutrition and exercise, and it became apparent to me what was causing his weight gain. His meals were unbalanced (incorrect protein, fat, and carbohydrate ratio), the intervals between them were too long, and he was eating too many calories at lunch and dinner. In addition, his exercise was inefficient. He wasn't maximizing his workout time. Tom began to understand what he could do better and got fired up to start the program.

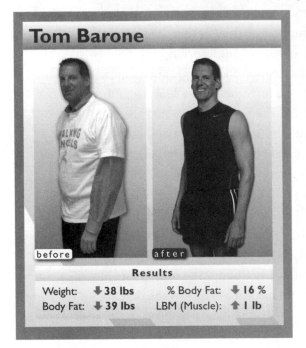

Tom Barone

before

after

Results

Weight:	⬇ 38 lbs	% Body Fat:	⬇ 16 %
Body Fat:	⬇ 39 lbs	LBM (Muscle):	⬆ 1 lb

I then asked Tom the big questions: Why do you want to be healthy? What are you going to "get" from it? You see, Tom's life is structured, and he is very driven; I knew he could make the nutrition and exercise adjustments. The thing I had to ask him was: "What is your motivation?" He answered, "I want to drop forty pounds." I replied, "That is your goal. *Why* do you want to lose forty pounds?" Tom followed with: "So I can look and feel better. I do not like having this extra body fat." I then asked, "What happens once you drop the forty pounds and look and feel better? What will keep you moving forward with your health?" He replied, "I have two boys, Jack and Joey, and we love to play sports together. Getting in shape is important to me mostly so I can be great for them. I love coaching their teams and playing sports with them. We have such a special relationship, and I know that the healthier I am, the more we can enjoy our time together." Being great for his sons is what will keep Tom motivated to lose the forty pounds and will keep him inspired not only during the easier times in life but also during the more challenging times. He will always have a clear picture of what his health means to him and what he will "get" from it.

Tom's next step was implementing the program. We began working together and immediately corrected his nutrition, revised his exercise, and developed his complete Body Confidence Plan (your Body Confidence Plan will be presented in chapter 4). Tom's new health knowledge provided him with the motivation and education to rapidly achieve his health goals. He dropped weight and fat like clockwork. Every week he became more and more inspired by how great he felt. For me, the highlight of Tom's journey was the day he took his "after" photo. Tom brought Jack and Joey with him, and the look of pride they had in their eyes for their father was special. As a father, I know this look; it is the one we all want from our children. In five months, Tom went from being the most frustrated with his health he'd ever been to feeling the best he'd ever felt in his life. He finally had complete Body Confidence. Most important to Tom, his actions are now leading his boys to live a healthy lifestyle.

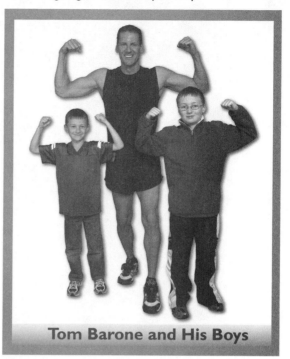

Tom Barone and His Boys

Shana's and Tom's stories show that the answers are there and that taking your Body Confidence to the next level is your choice. You do the work or you do not. The moment is here and now, waiting for you to seize it. Every chapter from this point on will guide you through the process of understanding your body, learning the Venice Nutrition Program, and then implementing the program into your world.

It is time for a new path that that empowers you to look and feel your best, a new level of thinking that provides you with the tools you need to unlock your body's full potential and permanently achieve your own Body Confidence.

The real answers and solutions are yours for the taking.

It is up to you. . . . Now let's go get them together.

2

FINDING YOUR
STARTING POINT

You must first know where you are starting before you can
determine where you are going and how fast you will get there.

How quickly will I achieve my goals?" This is the first question we ask
ourselves when we start any type of health plan. It seems like a fairly
straightforward question and should be easy to answer. By simply applying logic, we can determine at exactly what speed each health goal can be
achieved, right? If it were only that easy . . .

The first component in achieving your goals and taking your Body Confidence to the next level is to learn your metabolism's starting point. Your
starting point is the current speed of your metabolism (defined as the rate at
which your body processes energy). It is a concept that the dieting world has
long forgotten, replaced with the "quick fix" mind-set, which yields empty
promises and temporary results. We live in a state of instant gratification, and
many of us think that if we are going to put the time in on our health, we'd
better get rapid results. We remember how fast our results came in the past,
or we compare ourselves with a friend who is dieting and dropping pounds

by the day, or we believe that since we made improvements in our nutrition and exercise, our fat should just melt away. We expect our efforts to get immediate, matching results—discounting the physiological factors that truly determine the time frame in which our goals can be achieved.

You see, each of us has a unique metabolism. Your metabolism is as individual as your fingerprint. Just think about your circle of friends and family; most likely you can name the people who can eat whatever they want and never gain weight, the ones who seem to "look at food and gain weight" (likely yo-yo dieters), and those who can't seem to lose those last ten to twenty pounds no matter what. Each of these people has a specific metabolism, dictating their starting point and the rate at which their goals can be achieved.

Think of a game of poker: You are dealt five cards. Sometimes you get three of a kind, and sometimes you only have a pair of twos. Either way, whatever hand you are dealt is the one you must play. Regardless of the strength of your cards, if you play your cards well, you can win the hand. The same analogy can be applied to your metabolism. You are genetically dealt two "metabolic cards." These "metabolic cards" determine the speed of your metabolism. Regardless of the speed of your metabolism, if you implement the right strategies, you will win rewards in terms of your body and your health.

Your two "metabolic cards" are:

- Your body type

- Your set point

Let's first discuss your body type.

Your Body Type

Growing up, I watched my sister Laurie struggle with weight while my other sister, Chris, stayed naturally lean. It always puzzled me, since they both ate the same foods and had similar activity levels. Everything regarding weight and body-fat loss was just harder for Laurie than it was for Chris. I can remember the frustration it caused Laurie, wondering why she had such challenges with her weight and Chris did not.

It all became clear as I got older and began to understand the different body types and how each directly affects the speed of a person's metabolism. You see, Laurie had a body type like my mom's (slower metabolism, and more prone to store body fat), whereas Chris had a body type like my dad's (faster

Three Body Types

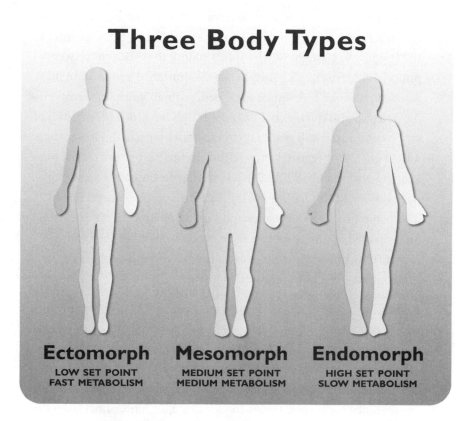

Ectomorph
LOW SET POINT
FAST METABOLISM

Mesomorph
MEDIUM SET POINT
MEDIUM METABOLISM

Endomorph
HIGH SET POINT
SLOW METABOLISM

metabolism, and more prone to burn body fat). Both my sisters came from the same gene pool, but each inherited a different body type and speed of metabolism from our parents. This is why Laurie struggled with weight much more than Chris.

Among all of us, there are three body types:

Ectomorph: Most food lovers have been envious of an ectomorph at some point; I know I have! An ectomorph is the person you know who can eat whatever they want and never gain weight. Ectomorphs are very lean and have a difficult time gaining weight. I often compare an ectomorph's metabolism to a road bike. Everything about a road bike is designed for speed—from efficient hill climbing to blazing downhill to exploding on the flats. A road bike is built light, lean, and lightning quick, just like an ectomorph's body type and metabolism.

Mesomorph: My metabolism is typical of a mesomorph. Meso-morphs have the ability to be lean and muscular, but they can also gain a good amount of excess weight and body fat. I know this well, since I have experienced both extremes. Because of the vast range, mesomorphs can vary greatly—from a world-class track sprinter to the friend you thought of who wants to lose that last ten to twenty pounds. A mesomorph's metabolism is similar to a mountain bike. A mountain bike is designed for speed, with an additional emphasis on strength and durability to handle tough terrain. This additional emphasis on strength makes the mountain bike a little slower than a road bike, so it requires more effort on the part of the cyclist to keep up with the road bike. This is similar to the way a mesomorph needs to work a bit harder to stay lean than an ectomorph does. The real plus side to a mesomorph's metabolism is that it provides an increased ability to gain muscle mass. Remember that your fat is primarily burned in your muscle, so more muscle equals a faster metabolism—for both men and women.

Endomorph: My mom's body type most resembles an endomorph. An endomorph has a slower metabolism and has a higher capacity to gain weight and store body fat. Your friend or family member that seems to "look at food and gain weight" is an endomorph. I compare an endomorph's speed of metabolism to a beach cruiser bike. Beach cruisers are designed for leisurely rides and require a lot more effort from the cyclist to keep up with a road bike or a mountain bike. When riding a beach cruiser you can ride the same distance that you can on a road or mountain bike, but the time it takes to arrive at your destination is typically longer. This is similar to an endomorph's metabolism. Through the years, many of my clients have thought that being an endomorph meant they were destined to forever struggle with weight and body fat. This is not the case, as Shana's story (told in chapter 1) clearly shows. Endomorphs can increase the speed of their metabolism. It just takes more effort for them than it does for an ectomorph or a mesomorph.

Now think of the body type that you best relate to, and then see whether you can think of one of the other types that you share some characteristics with. You may be an identical match to a particular body type, or you may be somewhere in between two of them. For example, my sister Chris is not a pure ectomorph; instead, she is a mixture of an ectomorph and a mesomorph. My sister Laurie, on the other hand, is a mixture of a mesomorph and an endomorph. Knowing your body type provides you with a strong initial understanding of the speed of your metabolism. No matter where you find yourself, you *will* be able to reprogram your metabolism. Again, this is similar to how a road bike, a mountain bike, and a beach cruiser will all reach the same destination, the only two variations among them being the amount of effort the cyclist expends and the amount of time it takes each bike to arrive at the final destination.

Your Set Point

Have you ever gained weight during the holiday season? It's hard not to; it feels like a six-week festival of eating: first Thanksgiving arrives, then there is party after party in December, and finally New Year's Eve tops it off. When January comes, you have a reality check and get back to your routine, and typically whatever weight you gained during the holidays is gone by February. Now, the weight you gained temporarily was an "inflated weight," a weight higher than your body normally carries, caused by eating too much food and possibly consuming extra alcohol. The weight that you get back to by February, after eating more moderately, is your "true weight," the weight your body maintains. This is why diets work so well for the first couple of weeks. We typically start diets at periods of frustration, when we are carrying a lot of extra inflated weight. We initially experience fast weight loss, and then as we approach our true weight, the diet seems to stop working . . . and then, *bam!* We reach an immovable plateau.

Now think about the weight you reach at that immovable plateau: that weight is your "true weight," also known as your *set point*—the weight your body wants to physiologically maintain due to your body type, speed of metabolism, and past nutrition and exercise history. Your weight-regulating mechanism, or WRM, is what decides whether your body burns or stores energy in order to maintain your set point. Your WRM is located in a portion of your brain known as the hypothalamus. It is your body's appetite control center. Imagine a temperature-controlled room with a thermostat set at seventy-five degrees. If the temperature goes higher than seventy-five degrees, the air conditioner switches on to cool the room. If the temperature goes lower than seventy-five degrees, the heater switches on to heat up the room. Your set point is like the temperature that the thermostat is set to, and your WRM is like the thermostat itself (activating the air conditioner or heater to maintain the room's temperature at seventy-five degrees). Your WRM causes the body to maintain its set point by either burning or storing energy. This is why you can shed those holiday pounds so quickly. . . . Once you begin eating normally again, your WRM will work in overdrive to bring your body back to its set point.

Your set point is initially determined by your body type and speed of metabolism. The lower your set point, the faster your metabolism. Ectomorphs have low set points, mesomorphs have medium set points, and endomorphs have high set points. Regardless of your body type and current speed of metabolism, your set point will become lower or higher based on your choices. Let me explain. . . . Have you ever felt that one day your true weight (not your inflated weight) just seemed to shoot up? Had you seemed to be holding at a particular weight for a long time and then all of a sudden your new true weight seemed to be five to fifteen pounds heavier, or even more? This is by far the most frequent reason that people want to start a diet. They feel that they were comfortably maintaining their weight and then *poof!*—new body fat appeared. Typically, we blame age or hormones. I have heard it countless times: "When I turned forty, my metabolism seemed to shut down." Now, it's true that age and hormones could be part of the cause. However, the reality is that the body rarely raises its weight and body fat overnight. (Water weight is the exception.) As I discussed in chapter 1, every time you have low blood sugar (typically caused by missing meals or eating too few calories), your body burns muscle to provide the glucose it needs to create energy, and every time you overconsume calories or carbohydrates, you spike your blood sugar, and your body stores fat. Remember, fat is primarily burned in muscle. The more bouts of unstable blood sugar you experience, the more muscle your body burns for fuel, which in turn decreases the size of your fat-burning engine. This loss of muscle directly slows the speed of your metabolism, making it harder for your body to burn fat. When this situation (loss of muscle and increase of body fat) occurs often enough, your set point rises.

This rise in set point is what causes the jump in weight and body fat. The more times this jump occurs, as described by the Yo-Yo Syndrome, the more challenging ("stickier") it will be to lower your set point, and the slower your metabolism will become overall. The Yo-Yo Syndrome makes your set point stickier because every time you diet and then rebound, you lose more muscle and store more fat, causing your metabolism to eventually move at turtle speed. The more you diet, the more resistant your body will be to diets, since your metabolism is much slower because of the damage that your previous diets caused. Yes, a "sticky" set point can be lowered; it just takes more effort and time to undo the damage that's been done to your metabolism. The solution to stop the rising of your set point is simple: just stabilize your blood-sugar levels. As I pointed out earlier, your body is a "refuel as it goes" machine, meaning that by feeding your body frequent, balanced meals in the optimal caloric range, your blood sugar will remain stable, causing your body to protect its muscle (your metabolism) and release its stored body fat. With stable blood sugar, you immediately take charge of your set point. Your next step is, then, lowering your set point. You accomplish this by stabilizing your blood sugar and optimizing your exercise. Your exercise is what activates your muscle. Stable blood sugar creates balance in your body, and your exercise strengthens your body and increases your muscle. More active muscle equals a faster metabolism, and a faster metabolism lowers your set point. This is how you will reprogram your metabolism and permanently lower your set point.

Now think about your set point, and ask yourself these questions:

What is your true weight?
Do you think you are at your set point or at your inflated weight?
Have you noticed your metabolism getting a little slower each year?
Have you dieted a lot in your past, and if so, do you think it has
    slowed down your metabolism?

The answers to these questions will help you set your goals in chapter 3 and determine how quickly these goals will be achieved. Knowing if you are above your set point is extremely important, it will provide you with the insight on how much "inflated weight" you will immediately drop on the program. It will also provide you with a glimpse of the moment when your first plateau will hit, so you can make the necessary adjustments to burst right through it. (Breaking through plateaus is explained in chapter 7.)

I always find with my clients that sharing success stories of people with similar body types, speeds of metabolism, and set points creates a strong connection that allows them to envision their starting point. For this reason, I am sharing Don's (ectomorph), Amy's (mesomorph), and Eric's (endomorph) stories with you. Let's start with Don.

Don Maclellan has the body type and speed of metabolism of an ectomorph. Don's body is an energy-burning machine. Like most ectomorphs, Don has struggled not with weight loss but with weight gain. The common term for people who struggle to gain weight is "hard gainer." Unfortunately, there is little sympathy for hard gainers. The majority of the population would, if given the choice, happily take on the "burden" of being able to eat practically anything they wanted and never gain weight. However, what I have learned by working with ectomorphs is that even though they do not have to worry much about gaining body fat, they are passionate about gaining weight. An ectomorph's desire to gain weight is similar to an endomorph's desire to lose weight. We have discussed the frustration dieters feel with the challenge of permanent weight loss. Well, ectomorphs feel a similar frustration with the challenge presented by permanent weight gain. You see, we are all different. All of us have different health goals and our own definition of what Body Confidence means to us. Most likely, if a person looks lean, fit, or skinny, the rest of us are under the impression that they are happy with their body, without ever actually knowing the goals they strive for. The dieting world alienates anyone who is not focused on losing weight. Why is that? Well, now you know the answer. Diets are not designed for a person whose goal is to gain weight.

This left Don in a similar place to where I found myself for years: searching for the right answers without knowing where to look. Growing up, Don was always called the "skinny" guy. (I know many women may like being called "skinny," but men *hate* that word. Men relate "skinny" to "scrawny," and there is nothing endearing about being called "scrawny.")

Over time, continually being called "skinny" began to eat at Don and started to affect his self-confidence. One day he decided enough was enough and went on a quest to build muscle mass. (Don hit his ectomorph tipping point.) He began reading every fitness magazine he could find, looking for the nutrition plan, workout, or supplement that would be the special ingredient to help him increase his size. Each magazine had its own version of a miraculous weight-gaining supplement, and after reading about it, Don would get excited, thinking this could be the answer for him. After thirty days with no results, his disappointment grew. And with each failed attempt, his disappointment grew even more. (Just like in the dieting world, the world of gaining weight is overhyped and full of false hope.) Don then started asking people at his gym for advice, many of whom just told him to eat more food. He thought that was easy enough and tried eating over five thousand calories per day. Doing this would temporarily help him put on a little weight, though the moment he missed a meal or ate less one day, every pound he gained was lost. So there Don was, lifting weights every day, trying a new supplement each month, and eating whatever he could, whenever he could. Every morning he would step on the scale, hoping for an increase in weight, for validation . . . that he hadn't done all this hard work for nothing. Unfortunately, his weight just stayed the same.

When I met Don, he was on the verge of giving up, feeling like there was no solution. He was looking at some supplements and asked me what I thought of a particular product. He told me that nothing he had done had worked to gain weight and he did not understand why. One of his dreams in life was to become a fitness model, and he felt that this dream was becoming impossible. I then proceeded to ask him some questions about his current nutrition and exercise, and immediately it made sense to me why Don could not gain weight. Since I had coached so many hard gainers to gain weight, it was pretty simple for me to figure out why Don was not gaining.

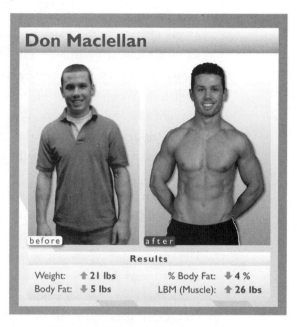

First off, Don did not have any structure in his meal plans. There was no balance to his nutrient ratios, meal intervals, or calorie intake. This imbalance left his blood-sugar levels unstable, regardless of the quantity of food he ate. Due to his metabolism, his body would waste the excess food he ate and then trigger bouts of low blood sugar, consuming muscle mass. . . . This is why Don was having such a hard time putting on weight. We quickly dialed him into the right meal structure, stabilizing his blood sugar and stopping his body from consuming its own muscle mass. In addition, Don focused on improving the quality of his food, especially his protein. Don was eating a large proportion of protein shakes and protein bars relative to the total number of meals he consumed. These food items are lower in quality than "real food." (I explain this in chapter 5.)

You see, protein is the only nutrient that contains nitrogen, and nitrogen is a main factor in whether our bodies are in a positive or negative state. Consuming a larger amount of nitrogen than what leaves our bodies puts us in a positive state. Keeping our bodies in a positive nitrogen state assists us in functioning optimally and building muscle mass. (I also explain this in chapter 5.) Don began eating higher-quality protein (which has more nitrogen per serving than protein shakes and bars), creating a greater ability for his body to build muscle. The final adjustment Don made was in his weight training. Hard gainers need to utilize a particular weight-training protocol to build muscle mass. (I discuss this concept in chapter 6.)

Once Don made these three adjustments, his weight and muscle mass began rapidly increasing. He put on five pounds the first month, and then over the next eight months he gained an additional sixteen pounds. Within a year of starting the program, Don gained twenty-one pounds and transformed his once "skinny" body into a muscular masterpiece! What I love most about Don's story is that he is now living one of his dreams: he is fitness-modeling. We spoke after his first photo shoot, and he said, "I really never thought this would happen . . . and it actually has. I can now call myself a fitness model." Don now has the knowledge to continue gaining weight, and he never has to worry about being called "skinny" again.

When Amy was five years old, her pediatrician told her mom that he thought Amy would grow up chubby. The pediatrician came to that conclusion because Amy was "big-boned" and had a mesomorph body type. Her sister's body type was more that of an ectomorph. All it took was one comment to start Amy's thirty-year journey of food deprivation and restriction. From that point on, her parents watched what she ate, sending her to school with carrots and celery while her friends were eating cookies and chips. She remembered feeling different from everyone else, wanting to eat what the rest of the kids ate. But she quietly put on a brave front and ate her rabbit food instead. Her family was Italian, and in their house, eating was always an event. Of course, this was at odds with her forecast of chunkiness. As her family celebrated by eating, she was always told, "That's enough" and "Kitchen's closed," while her older sister was given free use of the kitchen and her younger brother was encouraged to eat, eat, eat because he was a boy and he needed to be big and strong. The fact that Amy was big and strong was seen as a negative.

Amy was always active and engaged in sports, from swimming to dance to basketball. As her activity increased, so did her appetite and cravings. Her discipline was strong, and she continued to eat "healthy" foods; unfortunately, those foods were mostly carbohydrates. Amy was never taught what to eat; she was just told not to eat too many calories and to avoid fatty foods. That combination yields many blood-sugar spikes and the consequent fat gain. As the years progressed, Amy's constant battle with weight, body fat, and energy crashes would only get worse. She began to hate her body type, feeling that she was destined to be "the big girl." She became a chronic dieter, trying every program she got her hands on, only to find that nothing worked. As with most dieters, she would always lose a few pounds, only to gain it all back, plus more.

Amy hit her tipping point after returning from her honeymoon. She worked so hard to get leaner for her wedding, and on her honeymoon she gained seven pounds in seven days. That was it: from then on, she permanently eliminated the word *diet* from her vocabulary. It became "the D-word" to her. Over the next few years she had two wonderful children and chose to accept that she would be "the big girl" for the rest of her life. She felt that this destiny was in her genetic makeup.

When I met Amy she was overexercising and undereating, because that is exactly what she thought she was supposed to do. Back then, she was teaching a spin class, running marathons, and performing resistance training, all the while continuing in her struggles to get leaner.

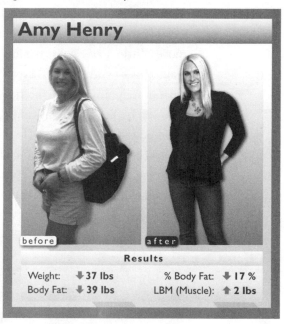

Amy Henry

before   after

Results

Weight:	⬇ 37 lbs	% Body Fat:	⬇ 17 %
Body Fat:	⬇ 39 lbs	LBM (Muscle):	⬆ 2 lbs

Even though she did not feel she was dieting, her body stayed in complete deprivation and restriction. She shared with me how she was struggling with low energy, how upset she was that she did not have enough energy to play with her two kids every afternoon, and how guilt was eating at her. Being a father, I could relate to how hard on her the lack of energy to play with her kids must be. It seemed crazy to me that this strong woman had struggled with her body for thirty years, willing to do the work but just not knowing what to do. She thought she was stuck in a body she did not want and that she just had to accept that fact. Amy and I dived right in; together we balanced her nutrient ratios, increased her meal intervals, and diversified her exercise so she was working out smarter and more efficiently. Her body was quick to respond: she began dropping body fat, her weight decreased, and she finally had energy in the afternoon. Her body just needed to be pointed in the right direction.

A few months later, I met with Amy and asked how she was doing. Her response made my day. She said, "I never thought I would love my body type, yet now I do."

Eric Standridge experienced the rise of his set point countless times, fighting weight ever since he could remember. He was embarrassed about his size, always avoided having his picture taken, and continually put on a happy face while deep down he was extremely disappointed in himself for being fat. He would look at people who were, in his words, "genetically blessed with a fast metabolism" and ask himself, "Why not me?" He followed in the footsteps of Shana and Amy, giving every diet a shot. He would start out strong, dropping weight quickly . . . and then his weight loss would slow down by the third week, move a little slower come the fourth week, and by the fifth week he would plateau. This is when he would reach his set point (even though he did not know what a set point was at the time). These plateaus would trigger frustration followed by Eric giving up and gaining all the weight back along with a little extra poundage, of course. He lived in the yo-yo dieting world. (It is interesting to think about how predictable dieting actually is; anyone who's tried it has gone through the same cycle!) So there he was, a classic "couch potato," over one hundred pounds overweight, and with a not-so-promising health future. Eric was scared; he knew that no one drops one hundred pounds quickly

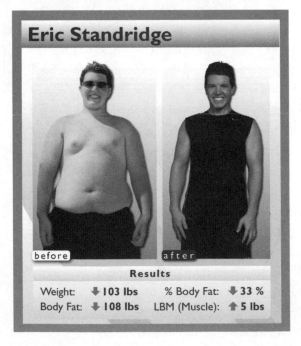

Eric Standridge

before — after

Results

Weight:	⬇ 103 lbs	% Body Fat:	⬇ 33 %
Body Fat:	⬇ 108 lbs	LBM (Muscle):	⬆ 5 lbs

(at least, not permanently), that it would take a lifestyle change. There were three huge obstacles standing in Eric's path: his hatred of eating "healthy"; his lack of motivation to exercise; and the damage years of dieting had done to his set point (causing his results to appear at a slower pace, affecting his motivation).

I met with Eric, and we spoke about creating solutions for his three big obstacles. First, he could eat the foods he loved; he just needed to commit to correctly working them into his program and to eating them in moderation. Then, we looked at the importance of enjoying exercise . . . of his finding an activity that he was excited to engage in. I explained to Eric how his years of dieting had affected his set point and that his progress would come in waves . . . that he would have moments of weight loss and body-fat loss followed by his body plateauing for a short period of time (one to three weeks). The reality was that Eric needed to lose over one hundred pounds. His body would release weight in specific amounts (about twenty pounds at a time) and then recalibrate to his new set point before he could once again drop more weight. This process is how his set point would be reprogrammed—speeding up his metabolism and reversing the damage that years of yo-yo dieting caused. I also expressed to Eric that I understood that he wanted the weight off as fast as possible but that the body, in its wisdom, just does not work like that. He needed to learn to work *with* his body, not against it, remembering that it took him years to put the weight on and that it would be a gradual process to *permanently* get it off.

Now, Eric chose to start . . . and over the next fourteen months, he built momentum each day. He focused on being consistent with his daily meals and meal intervals while simultaneously learning how to enjoy his food. He was eating the foods he loved; he finally understood what "moderate" actually meant. He was in shock that he did not have to give up the food he liked to eat. As his nutrition improved, so did the joy he found in exercise. He initially started walking three times a week, then four, then five. Walking improved how he felt, though he was still not "loving" to work out. Then a few months into the program we shifted from walking to running . . . and he found his exercise passion. Eric Standridge discovered that he loved to run . . . and he was off. The combination of his improved nutrition and his love for running caused his body fat to begin melting away alongside his weight. Each month his metabolism became faster and faster, and his set point lowered. He was making permanent lifestyle changes. His three huge obstacles were a thing of the past, and his hatred of exercise shifted into one of the greatest passions in his life. I watched Eric first run a 10K race, then a half marathon, and now he is training for his first full marathon—a great distance from his couch potato days.

Throughout our journey, my most memorable moment with Eric was when he broke the one-hundred-pound mark in weight loss. When we started our work together, he said, "This has to be the answer for me. I can't handle the feeling of failure with my weight again." Every time I see Eric it is like looking at a different person. The newfound pride and confidence he walks around with are inspiring. I think this is because he finally knows how to make his body work for him and actually feels in control of his health. In addition, Eric reprogrammed his set point. He lost 108 pounds of fat and put on 5 pounds of muscle. This increase in muscle mass and loss in body fat increased the speed of his metabolism and permanently lowered his set point.

Your Starting Point?

As you have learned, your starting point is the combination of your two "metabolic cards"—your body type and your set point—along with every choice you made that affected your metabolism in a negative or positive way up to this moment in time. This is where you sit, right now, and accepting it is crucial. Long-term success and True Confidence in your body are within your grasp. It is time to take control of your set point and reprogram your metabolism into a fat-burning machine.

When you are ready, let's move on to chapter 3 and set your Body Confidence goals!

3

CHARTING YOUR COURSE TO BODY CONFIDENCE

*Our goals are living and breathing pieces of us.
They provide us with clarity, purpose, and direction.
We must always remember that we control
the goal, the goal does not control us.
As we change, so will our goals.*

Picture this: you wake up every day and let the number on a scale determine your mood, the amount of energy you have, and even your motivation for the rest of the day. You let that number be the sole determining factor as to whether or not you are a step closer to achieving your goal. Millions live with that torment every day. Imagine living for a goal without any real plan, understanding, or direction regarding how to get there—being attached to an outcome that you have little control over. This is how most people set their health goals, and it can lead to an overwhelming feeling of failure when they fall short of that goal.

Now think about how you set your health goals in the past. Did you say something like, "I am going to lose *X* pounds"? At the time, did you know your starting point (speed of metabolism)? Did you set multiple short-term goals, or only one big goal? Was your weight your only measurement? Did you have any real plan for how you were going to achieve your goal? Did you feel like you were making permanent internal and external body changes on your way to your goal, or were the changes simply temporary?

The reality is that we have been trained for years to focus solely on our weight and to let that number determine every adjustment we make. Whether your goal is to lose weight, gain weight, or maintain it, your weight, wherever you wish it to be, is only part of your goal equation. Your actual focus should be your *body composition*. The accurate way to set your goals is through knowing your body composition, which in turn will take your Body Confidence to the next level.

Body Composition: Your Body's Makeup in Percentages

Body composition is divided into two main categories: *body fat* (all the fat in your body) and *lean body mass* (everything minus the fat in your body—primarily muscle, bone, and water). The easiest way to find out your body composition is to measure your body-fat percentage.

For example, if Jane weighs 150 pounds and has 20 percent body fat, she would have 30 pounds of body fat (150 × 0.2 = 30). Then, by simply subtracting Jane's 30 pounds of body fat from her overall weight of 150 pounds, we find out that Jane has 120 pounds of lean body mass (150 − 30 = 120). These calculations show that Jane's body composition is 30 pounds of body fat and 120 pounds of lean body mass.

The Two Types of Body Fat

One type of body fat is between your skin and muscle (*subcutaneous*), and the other type is found underneath the muscle that surrounds your organs (*visceral*). All body-fat tests will estimate both types of fat in your body, so all you really need to know is the overall estimated percentage of your body fat. There are multiple ways to have your body fat measured, and for consistency and convenience I recommend two types of testing (the methods that our nutrition centers use to measure body fat). You should get your body fat measured every two weeks until you reach your Body Confidence goals.

The methods that I recommend are the following:

1. **Skin caliper.** This is the type of testing I use with my clients. Skin calipers measure folds of skin and fat at various points of the body. Afterward, these measurements are put into a formula to determine body-fat percentage. Many health clubs, fitness centers, and health professionals can measure your body fat with a skin caliper. Your local health facilities may offer this either as a complimentary service or for a nominal fee.

2. **Body-fat scale.** A body-fat scale uses technology called *bioimpedance,* which involves passing a safe amount of electrical current through your body. Body-fat scales can be purchased online or at many retail stores. Body-fat scales are extremely convenient, since they let you measure your body fat at home. This convenience allows consistent body-fat measurements. A good-quality body-fat scale costs between one hundred and two hundred dollars. The brand I recommend is Tanita.

   Recommendation: Note that obtaining your body-fat percentage is not required for the program. However, knowing your body-fat percentage will be extremely helpful in setting your goals. Your ability to consistently measure your body fat every two weeks will be important in determining whether your body composition is improving.

   In addition, there are three other advanced methods of body fat testing: Hydrostatic (underwater), BodPod (air chamber), and Dexa Scan (x-ray). Each of these methods is very precise, but access to them is difficult to obtain. If you are near a facility that does use one of these methods, you can use that method to measure your body fat percentage.

Envisioning Your Body Confidence Goals

Ask yourself this: if you were able to achieve the look and size that you want and that would let you feel great, would you care how much you weighed? Think about that. . . . Many times clients enter my office with a number in mind—their perfect weight—because they believe that is the weight at which they can look the way they want to look. No one really cares about the weight itself; it is simply the only method of measure that they are taught. I ask each of my clients, "Does your weight really matter if your size, look, and energy are all fantastic?" The response is always the same: their weight is insignificant if they can achieve the look they want. This is a big shift from the dieting mind-set. Dieting teaches us to focus on weight, yet when someone wants to own a truly healthy body, they don't envision numbers on a scale; they envision themselves fit, lean, and healthy. If they look and feel like they want to look and feel, the numbers become irrelevant.

This is what Body Confidence is all about. Body Confidence is the true goal we each strive for, internally and externally. The numbers are just part of the goal-setting process. This is why your Body Confidence goals must be based on your body-fat percentage. By focusing on body-fat percentage, you will reprogram your metabolism through an improved body composition (less fat, more muscle). Now of course if your goal is to lose weight, you *will* lose weight, as the success stories in this book have shown. The point I am making is that focusing solely on weight is an outdated concept. By shifting your mind-set to focus on your *body-fat percentage,* you will do much more than lose weight: you will make your body work for you and achieve permanent results.

None of us just want to be "healthy"; we want an extra step—a sense of invincibility and a look and feel that breed Body Confidence. We want a higher quality of health, both internally and externally. Our health industry sets standards for people to achieve average health, and who wants to be average? When did being in "average health" become the goal? Maybe this is why our population is regressing so much. We have simply set the bar too low. Every client I have ever coached had a desire to take their Body Confidence to the next level, and the only way they could truly reach that next level was to raise the bar. This is exactly why I created Venice Nutrition's Four Levels of Health. The Four Levels of Health provide optimal body-fat standards and ensure that whatever your goal is, you will reach a body-fat percentage that yields optimal health while achieving a great, lean look. Before we dive into the Four Levels of Health, there are two important points about body-fat percentage to consider:

- First, there is a difference between essential body fat for men and for women. Essential body fat is necessary to maintain life. Essential fat is 1 to 3 percent in men and 10 to 12 percent in women. (This is not your body-fat recommendation; it is just the essential fat you need to survive.) This difference in essential fat is due to the fact that women's bodies, for multiple reasons (childbearing, hormone functions, and so forth), require more body fat for survival than men's.

- Second, due to this difference in body fat between genders, there are different "ideal healthy ranges" of body fat for men and for women. A healthy range for men is 12 to 16 percent body fat, and a healthy range for women is 20 to 25 percent body fat.

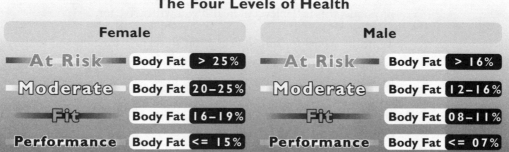

The Four Levels of Health

Female		Male	
At Risk	Body Fat > 25%	At Risk	Body Fat > 16%
Moderate	Body Fat 20–25%	Moderate	Body Fat 12–16%
Fit	Body Fat 16–19%	Fit	Body Fat 08–11%
Performance	Body Fat <= 15%	Performance	Body Fat <= 07%

The Four Levels of Health are designed to provide you with a device to gauge where you are and know where you want to take your body. Here are descriptions of each level of health.

At Risk

- Body-fat percentage is too high.

- There are many challenges that occur at this level of health: lower energy; slower metabolism; muscle loss; increased risk of potential health complications like diabetes, high blood pressure, high cholesterol, and so on.

- Typically, someone at this body-fat level has a goal of losing more than twenty-five pounds of body weight.

- If you are "At Risk," your goal is to get your body-fat percentage down to a "Moderate" level.

Moderate

- This is a healthy body-fat percentage.

- It is better to be below 15 percent for men and 23 percent for women. This figure provides a body-fat cushion that will prevent entering "At Risk" territory.

- Typically, a goal for someone at a "Moderate" level is to tone up and drop about ten to twenty pounds of body weight and take their body fat percentage to a "Fit" level.

Fit

- This is the body-fat percentage that provides a nice, toned physique.

- If your goal is to eliminate excess body fat and really tighten up your physique, this is the level of health you will strive for.

- Typically, a goal for someone at a "Fit" level is to tone up and to drop possibly five pounds or gain muscle to have more definition in their body.

- If you are at a "Fit" level, you may strive for a "Performance" level or choose to maintain in this level.

Performance

- This is an elite body-fat level.

- Typically, someone at a "Performance" level is looking to fine-tune their current body composition or enhance their skill set in athletics.

Taking Your Beginning Measurements

We each have external and internal Body Confidence goals. External goals are anything having to do with the "look" of your body—for example, losing weight and body fat, gaining muscle, and toning up. Internal goals are anything to do with how you "feel"—for example, increasing energy, reducing sugar cravings, having better-quality sleep, and lowering stress levels. As I have mentioned, both can be achieved simultaneously. Before we dive into goal setting, we need to take some measurements to provide the necessary data we can use to optimally set your external Body Confidence goals.

These measurements will be taken on a weekly basis (every two weeks for body-fat percentage), so it is important that you duplicate the environment in which you take them each week, meaning you should wear the same clothing, use the same scale, and, of course, use the same measuring device. Then, fill in your beginning measurements on page 66.

1. **Weight.** Weigh yourself *only* once a week, first thing in the morning, and always in the same clothing. There are many factors that can influence your weight, a few being stress, alcohol, lack of sleep, menstrual cycle, and too much sodium or too many carbohydrates at a meal. This is why weight is only part of the equation; it does not always tell the real story of progress. By weighing yourself only once a week in the same controlled environment, you are positioning yourself for the most accurate weight. This consistency will help minimize the day-to-day fluctuations your weight can undergo.

   One important note regarding weight: For women: Each month during your menstrual cycle, hormone changes will typically cause water retention and additional bloat, which cause a temporary increase in weight. This weight fluctuation varies for everyone. You should still weigh yourself; just be aware of the additional bloat you may experience at this time each month.

2. **Body-fat percentage.** Choose the measuring device that is more convenient for you—either a skin caliper or a body-fat scale. Once you choose your measurement method and know your starting body-fat percentage, you can calculate your pounds of body fat and pounds of lean body mass. It's a simple math formula. Here it is again for your reference:

   (Your weight) × (your body fat percentage) = your pounds of body fat

   (Your overall weight) − (your pounds of body fat) = your pounds of lean body mass.

   This information will provide your beginning body-composition numbers. Measure your body fat every two weeks until you reach your Body Confidence goals.

3. **Body-part measurements.** There will be moments when a week goes by and the scale does not move . . . yet your clothes fit better. This is why you take body-part measurements: dropping inches is a clear sign of progress. Use a tape measure, and measure these parts of your body at the same spots each week. For the most accurate measurements, measure each body part without clothing.

   - **Neck**—measure around the middle of your neck.

   - **Hips**—measure your widest point.

   - **Waist**—measure across your belly button.

   - **Thigh**—measure the top of your thigh.

Your Body Confidence Goal-Setting System

For many, the territory you are about to enter is uncharted, a place where your Body Confidence goals can be set based upon accurate information rather than emotion. It is a place where dieting can never take you.

There are two parts to your Body Confidence goal-setting system:

1. Choosing your Body Confidence goal type

2. Charting your course to Body Confidence

Part 1: Choosing Your Body Confidence Goal Type

There are two main goal types. Choose the one that best fits your needs.

Goal Type 1: **Lose Body Weight / Body Fat and Tone Up.** This is the main goal of the majority of our population. The main focus of this goal is on losing weight and body fat while toning up. Note that because your blood sugar will be stable, you will also increase your lean body mass (muscle mass) when you choose this goal.

Goal Type 2: **Gain Weight / Increase Strength / Build Muscle Mass.** This goal is designed for people at a Performance level of health only. The main focus of this goal is to gain weight, increase strength, and build muscle mass. If your body fat is higher than the Performance level of health, choose Goal Type 1 to start the program. Goal Type 2 is not designed to lose body fat, just maintain it. With Goal Type 1 you will lose the necessary body fat and still build lean body mass. Once your body fat falls within the Performance level parameters, you can shift to Goal Type 2 and maintain your Performance level body-fat percentage.

YOUR INTERNAL GOALS (FOR *BOTH* GOAL TYPES)

No matter what your external goals are, internal results are the same for both goal types. Since you will be stabilizing your blood sugar and creating a balanced environment in your body, both goal types will achieve an increase in energy, clearer focus, reduced sugar cravings, better-quality sleep, lower stress, optimal digestion, an improved balance of hormone levels—basically, an overall higher quality of health.

Part 2: Charting Your Course to Body Confidence

Now that you've identified your goal type and have an overall picture of what you want to achieve, it's time to put some time frames around your goals. As we set them, I would like to introduce a concept called the *Kaizen method*. (*Kaizen* is a Japanese term defined as "continuous improvements in small increments.") It is a method that I have personally experienced and witnessed work wonders when setting Body Confidence goals. Regardless of how long we have chosen to neglect our body when we hit our tipping point, we are all under the impression that our excess weight and body fat need to leave immediately. We forget the core principles of progress and the reality that everything takes time. We choose to ignore the word *patience* and instead set a big goal, expecting to get there the next day. As each day passes, our patience shrinks, causing us more frustration that our health results are not coming fast enough. Then one day we decide to just quit, telling ourselves that whatever we were doing for our health is not working, or that the goal we set was unrealistic.

Does any of this sound familiar? It may, since this example is typical of how health goals are set in our society. We are trained to set one big number as our goal and go for it (the "Big Goal" mind-set). . . . We focus solely on the destination and forget about the journey we must take to achieve it. When I was introduced to the Kaizen method, it changed the way I looked at my health. In fact, the example I just shared was me. I was the classic "Big Goal" setter—working hard to achieve that one goal. I never felt it could be achieved fast enough, and I was not enjoying the process I underwent as I worked toward the goal. This mind-set was exhausting. Whether I achieved the goal or not, I always felt like I was chasing something, never content with what I accomplished. By shifting my mind-set to one where I set incremental goals, I began achieving them one by one on a short-term basis, and each achievement felt like a victory. This provided me with a sense of accomplishment each day.

Imagine that you're standing on a map to Body Confidence, with your current health being point A (your starting point). Now visualize exactly what you want your body to look and feel like, placing your newfound Body Confidence on the other side of the map at point Z (your long-term goal). Your map now has a long-term goal established, point Z being quite a ways from point A.

What if you set additional short-term goals along the map? Doing so would help illustrate a clear path and enable you to see continual progress along the way to your long-term goal destination. This mind-set would allow you to win again and again, feeling successful on your path to achieving your long-term goal. Think about driving cross-country from Los Angeles to New York

City. In this example, Los Angeles would be point A (your starting point) and New York would be point Z (your long-term goal). Since the distance is lengthy, approximately twenty-eight hundred miles, you have a choice between driving with one of two different mind-sets on your road trip—the "Big Goal" mind-set or the Kaizen mind-set. If you focus solely on driving an insane number of miles each day in an attempt to arrive in New York as fast as possible, you will be exhausted to a point that you will probably not enjoy any of the drive. Not only that: once you do get to New York, you will be too tired to have any fun. The scenario I have described reflects the "Big Goal" mind-set I had for many years. In this mind-set, you live for the destination, and since getting there is such an unpleasant experience, you end up not being able to really enjoy it.

The Kaizen mind-set, on the other hand, provides a whole different experience. Returning to the trip scenario, what if you pulled out a road map and chose a route that had the most interesting and fun cities to visit on your way to New York? You would pick places you have always wanted to see, giving you something to look forward to each day you spend on the road. These cities would be your short-term goals, and each one you reached would bring you one step closer to your long-term goal (New York). Both mind-sets will get you to New York (your destination), true, though the Kaizen mind-set will yield a much more enjoyable path. This is why your goal-setting mind-set matters. In the end, your long-term goals can be achieved by utilizing either mind-set.

However, there is one more thing you should remember: achieving your long-term goal is only the first objective; maintaining that long-term goal is the second objective. Keep in mind that maintaining anything that is not an enjoyable experience is not easy. The "Big Goal" mind-set I have described is a big reason for burnout, causing many to fall off their health plan, as shown in a study by UCLA in 2007. According to this study, 83 percent of obese patients who started a weight-loss diet based on deprivation and/or restriction (calories in/calories out, low carb, etc.) gained more weight back than they had lost within two years of ending their diet. I think a big part of why diets fail in the long term (aside from the fact that they are based on incorrect theories of permanent weight loss) is due to the mind-set focused on the "big goal" and the dieter not enjoying the experience while on the diet.

By setting your goals in stages, you will be continuing to win as well as staying present throughout the entire process. This is what the Kaizen method is all about: acknowledging your continual improvements in small increments. We will use this method for both your external and internal goal-setting processes. The important thing to remember on your map to Body Confidence from A to Z is that your overall health momentum will be fueled by experiencing the achievement of accomplishing your short-term goals, and it will prove that you are getting closer each day to reaching point Z. Setting your goals in this way will maintain your presence along the journey as well as when you reach the destination. You will also make permanent lifestyle shifts that will ensure permanent results.

Goal Setting for Goal Type 1: Losing Body Weight / Body Fat and Toning Up

Whether you want to lose five pounds, twenty pounds, fifty pounds or more . . . the goal-setting system is the same for all weight and body-fat loss. In order to provide sufficient clarity in this process, before we set your goals, I would like to share the goal-setting process of two clients, a female and a male: Jennifer Oppenheimer and Scott King. Their results will provide you with a clearer picture of how to set your goals in your own goal-setting chart. Let's start with Jennifer.

Jennifer is in her mid-forties, and she felt her metabolism was slowing down due to her age and hormones. To make matters worse, she was struggling to find the time to eat well and exercise. You see, Jennifer has a full life as a wife, mom of two children, and owner of a baking business. She knew she wanted to lose her extra thirty pounds and make the journey from a size 10 to what she used to be, a size 4. . . . The task, however, seemed too daunting. There were three main obstacles that always seemed to get in Jennifer's way when she attempted to drop the weight. First, there was her busy lifestyle; she was always feeling that taking care of her health was just a lower priority than all of her other responsibilities. The second obstacle was her horrible sugar cravings. Jennifer is a baker, primarily of pastries. Whenever she would diet, she would eventually succumb to her cravings. They were uncontrollable; she was surrounded daily by her favorite desserts. Her final obstacle was her goal setting. Jennifer always focused on the goal of dropping thirty pounds, which would put her once again in a size 4. Every diet she did would yield initial results—ten, fifteen, even twenty pounds—but she always became frustrated with how hard

Jennifer Oppenheimer — Goal-Setting Chart

GOAL TYPE 1 Lose Body Fat / Body Weight & Tone Up

	Starting Point	1st Goal	2nd Goal	3rd Goal	4th Goal	Results
Level of Health	At Risk	Still At Risk	Moderate	Fit	Performance	Performance
Weight (lbs)	162	150	138	128	123	↓39
Body Fat (%)	38	32	25	18	15	↓23
Lean Body Mass (lbs)	100	102	103	105	105	↑5
Body Fat (lbs)	62	48	35	23	18	↓44

before   after

On average, the first short-term goal takes 2–4 weeks to achieve. From then on, each short-term goal takes approximately 4–6 weeks.

it was to drop the last ten pounds. This is where she would always fall off the diet, thinking there was no way to overcome her obstacles, and hence putting all the weight back on plus a little more. When I met Jennifer, she showed me photographs of a time when she was not carrying the extra weight. She shared how much she wanted to get back to that place and how much better her Body Confidence was then. She truly thought she was a victim of age and hormone changes . . . and that she was forever cursed with that extra weight.

Jennifer was committed and ready to start the program immediately; she just needed to learn how to overcome her three obstacles. In our work together, she and I quickly tackled each one. We started by shifting Jennifer's goal-setting mind-set. Ever since she put on the extra thirty pounds, all she wanted to do was get it off. The problem with that was that she never recognized the positive results she would achieve along the path to losing those thirty pounds. After we set her new short-term external goals, Jennifer was able to see her progress constantly and began to feel that she was on her way to achieving the long-term goal of losing those stubborn thirty pounds.

The next step was to eliminate her sugar cravings. She began eating to stabilize her blood sugar, and immediately her cravings became a nonissue. She could bake cookies, cakes, pies, and muffins without physiological cravings. Of course, Jennifer still loved her desserts, but at that point she regained control over her cravings. In Jennifer's past dieting history, every day on which she attempted to lose weight was more difficult than the previous one. This time, though, while on the program, each day became a little easier. A clear vision of her goals, and control of her sugar cravings, increased Jennifer's confidence. This new confidence empowered Jennifer to work her health into her busy lifestyle without feeling she was neglecting her family. Jennifer chose to include her family in the process and began cooking Venice Nutrition–

approved recipes and going on family walks. This allowed Jennifer to stay on plan and spend time with her family. (How to include your family and friends is covered in detail in chapter 8.)

Jennifer found the answers to regaining her Body Confidence and took her body from an At Risk level of health all the way to a Performance level. Ultimately she dropped well over her long-term goal of thirty pounds and returned to a size 4. She finally learned how to take control of her health and work it into her world.

Scott King also started at an At Risk level of health. Scott is a veteran of the air force, and for most of his life he has been lean and fit. He has always been active, being both a runner and a cyclist. Scott is similar to most men in that he always used exercise to stay lean. Scott would eat pretty much whatever he wanted, and his activity level would then allow him to burn off the extra calories. This continued to work for Scott until he entered the corporate world of finance management. Each week his exercise time dwindled, while his nightly business meetings increased. Scott was encountering a dilemma that many people reach: his poor nutrition habits were no longer countered by his high exercise level, and his weight started creeping up.

For the next few years, Scott's business continued to expand, and unfortunately, so did his waistline. He would get moments of inspiration and attempt to eat better and start working out. These moments would last for a few weeks, and then his business obligations would derail him. He would have an unexpected business trip, a new proposal deadline, or a late-night meeting. He would encounter an event that would cause him to fall off his routine and regress to his unhealthy habits. Scott hit his tipping point when he got a new driver's license. When his license was handed to him, he could not believe how big his face had become. He thought he looked like a chipmunk. It was at this moment that Scott knew something had to change. His waist size had gone from a 33 to a 38, he was at an all-time high in weight, and the additional weight was causing stress on his joints and lower back.

When I met Scott, he told me how he was very goal oriented and wanted to be clear on his progress points. Since Scott was in finance, he was well aware of the concept of small incremental changes and how they end up yielding big overall results. We started with laying out his map to Body Confidence, and we set his long-term goals of getting his weight below two hundred pounds, his body fat below 10 percent, and his waistline back to a 33. Based on his beginning stats, he had four short-term goals to achieve before reaching his long-term goal.

Scott King — Goal-Setting Chart

GOAL TYPE 1 Lose Body Fat / Body Weight & Tone Up

	Starting Point	1st Goal	2nd Goal	3rd Goal	4th Goal	Results
Level of Health	At Risk	Moderate	Moderate	Fit	Performance	Performance
Weight (lbs)	237	222	212	202	197	⬇40
Body Fat (%)	23	18	13	9	7	⬇16
Lean Body Mass (lbs)	182	182	184	184	184	⬆2
Body Fat (lbs)	55	40	28	18	13	⬇42

On average, the first short-term goal takes 2–4 weeks to achieve. From then on, each short-term goal takes approximately 4–6 weeks.

Scott was very structured and willing to do the work; he just never knew how to stabilize his blood sugar. Once Scott knew his nutrient ratios, calorie intake per meal, and meal intervals and received his meal plans, he integrated them into his daily routine. His waistline began to shrink immediately. As he progressed, Scott's energy increased, and the time he used to spend being inactive was now filled with exercise. Scott started walking, cycling, and eventually running again—all without joint or lower-back pain. At each meeting we had, you could see him gaining confidence in his ability to achieve the look and feel he wanted. His Body Confidence reached the ultimate level when he achieved his long-term goal of dropping below two hundred pounds, with a body fat below 10 percent and a waist size of 33! He looked up at me and said, "I finally feel like I have my life back."

Jennifer and Scott both provide examples of using the goal-setting system. Now it's time for you to read the goal-setting guidelines and time frames, and then proceed to your own goal-setting chart on page 66.

Here are the goal-setting guidelines and time frames for Goal Type 1.

Body Confidence Goal-Setting Guidelines

1. First, enter your initial measurements in your goal-setting chart: weight, body-fat percentage, pounds of body fat, and pounds of lean body mass.

2. Now it's time to set your short-term goals. In the goal-setting chart you will see columns. Take your starting weight, and drop approximately two pounds for every 1 percent body fat; for example, losing 10 percent body fat means losing twenty pounds of weight. To achieve this result,

you would set a long-term goal of twenty pounds and 10 percent body fat, along with a short-term goal of ten pounds and 5 percent body fat. This ratio of weight to body-fat percentage will keep your body composition within a good range. Feel free to refer to Jennifer's and Scott's goal-setting charts as examples. One important note: *Your long-term goal must reach at least a Moderate level of health.*

3. Calculate the pounds of body fat and pounds of lean body mass for each of the incremental goals you have set. This will provide you with a better overall picture of your goals.

   Weight × (% body fat) = pounds of body fat

   Weight − (pounds of body fat) = lean body mass

4. Remember, this is an approximation; for example, you may lose fourteen pounds for every 5 percent of body fat. The important things are that you are confirming that the weight you are losing is body fat and that you are maintaining or increasing your lean body mass.

It is important to give yourself a cushion of plus or minus four pounds and 2 percent body fat for your long-term goal. With life, it is almost impossible to stay exactly at a particular weight and body fat. This cushion will provide you with a range to stay within and will keep you dialed in without the stress that maintaining an exact number would bring.

Goal-Setting Time Frames

- In order to achieve permanent results, your body must be in homeostasis. You should begin to achieve internal goals before or at the same time as you achieve your external goals.

- If you are at an inflated weight (a weight higher than your normal weight—explained in chapter 2), you will most likely drop weight, body fat, and inches at a quick pace until you reach your true weight, or set point.

- Here are the average losses of weight, body fat, and inches in the *first two to four weeks* on the program.

   Lose 10–20 pounds in weight.

   Drop 5%–10% in body fat.

   Lose 2–4 inches in measurements.

- Spot-reducing is a *myth:* I have been asked many times about "spot-reducing," which means losing body fat in a particular region of your body. The reality is that spot-reducing is not possible. Unfortunately your "trouble areas" are typically the last place you get lean and the first place that stores fat (life just is not fair). The body typically follows this pattern when dropping weight and body fat. Your body will initially release body fat and bloat from your face, neck, legs, and arms. After that, you will continue to lose in those areas while continuing to get leaner throughout your core (chest, stomach, hips, butt, and upper thighs). You will notice that this cycle repeats every time you lose another eight to ten pounds.

- Once you reach your set point, the following list provides a reasonable set of short-term goals for you to achieve every two weeks until you reach your long-term goal level of health.

  Lose 2–4 pounds every two weeks.

  Drop 1%–2% of body fat every two weeks.

  Lose 0.5–1 inch per body part every two weeks.

Goal Setting for Goal Type 2: Gain Weight / Increase Strength / Build Muscle Mass

This goal type is designed to focus purely on increasing muscle mass. This goal type is chosen primarily by three groups of people: ectomorphs, athletes, and those who achieved their goal weight and body fat from Goal Type 1 and still want an increase in lean body mass. Here, you'll meet Kati Duwa and Dave Stockton. Both Kati and Dave started in Goal Type 1, and once they achieved their results, they shifted their goals to gaining strength and muscle mass. We will use their initial goal settings as well as their new goal settings as examples for you.

When I first met Kati, she was very clear about her goals. She wanted to lose body fat and gain lean body mass. One of her dreams was to have the body of a fitness model. She was already in good shape, read all the health magazines, ate "healthy," and even worked out five or six times a week. Kati

Kati Duwa — *Initial* Goal-Setting Chart

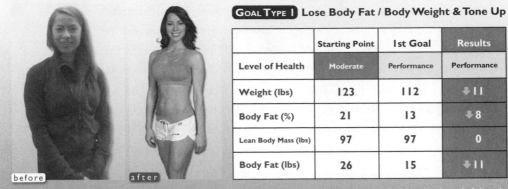

GOAL TYPE 1 Lose Body Fat / Body Weight & Tone Up

	Starting Point	1st Goal	Results
Level of Health	Moderate	Performance	Performance
Weight (lbs)	123	112	↓11
Body Fat (%)	21	13	↓8
Lean Body Mass (lbs)	97	97	0
Body Fat (lbs)	26	15	↓11

before   after

On average, the first short-term goal takes 2–4 weeks to achieve. From then on, each short-term goal takes approximately 4–6 weeks.

Kati Duwa — *Current* Goal-Setting Chart

GOAL TYPE 2 Gain Weight / Increase Strength / Build Muscle Mass

	Starting Point	1st Goal	2nd Goal	3rd Goal	Results
Level of Health	Performance	Performance	Performance	Performance	Performance
Weight (lbs)	112	114	116	118	↑6
Body Fat (%)	13	13	13	13	0
Lean Body Mass (lbs)	97	99	101	103	↑6
Body Fat (lbs)	15	15	15	15	0

On average, the first short-term goal takes 2–4 weeks to achieve. From then on, each short-term goal takes approximately 4–6 weeks.

felt she knew what to do based on all the diet books and magazines. Yet even with all her knowledge and effort, fine-tuning her body still presented her with a great challenge. As our conversation progressed, Kati spoke about how she avoided foods with fat and too many carbohydrates and how she also tried to not eat past 6 P.M. This is what she had learned through her reading and research. She shared how her cravings were extremely intense and how she would weekly binge-eat because of the unbearable food restrictions she felt. Every binge triggered another bout of exercise as she attempted to counter the damage her excess caloric intake had caused.

Getting Kati on the right path was a simple process. She was already consistently preparing her food and working out. . . . She was simply implementing faulty concepts. When Kati started the program, she was introduced to stabilizing her blood sugar and exercising efficiently, leading her to achieve her Body Confidence goals. She learned that avoiding fats and carbohydrates and not eating past 6 P.M. were all old-school thinking and based on highly inaccurate information. With her newfound knowledge, in a six-week period Kati took her body to another level and achieved the look of a fitness model.

Reaching her external goals was only part of Kati's success. For many years she felt embarrassed about her binging, and had no understanding of why she couldn't control herself. She would continually ask "What is wrong with me?" Once she started the program, Kati quickly discovered that nothing was wrong with her, she just had low blood sugar. The moment that resonates most with me about Kati's journey was the day she took her after photo. We were sitting in my office and she told me "Mark, I feel so strong. For the first time in my life, I finally have control over my cravings."

When Kati took her body to a Performance level of health she discovered what was truly possible with her body. The results she achieved increased her motivation. Kati decided she wanted to begin competing in fitness shows and knew adding additional lean body mass would give her a better chance at winning when on stage. Her goal shifted to gaining weight, six pounds of muscle to be precise, while keeping her body fat at 13 percent.

Dave Stockton was similar to Kati in the sense that he worked out consistently and was unhappy with his progress. No matter how hard he tried, he could not obtain the cut, muscular look he saw on the covers of the fitness magazines he read. Dave is a father and traveling working professional. Even with his busy schedule he made his exercise a priority; he just did not understand the importance of his nutrition. When I first met Dave, I asked him, "What is your nutrition plan?" He replied, "I really don't have a plan, I just eat when I can." Dave thought that as long as he ate healthy and had a good amount of food at each meal, his body would progress because of his exercise. This type of eating had Dave's physique appearing "soft"; he was not getting the "hard" look he wanted. That's why he classified himself as "not overweight and definitely not in shape." Dave desperately wanted to put on muscle and learn the best way to make his nutrition work for him. He was already making positive health choices; as with Kati, he just needed to be led in the right direction.

Dave Stockton — *Initial* Goal-Setting Chart

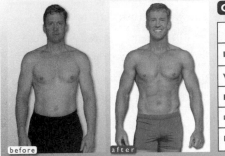

before / after

GOAL TYPE 1 Lose Body Fat / Body Weight & Tone Up				
	Starting Point	1st Goal	2nd Goal	Results
Level of Health	Moderate	Fit	Performance	Performance
Weight (lbs)	187	176	164	↓23
Body Fat (%)	18	11	4	↓14
Lean Body Mass (lbs)	153	156	158	↑5
Body Fat (lbs)	34	20	6	↓28

On average, the first short-term goal takes 2–4 weeks to achieve. From then on, each short-term goal takes approximately 4–6 weeks.

Dave Stockton — *Current* Goal-Setting Chart

GOAL TYPE 2 Gain Weight / Increase Strength / Build Muscle Mass						
	Starting Point	1st Goal	2nd Goal	3rd Goal	4th Goal	Results
Level of Health	Performance	Performance	Performance	Performance	Performance	Performance
Weight (lbs)	164	168	170	172	175	↑11
Body Fat (%)	4	5	5	5	5	↑1
Lean Body Mass (lbs)	158	160	162	164	166	↑8
Body Fat (lbs)	6	8	8	8	9	↑3

On average, the first short-term goal takes 2–4 weeks to achieve. From then on, each short-term goal takes approximately 4–6 weeks.

Dave stabilized his blood sugar and learned how to work out more efficiently and effectively. With these new adjustments, Dave sculpted his body and created a system to make his plan work while he travels. He achieved his initial long-term Body Confidence goal of shedding his unwanted body fat and gaining five pounds of muscle, and in my opinion, he looks perfect for the cover of a fitness magazine. Now the sky's the limit for Dave.

Dave's newfound Body Confidence showed him what is possible. For as long as he could remember he always wanted to build more muscle; he just never knew the tools to use to unlock his body's full potential. He now has these tools, and his new long-term goal was to gain ten additional pounds of muscle. This is his new goal-setting chart for his next long-term goal.

Kati's and Dave's *current* goal-setting charts provide you with great examples of how to set your goals for Goal Type 2. Your own goal-setting chart can be found on page 66.

Guidelines for Goal Type 2

1. Enter your beginning measurements in your goal-setting chart.

2. Now it's time to set your short term-goals. In the goal-setting chart you will see columns; these columns are for your different short-term goals. Take your starting weight and increase it by two pounds per column. Your body-fat percentage will remain the same throughout your weight-gaining phase. You may notice that your pounds of body fat may go up a little (one to three pounds, depending on how much weight you gain). This is inevitable. If your body fat remains at the same percentage and your weight goes up, naturally you will have an increase in pounds of lean body mass and pounds of body fat. The minor increase in pounds of body fat is unnoticeable. More lean body mass actually makes you look leaner and tighter. Feel free to refer to Dave's and Kati's goal-setting charts as examples.

3. Only those at Performance levels of health should focus on gaining weight.

4. Calculate the pounds of body fat and pounds of lean body mass for each of the incremental goals you have set. This will provide you with a better overall goal picture.

    Weight × (% body fat) = pounds of body fat

    Weight − (pounds of body fat) = lean body mass

5. It is important to give yourself a cushion of plus or minus 4 pounds and 2 percent body fat on your final long-term goal. With life it is almost impossible to stay exactly at a particular weight and body fat; this cushion will provide you with a range to stay in and keep you dialed in without the stress that maintaining an exact number would bring.

Goal-Setting Time Frames for Goal Type 2

-   In order to achieve permanent results, your body must be in homeostasis. You should begin to achieve internal goals before or at the same time as you achieve your external goals.

-   *Due to the anabolic (growth) environment created from stable blood-sugar levels and high-quality protein, you should quickly gain two to four pounds of weight.*

Your Goal-Setting Chart

GOAL TYPE _____

EXTERNAL GOALS

Body Composition Goals						
	Starting Point	1st Goal	2nd Goal	3rd Goal	4th Goal	Results
Level of Health						
Weight (lbs)						
Body Fat (%)						
Lean Body Mass (lbs)						
Body Fat (lbs)						
Body Part Measurements						
Neck Meas. (in)						
Hip Meas. (in)						
Waist Meas. (in)						
Thigh Meas. (in)						

You may have more or less than four short-term goals.
This all depends on your long-term goal.

INTERNAL GOALS

e.g. "Increased Energy" or "Reduced Sugar Cravings"

1
2
3
4
5
6

On average, the first short-term goal takes 2–4 weeks to achieve.
From then on, each short-term goal takes approximately 4–6 weeks.

- Once you reach your set point, the following is a reasonable progression every month:

  Gain 1–2 pounds every month until you reach your goal.

  Gain inches in areas where you want to build muscle mass. (Measure those body parts on a monthly basis.) The specific amount gained per month depends completely on the individual.

Your Map to Body Confidence Is Set

Your starting point is established, your destination is determined, and your course is clear. You are geared up and ready to take your Body Confidence to the next level. It's time to press down the accelerator and speed into the Venice Nutrition Three-Step System to *unlock your body's full potential!*

Chapter 4, here we come. . . .

4

YOUR BODY CONFIDENCE FOUNDATION

Knowledge is knowing. Wisdom is applied knowledge.

—Dan Millman

It is one thing to acquire knowledge; it is another to actually apply it. It's time to take the knowledge you just learned and apply it to your own personal health and lifestyle. The next three chapters will provide you with the tools you need to develop a rock-solid Body Confidence Foundation that will unlock your body's full potential.

Think of the process of buying, building, and living in a house. Think about it: where our home is located determines many things—our commute to work, where our children go to school, how safe we are, what we do for entertainment, which social events we attend, plus so much more. Our home is located in the center of our personal world, since it affects so many aspects of our daily life. So far what I've been talking about is just our home's location, though. . . . What about the square footage, the layout, the type of flooring, its functionality, what the view looks out on, how large a backyard it has, and so on? . . . I think you get my point. Where we live is an extremely important choice, and what we "get" from our home plays a huge part in our happiness.

Because of the magnitude of this decision, we spend an abundance of time choosing our home. I think many of us know the consequences of quickly choosing your living space. Simply put, you end up regretting it or, at the very least, becoming all too familiar with its limitations. Add to that the fact that this is not a decision that can easily be reversed. Because choosing a home is so important, it is what I call a powerful "why." We have a "why" in everything we do. . . . "Why" is defined as the reason we do something. The time we choose to invest in the process along with our commitment to stay the course, is dependent on the strength of our "why." This is why choosing a home is considered a very strong "why."

Now we must think about the actual infrastructure that went into building our home: leveling the land; laying the foundation; building the frame; installing the plumbing, electricity, and gas lines; painting the outside and inside; and so on. It had to be built to last, and it has to withstand all types of weather. A good house has a strong infrastructure.

Once you choose your house and are confident in its infrastructure, it's time to live in it. The work isn't over, though. Think about all the things you must do to maintain your home: cleaning, doing minor repairs, adding a new feature, purchasing additional furniture—the examples are infinite. Ask

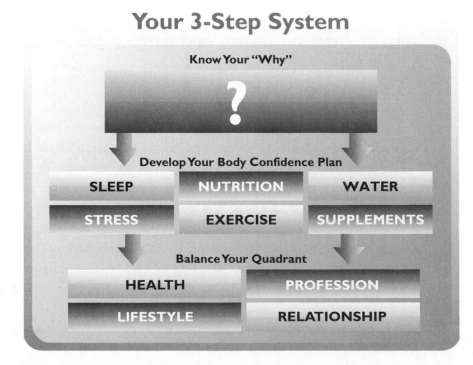

yourself how much time you spend each day, week, or year maintaining your house. What happens when you get busy or sick for a week and you don't have time to clean the kitchen, do laundry, or, if you have children, pick up toys? (My son, Hunter, like most six-year-old boys, is a daily tornado inside our house.) We all know what happens: the house becomes a mess. Maintaining an organized and clean house takes a daily effort.

Now it's time to ask yourself whether you spend the same amount of time on your health as you do on your home. How is the process of choosing your home, building your home, and maintaining your home any different from how you maintain your health? Think about it: our true home is our body, and just as we know a neglected house when we see it . . . we also know when we neglect our bodies. The reality is this: just as there are criteria determining the process that goes into your home, there are criteria for your health. The Venice Nutrition Three Step System provides the criteria necessary to solidify your Body Confidence Foundation.

Step 1: **Knowing your "why"**—your reason and purpose for Body Confidence

Step 2: **Developing your Body Confidence Plan**—your game plan to achieving Body Confidence

Step 3: **Balancing your Quadrant**—working your Body Confidence plan into your world

Step 1: Knowing Your "Why"

Ask yourself, *"Why" do I want to be healthy?* Really think about this one; it will be the most important health question you will ever ask yourself. Then follow up with this question: *What happens once I achieve my "why"?* For example, let's say you're reading this book because your Body Confidence goal is to lose thirty pounds. Your "why" is the reason you want to lose thirty pounds, which is to look and feel great for a wedding in three months. Your motivation is high, so you dive right into the program, set realistic and attainable goals, and three months later, you did it! You lost thirty pounds and 15 percent body fat. You achieved your goals, and when the wedding came, you looked and felt amazing.

Now what? What is going to keep you moving forward and progressing with your health? Your "why" and goals were both achieved. You tell yourself,

"I worked hard, so I will take a week off, then jump right back on." A week passes, and the motivation is not there anymore. Instead of advancing or maintaining, you begin to regress with your health. Even though you stabilized your blood sugar and really enjoyed the three months you lived the program, you are simply having a hard time jumping back on. . . . Why is that? The answer to this question is a simple one: you didn't have a "why" strong enough to carry you through. The reality is that no matter how physiologically sound a program is—whether it gets you great results and works into your lifestyle—if you are unclear on *why* you want to be healthy, you will always struggle.

Finding your "why" is like choosing where you want to live. Finding a strong "why" will play a big part in your daily happiness. This same type of thought process needs to be applied to "why" you want to be healthy. The truth of the matter is that short-term "why"s—like looking and feeling great at a wedding in three months—are very powerful and do work. The challenge with using a "why" that lasts you only three months is just that: it lasts only three months. In the short term, "why"s like this are great to have as long as there is a powerful long-term "why" already in place. . . . It will be your reason to keep going once you achieve your short-term "why."

My client Rachel is a great example of having powerful short- and long-term "why"s. Rachel came to me because she was a collegiate tennis player and wanted to drop body fat, increase speed, and maximize her recovery. Her short-term "why" was strong and clear: she wanted to get great results so she could be better on the tennis court and have an edge over her competition. This "why" would keep her disciplined and lead her to achieving her Body Confidence goals. The big questions I asked Rachel were: What happens after the season and you have achieved your goals? What will keep you moving forward with your health? Fortunately, she had a even more powerful long-term "why." You see, Rachel is a type 1 diabetic. Her long-term "why" was to minimize her daily insulin intake. Less daily insulin would keep her body and blood-sugar levels optimally balanced and efficiently manage her diabetes for life.

Type 1 diabetes is a condition in which the pancreas does not produce insulin. Since insulin is essential for the body to maintain balanced blood sugar (as discussed in chapter 1), a type 1 diabetic needs to take insulin. The technology these days is amazing. Most type 1 diabetics now have an insulin pump (instead of needing to give themselves shots throughout the day) that provides their body with the correct amount of insulin depending on their nutrition. Remember, the purpose of insulin is to lower the blood sugar, so the amount of insulin a type 1 diabetic needs is directly determined by their quality of nutrition. Type 1 diabetics are exactly like anyone else, with one exception: most people's pancreases make insulin, and theirs does not. Both diabetics and nondiabetics still need insulin.

When I started working with Rachel, she was taking an average of 70 units of insulin per day. Within two weeks of starting the program, the amount of insulin she needed dropped to only 48 units per day. Her body needed 22 fewer units of insulin per day! Even though she was eating healthy and exercising before she started the program, her blood sugar was still spiking, which is why she needed extra units of insulin. This extra insulin would lower her blood sugar and also end up causing her to store fat. (High blood sugar causes fat storage.) The moment we correctly stabilized her blood-sugar levels by focusing on meal intervals, nutrient ratios, and calories per meal, her blood-sugar elevated far less, and therefore her body required less insulin. This in turn released her stored fat and maximized her energy and performance on the court. Her stored fat was then burned in her muscle during her training on the tennis court. Within six weeks Rachel dropped fifteen pounds of fat and added 3 pounds of lean body mass! This positive shift in her body composition took her tennis game to the next level. She was quicker, stronger, and had much better endurance during matches.

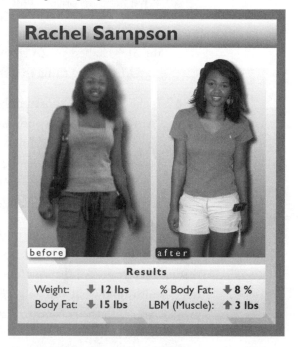

Rachel Sampson

before   after

Results

| Weight: | ↓ 12 lbs | % Body Fat: | ↓ 8 % |
| Body Fat: | ↓ 15 lbs | LBM (Muscle): | ↑ 3 lbs |

Rachel used her short-term "why" as the driving force to achieve her Body Confidence goals. Once her goals were achieved, her long-term "why" of optimally managing her insulin levels was what kept her consistent with her Body Confidence plan each day. She will always be a type 1 diabetic. She will always need additional insulin. Rachel may have many short-term "why"s throughout her life, but her long-term "why" is what will always keep her moving forward and progressing with her health.

Rachel came to know both her short- and long-term "why"s. Now it's time for you to think about *your* short- and long-term "why"s. You have set your

Body Confidence goals; now let's figure out the reason you want to achieve those goals.

Ask yourself these five questions:

1. "Why" do I want to achieve my goal(s)?

2. What will I "get" from achieving my goal(s)?

3. What happens once I achieve my goal(s)?

4. Is my "why" strong enough to keep me focused on my health during life's challenges? (A challenge can be moving, a new job, illness, traveling . . . anything that throws a wrench into your daily routine.)

5. Is the "why" I've chosen only short term? If so, what is my long-term "why"? (Losing thirty pounds to look and feel great for a wedding is an example of a powerful short-term "why." Tom Barone's "why" of becoming healthy so that he can be the father he wants to be for his boys—discussed in chapter 1—is an example of an excellent long-term "why." You should always have a short-term "why" and a long-term "why.")

Know that the short-term and long-term "why"s you have chosen may change through the years. All that matters is that you always know "why" you want to be healthy and what you will achieve by being so. Being clear on this will provide you with the reasons to stay the course and fully live with complete Body Confidence.

Step 2: Developing Your Body Confidence Plan

Think of when the home you live in was built. Do think the builders had a blueprint, or did they just wing it? If your house was built without a plan, it would most likely have a faulty structure and be ready to collapse at any moment. Now think about a business. Do you think a business with a plan has a greater chance at success than a business without a plan? Both of these analogies apply to your health. Following a diet is like building a house or starting a business without a plan. . . . They are all doomed to crumble. Now consider this: you have a Body Confidence plan designed to create a balanced internal environment in your body, a plan that will evolve with you and provide the necessary guidance and structure to keep you in tune with your body. A plan like this is like a blueprint for a house or a business—something you can always use as a reference point. It's also a point to return to and adjust if something needs to change. Your Body Confidence plan focuses on the six components that primarily determine your body's overall health.

THE SIX COMPONENTS OF YOUR BODY CONFIDENCE PLAN

1. Sleep—*your battery charger*
2. Nutrition—*your fuel*
3. Exercise—*your burner*
4. Vitamins, minerals, and omega fatty acids—*your protection*
5. Water—*your fluid*
6. Stress—*your X-factor*

In the introduction I discussed how and why I created the Body Confidence plan. It was the key to helping Abbi regain a vibrant body and mind. You see, each component has a direct effect on how your body functions. Correctly implementing each component of your plan will be the determining factor in achieving your Body Confidence goals. This section of the chapter is designed to provide you with a part of the plan. *Due to the depth of content and importance of your nutrition and exercise plans, these two components—nutrition and exercise—will be presented to you in chapters 5 and 6, respectively. Here, we'll focus on getting your sleep, vitamins, minerals and omegas, water, and stress dialed in.* Let's begin with your key component: sleep.

Component 1: Sleep—Your Battery Charger

That's right: sleep is the most important component of your Body Confidence plan! As I previously shared, "You are what you eat" should really be "You are what you metabolize." Without a consistent sleep schedule, it is a much larger challenge for your body to optimally metabolize its food, manage its stress levels, and have enough energy for you to exercise. Imagine a cell phone. It has a battery that needs to be kept continually charged. Most of us charge our cell phones each night so we can have full battery power for the following day. Have you ever forgotten to charge your phone and tried to take on the day with only half a charge? Every time you look at your phone, you watch as the battery bar dwindles away, knowing full well that it will soon run out of juice and you will be phoneless. Well, your body's battery is your *adrenal gland,* similar to the battery in a cell phone. The adrenal gland releases two hormones—adrenaline and cortisol. Both help keep your energy flowing throughout the day, just as your phone's battery releases energy to keep your phone running. The way you keep your battery (adrenal gland) charged is by getting enough sleep.

Your sleep recharges your body, just like a phone charger does with a cell phone. Sleep also allows your body to repair and renew tissue, nerve cells, and other glands, plus sleep allows your brain to reorganize its thoughts and memories, like organizing a file cabinet. In a perfect world, we would always get the proper amount of sleep and have enough energy for the day. As we all know, that world does not exist. The nights when you do not get enough sleep cause you to start half charged. There are many similarities between your battery (adrenal gland) and a cell-phone battery, but there is a big difference: When a cell-phone battery runs out of juice, it ceases working. This is not the case with your body. Your body will keep working—just at a less efficient pace. The more sleep deprived your body becomes, the harder it is on your body, because lack of sleep creates a hormonal imbalance of adrenaline and cortisol. This imbalance causes an energy deficit in your body, which triggers a universal metabolic slowdown. This cycle of slowdown and hormone imbalance creates a negative environment in your body, triggering water retention, digestive challenges, irritability, lack of clarity, and unstable blood sugar—to name a few.

Think of a time when you accumulated days of sleep deprivation. How did you feel? How was your digestion? How were your stress levels? Since lack of sleep can create havoc in your body's hormonal system, it is important to establish a real *plan* for sleep. Sleep deprivation is inevitable at times. At these moments, your sleep plan will give you the tools you need to get back on track and fully recharge your battery. Your sleep plan is composed of four strategies. These four strategies focus on optimizing both the quantity and quality of your sleep. Here they are:

1. **Learn the optimal number of hours you need to sleep.** We hear it all the time: get eight hours of sleep every night. The reality is that we are all different. Some people require more than eight hours of sleep, and some require less. Abbi needs a solid eight hours per night, and

I need about six hours. The easiest way to figure out the number of hours of sleep you need each night is to think back to a time when you consistently awakened to start the day rested. The number of hours that you slept then is the number of hours of sleep that you should aim for.

One important note: It doesn't matter the time of day or night that you sleep, as long as you follow the principles explained in each strategy. Meaning: if you work a graveyard shift and you sleep from 7 A.M. until 3 P.M. each day, as long as you implement these four strategies, you will be optimizing your sleep.

2. **Develop a sleep schedule.** Every parenting book recommends putting a baby on a sleep schedule. Why is that? It is because our bodies function better with consistency, and a schedule provides that type of consistency. Of course, as life gets busier it becomes more difficult to follow a sleep schedule. With late meetings, travel, sick children, and, basically, the reality of life, sleep itself can become a challenge. For this reason, your sleep schedule will derail at times. Here are three steps to developing your sleep schedule, including the adjustments to make when you fall off:

Sleep Schedule Steps and Adjustments

Step 1: Know the optimal number of sleeping hours you need each night.

Step 2: Choose a daily wake-up time and bedtime—preferably the same each day.

Step 3: Make up your sleep when you fall off your schedule. Sleep deficits can be made up! Let's say you need eight hours of sleep per night and you slept only six for two nights in a row. This would mean you are in a four-hour sleep deficit. It is important to keep the same wake-up time each day, so you would then go to bed earlier each night until the four hours you have lost are made up. This means that one night you go to bed two hours earlier than normal and still wake up at the same time the following morning. This would result in you making up two hours of your deficit. You could then do the same thing that evening or space it out over a few more days until you made up the remaining two-hour sleep deficit. The key in all of this is to keep the same wake-up time: this keeps your sleep/wake cycle intact. As much as we all enjoy sleeping in on the weekend, proceed with caution. Think of the last time you slept in: most likely you stayed up later that evening, and the following morning you wanted to sleep in again. Your body is a fast-adapting machine, and it will quickly adjust to your bedtime and your wake time. Inconsistency in both will lead to an erratic pattern, resulting in sleep deficits. Controlling your wake-up time will ensure that you are stabilizing your sleep/wake cycle.

3. **Maintain a quiet environment.** Many people fall asleep while watching a movie or television. Initially, this may help you fall asleep, yes. But then, as the night progresses, the noise and light will only disrupt your sleep cycles. Let me explain. Your sleep each night goes through cycles. It cycles between non-REM sleep and REM sleep. REM (Rapid Eye Movement) is a cycle that makes up approximately 20 to 25 percent of an adult's sleep. In REM sleep, your brain activity is similar to what it is during an awakened state, though your muscles remain in a state of paralysis. This is when most of your dreaming occurs. The muscle paralysis you experience simply ensures that you cannot act out your dreams. REM sleep renews the mind. During REM sleep your mind organizes its thoughts and memories, similar to putting files in a file cabinet. In addition to working as a filing system, REM sleep also replenishes your feel-good chemicals (serotonin and dopamine), which boost your mood throughout the day.

   Non-REM sleep has four stages and makes up approximately 75 to 80 percent of an adult's sleep. Stage 1 is considered light sleep, the easiest time to wake up. Stage 2 prepares your body for deep sleep. And stages 3 and 4 are considered deep sleep. Whereas REM sleep renews your mind, deep sleep renews your body. Deep sleep is the time when your body repairs tissue, stimulates growth, and strengthens your immune system. Once you go through these four stages of sleep (about 90 minutes from stage 1 through stage 4), you enter REM sleep (initially lasting around ten minutes, and typically increasing in length as your sleep progresses). Once your REM sleep is completed, the cycle repeats itself. This means you will then reenter stage 1, light sleep. This is why if you sleep with a TV on, the noise from that TV could wake you from your sleep or at the very least affect the quality of your sleep. (An exception to this is a situation in which you are sleeping with a noise device that has a consistent volume. This kind of noise does not have the volume ups and downs that a TV program would have.)

Many times people feel that watching TV is the only way they can fall asleep. If this pertains to you, I suggest focusing on strategy 4, since it will yield a much better result than watching TV as you drift off to sleep.

4. **Create proper downtime.** Think about your typical twenty-four-hour day. We wake up, and usually it takes about an hour to get in the groove of the day. After that, we take on the day at an intense level. Then our body begins to decompress and needs its downtime. At that point we sleep to recharge, and the cycle repeats itself. This has always been our sleep/wake cycle. Now think about the times when you go to bed without any downtime. . . . How well do you sleep? Do you toss and turn? If you are exhausted, you probably fall right to sleep. If not, you probably toss and turn. The way I create proper downtime is by viewing each day like a sport. When I wake up, I look at that part of my day as my warm-up; then as I enter the bulk of my day, I start playing the game; and then as the night approaches I shift to my cooldown, which is my downtime.

    My point is that it is very challenging to push and push through each day without any kind of decompression. Nightly downtime will greatly assist you in optimizing your sleep. Now, your downtime can be anything that relaxes you, that is healthy, and that you find joy in. Ideally you would have at least an hour of downtime before bedtime. A few examples: taking a bath; reading; a light, relaxing walk; listening to music; surfing the Web; watching a movie or TV (just make sure to turn off the TV before you go to bed).

Component 2: Nutrition—Your Fuel

As I have shared, your body is a "refuel as it goes machine." So the next question is, "What type of fuel should I feed my body?" In chapter 5 we will be diving into every facet of your nutrition plan. With this plan we will stabilize your blood sugar, consistently release your stored fat, and optimally balance your hormones, all as you eat the foods you love and successfully work your nutrition plan into your world.

Component 3: Exercise—Your Burner

Your exercise is what activates your engine (muscle) to burn your fuel. A common misconception is that all exercise is equal . . . the truth is far from that. In chapter 6 we will explore the two categories of exercise and then design a diverse plan that recruits of all your muscle fibers, which will maximize your fat-burning capabilities, increase your lean body mass, and speed up your metabolism.

Component 4: Vitamins, Minerals, and Omega-3 Fatty Acids—Your Protection

It seems like a new magic vitamin or supplement promising us great health appears every day. The manufacturers promise that all you need to do is take the supplement each day and your health goals will be achieved. When I was fitness-modeling, I bought into the hype. I was driven to achieve the best possible natural physique, so I went all-in on anything that magazines or TV commercials said would get me closer to the body I wanted. It got to the point where I was spending about four hundred dollars per month on supplements. I bought vitamins, minerals, fat burners, omega fatty acids, and even creatine (a product that helps with strength, muscle mass, and recovery). It got to the point where I was taking so many supplements that I had no idea what was working. Add that to the fact that my physique continued to improve each month, and I definitely did not want to stop taking any of them. I began to believe that the supplements were the reason I was getting results, that all of my hard work with nutrition and exercise was secondary to the supplements I was taking. Unfortunately, this is how the supplement companies (and pharmaceutical companies) condition us. They all claim that a pill is our solution and is more powerful than the daily choices we make.

It was then that Abbi once again brought me back to reality. I was reading an ad in a fitness magazine promoting a new vitamin-like substance that was being touted as the next amazing antioxidant (a substance that helps protect your body). I was very excited and immediately showed the ad to Abbi. She took one look at the ad and said, "Are you sure all these supplements you take even work? Your body might be just as good without them." *What was she was thinking!?!?* "Of course they work," I replied. "Why else would I take them?" She said, "Why not try a month without them and see what happens?" That was tough advice to hear, since I honestly thought all my results were due to the supplements I took, and fear told me that stopping would cause my results to disappear. Then I thought to myself, "What if she's right?" I paused for a while, thought about it some more, and then responded, "OK, I'll give it shot. But if I lose all of my progress, I'm blaming you!" We both laughed, and I immediately stopped taking 95 percent of the supplements. I kept taking two: a liquid multivitamin/mineral, and 5 grams of omega-3 fatty acids.

After a month passed, I was in a state of disbelief, since everything about me felt and looked the same as when I was taking the supplements. I quickly realized that all the supplements I was taking were a nonfactor. I was filling my body with unnecessary products, wasting four hundred dollars a month, and, most important, crediting all of my positive health results to supplements that didn't seem to do anything! The truth is that I was discounting all of my hard work. From that point on, I focused on understanding which supplements were essential to my body and which were not. I knew then, beyond the shadow of a doubt, that 99 percent of my health results were because of my hard work, not supplements.

In this part of your Body Confidence plan, my purpose is to focus on three essential nutrients that your body needs and that many times are delivered through taking supplements. These three nutrients are vitamins; minerals; and omega-3 fatty acids. All three are called essential nutrients, which means that each is essential for your body to function at optimal levels. *Essential* also means that your body cannot synthesize (make) enough of these nutrients or that it cannot synthesize them at all. I also want to make it clear that you can get the optimal amount of vitamins, minerals, and omega fatty acids by diversifying your food choices. This means you do not need to take any supplements if you eat the right foods. Yet the majority of us live very busy lifestyles and, because of this, lack the necessary diversity in our foods. So most of us do not get enough of the essential nutrients our bodies need. For this reason, I would recommend taking a multivitamin/mineral and omega-3 fatty acids.

Multivitamin/Mineral Recommendations. The marketplace is saturated with multivitamin/minerals. Instead of recommending one brand, I will recommend the *type* of multivitamin/mineral to purchase. Your multi will come in one of four different forms: liquid, capsule, chewable, or tablet. I suggest going to a local health-food store and looking over a few of the options. Your best choice is always the liquid, since this will ensure maximum absorption. The two things you want to watch for are the taste and expense of the supplement. A liquid is always more expensive and will typically last one month. Liquid is ideal for anyone who suffers from digestive challenges. Your second choice is the capsule form. Capsules are also absorbed nicely by the body. Your third and fourth choices are the chewable form and the tablet. The chewable form has a better absorption factor than a tablet. Tablets should be your last choice; many times they are not even digested by the body.

Your Multivitamin/Mineral Dosage. I would simply follow the recommended dosage on the bottle and make sure to take your multivitamin/mineral in the morning with food. You definitely want to be careful about overconsuming vitamins and minerals. Two important keys to the program are balance and quality, so just doing or taking more is not better. You need to make sure you get just the amount your body needs.

Omega-3. Ninety-five percent of my clients are deficient in omega–3 fatty acids when I begin working with them. Within two weeks of adding these essential fats to their diet, clients report noticeable improvements in their hair, skin, and nails. Studies show that omega–3s can lower blood pressure and cholesterol, improve brain function, and reduce joint pain and inflammation.

Since omega–3 is an essential fatty acid (your body cannot make it), it is crucial that you get it through food or supplementation. Here are three options:

- **Option 1.** Eat a fatty fish at least three times a week, preferably salmon. There is concern about mercury levels found in fish, though the topic is still under debate. (I do think salmon consumed in moderation is fine, however.) If this issue is of concern to you, I would choose option 2 or 3 to get your omega fatty acids.

- **Option 2.** Take 3,000 to 5,000 mg of fish oil. This works out to three to five gelcaps per day (depending on the brand). Here are some tips about fish oil:

    Avoid supplements that come in clear bottles: light can affect the potency of omega-3.

    If you suffer from acid reflux or have a sensitive stomach, fish oil can cause you to have burps that smell like fish (not exactly what you want). There are two ways to avoid this: you can purchase pharmaceutical-grade fish oil, or you can freeze your gelcaps. Freezing them will delay digestion and usually prevents any reflux.

- **Option 3.** Take 3,000 to 5,000 mg of flaxseed. Here are some tips:

    Flaxseed oil gelcaps typically do not cause reflux.

    Flax oil can be used in shakes as your source of fat.

    Flaxseeds can be eaten whole or ground and added to any meal as a topping.

MULTIVITAMIN/MINERAL / OMEGA TAKEAWAY

Simply take a multivitamin/mineral each morning along with omega gelcaps, and your body will be getting the essential nutrients that are typically lacking in most people's diets. Combine these two supplements with high-quality food (presented in the next chapter), and your body will have all the nutrients it needs to perform at optimal levels.

Component 5: Water—Your Fluid

Water is the most underestimated essential nutrient. Water is a core component in your overall health and a crucial part of achieving your goals. Your body is made up of approximately 60 to 70 percent water. You can live up to five weeks without food. However, on average you can live only three to five days without water! So to say the least, water is very important to your body. There are four main benefits of drinking enough water:

1. **Water keeps your metabolism humming.** After achieving stable blood sugar, you will be consistently releasing fat and toxins. Proper water intake flushes out the excess by-products that your body does not need. Solid hydration also allows your kidneys and liver to work at optimal efficiency. Last, water is necessary to maximize digestion and prevent constipation.

2. **Water maintains healthy blood and muscles.** Have you ever woken up with a cramp in your leg? We all know this is painful, and it is almost always caused by dehydration (not enough water in your body). An imbalance of two electrolytes (sodium and potassium) is what causes the cramping. You will be exercising on the program. If you make sure you stay hydrated and stretch as recommended (in chapter 6), middle-of-the-night scream festivals caused by cramping will be a thing of the past.

    Now, think about your blood. Your body's survival is based on its flow throughout your circulatory system. If you are dehydrated, your body may not have enough water to keep your blood flowing smoothly. If this is the case, your body will release a hormone called antidiuretic hormone (ADH), which triggers your kidneys to absorb available water (from any part of your body where it exists) to increase total body water. This then increases your blood pressure and blood volume. Your other bodily needs will suffer, because water is necessary in every bodily function. This is not a scenario that you want to occur. Lack of water directly affects your body's ability to metabolize your food, leading to bloating and constipation. There is an easy solution: stay hydrated.

3. **Water radiates your skin.** Hydrated skin has a "fresh" look to it, which combined with an intake of omega-3 fatty acids causes the "glowing look" we all strive for.

4. **Water eliminates bloating.** Every gram of sodium and carbohydrate (discussed in chapter 5) attaches itself to water molecules. This is why after you eat a salty meal with a lot of bread (or any heavy

carbohydrate), you feel bloated. Many times people think drinking more water will cause additional bloating. The truth is that this process works in the opposite way. Drinking more water when you are bloated actually causes your body to release water that's been stored while eliminating excess sodium, which in turn eliminates bloating.

The More Water You Drink, the Better

The standard recommendation is *at least* half an ounce of water per pound of body weight. This also depends on activity level and environment. Meaning, if you live in a hot and humid place, your body will require more water. (Males typically require more water than females due to weight and additional muscle mass.) Hydrated muscle contracts approximately 10 to 20 percent better than dehydrated muscle. This maximum contraction allows you to optimize your exercise and results. In addition, hydrated muscle is tighter and provides a more toned, firm body.

Here are my recommendations:

Females: Drink at least 8 cups of water per day (64 ounces / 2 liters). Drink at least 8 ounces with every meal and at least 8 ounces between each meal. This will ensure that you get 16 ounces every three to four hours. Ideally, work your way up to 12 to 16 cups per day (96–128 ounces / 3–4 liters).

Males: Drink at least 12 cups of water per day (96 ounces / 3 liters). Drink at least 12 ounces with every meal and at least 12 ounces between each meal. This will ensure that you get 24 ounces every three to four hours. Ideally, work your way up to 16 to 24 cups per day (128–192 ounces / 4–6 liters).

Note: 1 cup = 8 ounces

The Two Ways Your Body Tells You It Needs Water

First, you need more water if you are thirsty. Your body's way to tell you it needs water is through your thirst mechanism. If you are thirsty, you have waited too long to drink water. The key is to keep drinking water, so you never get thirsty. This will ensure that your body stays in a hydrated state. Second, if your urine is clear, you are in a hydrated state. The only exception to this occurs when you are taking a multivitamin/mineral and it is not being absorbed well or has a lot of water-soluble vitamins (B and C). Excess water-soluble vitamins are urinated out of your body and color your urine. If that is the case, you may want to take a different multivitamin/mineral, one that can be absorbed better.

WATER TAKEAWAY

Water is a key component of your Body Confidence Plan. It seems to be constantly neglected. I think this is because people just do not know why it is so important. It's easy to simply say, "Drink more water." But what will water really give you? Now you know. So drink up and you will see, feel, and experience the difference with a hydrated body!

Component 6: Stress—Your X-Factor

I think by now we all have heard about the negative effects of high stress levels. Most likely each of us has experienced these or is currently living at an uncomfortable level of stress. It can sometimes feel uncontrollable, given the fast pace and unpredictability of life. However, we cannot avoid the facts: stress is a part of life. We have two choices: learn how to manage it, or let it destroy our body. These two choices are why stress is your X-factor (unknown variable). You could be flawless with the first five components of your Body Confidence Plan, but if your stress (component 6) is left unchecked, it will sabotage your health and prevent you from achieving your goals. To learn how to manage stress, you must first understand the different types of stress and how stress affects your body overall.

Let's First Define Stress

Stress is defined as an emotional or physical response to change. There are two types of stress, *acute* and *chronic*.

Acute Stress Is Your Body's Way of Protecting Itself

Think about a brief stressful moment in your life—something that lasted for a short period of time. Maybe the event you are thinking of is a car accident. Maybe it's a fight, or even the act of getting ready for a huge presentation—

something that you felt caused a high level of stress. That experience was *acute stress*, and it activated a mechanism in your body called the *flight-or-fight response*. This response triggers your body to immediately release two main hormones: cortisol (your stress hormone) and adrenaline (your energy hormone). An increased level of cortisol and adrenaline in your body will accelerate your heart and lung functions, suppress your immune system (which causes inflammation/bloating), slow your digestion, and raise blood-sugar levels to make nutrients readily available—among other things. Basically, these two hormones are released to prepare your body for battle, whatever that battle may be. Once the stressor is removed, your body shifts into a relaxed state and the hormone levels return to normal. This is the moment of relief we feel once the stress dissipates. As I said, this is our body's response to stress. Obviously the intensity of the stressor determines the degree to which we respond.

Chronic Stress Will Prevent You from Achieving Your Body Confidence Goals

Chronic stress occurs when you experience too many moments of acute stress. The continual level of stress within your body causes your body to keep high levels of cortisol floating in the blood, which prevents you from relaxing. Chronic stress can be extremely detrimental to your body, especially in four areas. First, cortisol raises your blood-sugar levels, causing your body to increase its fat-storing capacity. Second, cortisol suppresses your immune system, dealing a double whammy, since you then become more susceptible to getting sick; in addition, a suppressed immune system triggers inflammation and bloating, so weight is also increased. Third, cortisol slows your digestion; this digestive slowdown affects how you metabolize food and may cause constipation or diarrhea. Last, if your body cannot reach a point of relaxation, your quality of sleep will be affected; this lack of sleep will make it much more difficult to escape from the chronic stress state.

Two Categories of Stress

OK, so your first goal is definitely to avoid chronic stress levels. Your next goal is to learn how to optimally manage your acute stress levels and work on minimizing their occurrences. I suggest breaking your stressors up into two categories. They are:

Category 1—Stressors in which you *can* control your reaction. A few examples:

- Being late for a meeting

- Getting cut off while driving

- Gaining unwanted weight

- Setting an unrealistic work deadline

- Your kids refusing to put their shoes on (well, maybe that is a stressor you cannot control)

Category 2—Stressors in which you *cannot* control your reaction. A few examples:

- Being in a car accident

- Getting injured

- Coming down with a serious illness

- The death of a friend or family member

The categories speak for themselves. There will be times when stress will occur. This is a constant. It is inevitable. Learning to control category 1 means that the only factors that consist of the X-factor for you are things you cannot control. This will make stress become a nonfactor in your Body Confidence results.

Years ago, stress and anxiety seemed to control every part of my life. At times I felt like I was losing my mind. I felt like the pressures of life were piling up without an end in sight. It was at this time that I chose to examine exactly how I reacted to the stressors in my life. I created five steps to minimizing stress. In the process of doing this, I realized that controlling stress is about staying present in your day-to-day life. The five steps that I describe here arise from common sense and will provide a system that allows you to first recognize the stressor and then create solutions. For years I have taught my clients these same five steps, and they have helped them all regain control of their stress.

If you are currently experiencing stress challenges, I suggest starting to implement the following five steps immediately. If you are managing your stress well, there is no need to implement these five steps, and you can use this section as a reference in the future if your stress levels begin to rise.

The Five Steps to Managing Your Stress

Step 1: Keep Your Body Confidence Plan in Balance

Think about a time when you had a bad night's sleep. Were you more irritable the next day? What about a moment when you had low blood sugar and were starving? Did you feel more on edge? How about a time you missed a few cardio workouts? Did you feel stress building a little more each day? These are examples of how an imbalanced Body Confidence Plan can increase stress levels. Remember how sleep is your battery charger? If you take on the day with a half-charged battery, it will run out of juice by midday, causing an increase in stress levels, which triggers your body to begin overreleasing cortisol and adrenaline. This hormone increase is what gets you through the day; unfortunately, your irritableness and exhaustion will build by the minute.

Now think about when you last had low blood sugar and were starving. Your low blood sugar caused your body to eat your muscle to create fuel for your brain and body to function. Imagine the added stress that this process put on your body. That added stress is what caused your edginess. In addition, stress slows your digestive system, in turn suppressing your appetite. This is why many people can go all day without eating if their stress level is high. Then, once the day ends, the "flood gates of food" open and they become ravenous. This point is important to understand, since many people think stress increases your appetite. Actually, stress suppresses your appetite. The aftermath of stress, once your body relaxes, is when your appetite returns. Unfortunately, it typically returns in an aggressive manner, attempting to replace the calorie deficit created by not eating during your stress episode.

I did not realize how important my cardiovascular workouts were to maintaining my stress levels until I had pulled a calf muscle and could not work out for a couple of weeks. You see, we all have stress build up within us each day. The goal, then, is to keep our stress level manageable. The fact is, no matter how well we deal with stress, it still exists. Each of us creates systems that help us alleviate our stress. Exercise was one of mine. I love cycling. When I am on my road bike, I feel at peace; it's just me, my bike, and the road. Riding is my greatest stress reducer. When I suddenly removed it from my daily routine; my stress had nowhere to escape. I removed my most effective stress reducer and did not replace it with another. This caused my stress to linger inside of me and make me tenser with each day that passed. Once I realized this, I created additional positive escapes (explained in step 4) until I could start riding again. These new escapes provided my stress with a daily outlet.

Another powerful thing that exercise does is cause the release of *endorphins* (neurochemicals that causes a feeling of well-being). Endorphins assist with improving your overall mood and creating a sense of happiness, similar to the "runner's high" you might have heard about. Endorphins are fantastic stress destroyers.

Your Body Confidence Plan is an extremely important part of providing your body with the proper environment to implement the remaining four steps in managing your stress. A balanced plan provides an intangible benefit. It puts you in a state where you see things differently, where you see that what seemed like an insurmountable challenge really is not. It creates a platform where you can think more clearly and remain sharp. With a balanced plan, your body and mind will be working optimally, assisting you to succeed with the four remaining steps.

Step 2: Start a Stress Journal

One way to get the overwhelming flood of worry out of your mind is to write down your thoughts. This will allow you to become present with your stressors. Too many times we lose touch with the exact reasons we've gotten into a stressful situation, and these stressors get blown way out of proportion. For this reason, I suggest keeping a Stress Journal—writing down when and why you get stressed. Keeping a journal will provide the necessary awareness you will need to succeed with step number 3.

Step 3: Create Solutions

By becoming aware of the triggers of the stress you experience, you can create solutions. I always like to use the worst-case scenario to begin with. If you immediately reveal to yourself what the worst thing could be, you become much more aware of the size of the challenge you actually face. This can help you come to terms with the source of your stress. Ninety-nine percent of the time, you will find that even the worst case is manageable. Understanding this will help alleviate your stress. Afterward you'll find it much easier to create a solution that will prevent a repeat of that stressor.

Step 4: Implement Positive Escapes

Many stressors lead to a desire to escape for a moment. This is a natural thing; because when a stressor is present your adrenaline and cortisol levels have increased, triggering the flight-or-fight response. Then, once your stress level is reduced, your body shifts to a relaxation mode. This relaxation mode typically triggers a desire for a temporary escape or a payoff. The challenge here is that many escapes are negative. For example, my escape used to be food. An adjustment I made was to change my escape. When stressed, instead of eating pizza, a negative escape (any action that works against achieving your goal counts as negative), I now watch a movie, go for a walk, or play ball with Hunter. All of these count as positive escapes (any action that brings you closer to your goal). I still get the escape I desire. And because it's positive, the escape actually benefits me.

Step 5: Keep Learning

Keep working on yourself, keep finding new positive ways to handle stress, and keep reading. The more you work on managing your stress, the better you will get at controlling how you react to your stressors.

STRESS TAKEAWAY

Stress is a vital part of your body's defense mechanisms. Just like every other component in your Body Confidence Plan, the key to dealing with stress is to keep it in a balanced state. Now you have the knowledge and tools to control your stress and prevent it from becoming the X-factor.

Paula Lippert is one client who embodies Body Confidence. Paula is a married mother of three and a working professional. She has a vast amount of knowledge about every diet on the market. When we first met, she shared with me that she had actually read almost every diet book and tried them all. She would start one for a little while and then choose to stop. Some of them temporarily worked for her, but her biggest reason to stop was that she hated the feeling of being "on a diet." She grew up in the South, and her mother was a fantastic cook. Paula loved food from her earliest moments and did not want to sacrifice that part of her life. She worked out fairly consistently and ate relatively healthy. She was also carrying about thirty extra pounds. Paula had three big genetic challenges—the first being that she had a meso/endomorph body type (slower metabolism), like her mom. Second, she had had a full hysterectomy, which put her on hormone-replacement therapy, which consisted of her taking estrogen and progesterone. Third, she had an underactive thyroid (the gland that controls your metabolism) and was taking thyroid medication. I shared with Paula that any time you need to take hormones, even if they create stable levels in your body, they are not nearly as productive as the hormones that your body creates itself. In addition to these challenges, she had a high set point due to all her years of dieting. This is why no matter what she did, her body was refusing to drop weight and body fat.

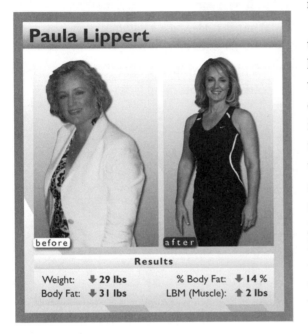

Paula Lippert

before

after

Results

Weight:	↓ 29 lbs	% Body Fat:	↓ 14 %
Body Fat:	↓ 31 lbs	LBM (Muscle):	↑ 2 lbs

Taking all of those metabolic factors into account, Paula's biggest challenge was her stress level. Her mom was her best friend, and over the last couple of years she had been suffering from Alzheimer's disease. This was tearing Paula apart emotionally. She was in a state of chronic stress, without any way to get out. When Paula and I started working together, our first objective was for her to become clear on her "why." She needed to remember what her health meant to her. It provided her with the confidence to be the best mother and wife she could be, and it gave her the strength to push through the tough emotional moments of seeing her mom regress daily from Alzheimer's.

Paula became clear on her "why," and our next objective was to work on each component of her Body Confidence Plan. Her nutrition, exercise, vitamins/minerals, omegas, and water were easy for her to implement. She already understood food and exercise; she just needed to be taught how to eat and exercise correctly. Once her blood sugar was stable, she did not feel like she was dieting. Paula's two biggest challenges were her quality of sleep and her stress levels. Since she was in a state of chronic stress, her sleep was erratic and she was unable to relax. She began working on the four sleep strategies and the five stress steps, and she began progressing each week. Paula needed to first get her body back to a balanced environment before she could start seeing external results. Her body slowly and steadily progressed as her stress levels reduced. The reduced stress levels helped improve her quality of sleep. Once she had all six components of her Body Confidence Plan working for her, the weight and body fat started dropping. What she once said was impossible began to happen. Over nine months, Paula actually dropped her extra thirty pounds. To Paula, losing that weight was just the icing on the cake. She got her Body Confidence back! One day we were having a conversation and she said, "You know, I still have tough days with my mom, but I now have the tools to pull myself out of that place. I finally found a way to make my health a priority."

What she said clearly shows the reason you identify a clear "why" and develop a plan. They both provide you with a purpose and evolve with you. Your health needs a strong structure and a plan, just like your home does. Now let's move on to the third step: balancing your Quadrant.

Step 3: Balancing Your Quadrant

Imagine a glass of water filled to the top; then picture adding more water to that glass. What happens? The water begins to spill and makes a mess. That's a perfect illustration of the way many people try to get healthy: they take an already full life and add a diet to it without making any adjustments to their other commitments. They simply neglect the other parts of their life for the length of the diet, and solely focus on achieving their health goal. Eventually, though, those neglected commitments push back. Life begins to resemble that glass of water and starts to spill over. And as they try to mop up the mess, the progress they have made with their health is too often the first thing to go. "There's just not time to be healthy" is a statement I hear all too often. Does it sound familiar?

It's no wonder we get caught up in the moment: so much of what we hear about diet and fitness promises quick fixes and fast results. But real success comes when we make permanent room for our health among all our other day-to-day tasks and relationships; that's what I mean when I talk about "Balancing your Quadrant."

Consider the four primary areas of your life: *health, lifestyle, profession,* and *relationships.* In a perfect world, each part of your life would be equally balanced—but we all know that's unlikely to happen! Your Quadrant will always be evolving, and that's OK. Just take the time to consider your commitments, and adjust accordingly. For example, this week you'll need to spend some extra time—say, ten hours—learning the concepts of the program and fitting them into your day. But after a couple of weeks, once you have a handle on it, a good portion of this time can go back into your Quadrant—let's say, seven of the ten hours. You can plan a fun weekend outing, for example, or give the health quarter some additional exercise time. Or let's say you've been doing amazingly well on the program for five weeks, but you just got slammed with a work deadline: you'll be working twelve-hour days for the entire week, and you typically only work ten hours a day. Where will you find two extra hours in an already packed day? A simple solution would be skipping your exercise that week. That's right: sometimes taking care of yourself means knowing when to ease up on exercise; this adjustment would keep your health stable, so you could get your work done without sacrificing sleep or overstressing yourself. As long as your blood sugar is stable, you will maintain your health until you can get back to those regular workouts. The goal here is to be reasonable with yourself. Don't try to do it all—that ultimately leads to burnout.

Balancing your Quadrant basically means adjusting your life to prevent spills (which is a lot easier than mopping them up after the fact!). As you begin your program, it's as important to consider how you'll juggle the hours of your day as it is to learn new fitness strategies and nutritional facts. Take some time to calculate how many hours you'll be spending on your health—and then be honest with yourself about which part, or parts, of the Quadrant you'll take those hours from. Give yourself time to regularly rethink that balance—weekly, monthly, or however often you need. New commitments arise all the time, and it's time for us all to stop trying to live as though there are limitless hours in the day.

Bill Murphy is an excellent example of how to balance a Quadrant. Bill and I belong to the same gym. I always saw how consistent he was with his workouts and that he ate pretty well. He was in good shape, and his goal was to get in great shape. The biggest challenge Bill faced was time. He owns a couple of hair salons and is one of the most requested and talented hair stylists in Atlanta. In addition to his busy work schedule, he is married, has two children, and coaches football for his son's team. One day we were talking and he shared that he wanted to do a bodybuilding show in the Masters Division (for people over forty). He spoke about how he could not find enough time in his life to take his nutrition and exercise to the next level. Bill was currently working out about four to five hours a week and was spending three hours a week on food preparation (a solid effort for his health). I asked him if he could make a commitment to giving more time to his nutrition and exercise for eight weeks; then he could go back to the same seven to eight hours he was currently spending on his health. Bill asked, "If I make this commitment, will my results be permanent?" I replied, "Most definitely. We can immediately improve your nutrition and exercise, and with eight weeks of hard work you can reprogram your metabolism and lower your set point. This will keep you in great shape."

At this point, Bill was all in, and our first piece of work was having him create more time in his Quadrant for health. For eight weeks he was going to need to get an additional three hours of exercise and probably another two hours of food preparation. This meant we needed to find five hours to swap. Bill adjusted each part of his Quadrant and focused on preparing his food in bulk during the days he took off from work. This would set him up for his busy workweek.

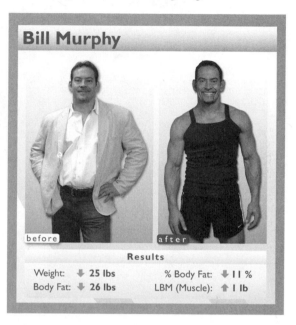

Bill Murphy

before

after

Results

Weight: ⬇ **25 lbs**		% Body Fat: ⬇ **11 %**
Body Fat: ⬇ **26 lbs**		LBM (Muscle): ⬆ **1 lb**

Over the next eight weeks, Bill gained a balanced Quadrant and took his body to an elite level. He dropped twenty-five pounds and 11 percent body fat, and he won first place in his bodybuilding competition! Bill and I met a week after his victory, and he went right back to his schedule before the eight-week drop. I am pleased to say his results have stayed. *When you correctly achieve your goals, the progress you achieved remains in place.* Even more impressive is that Bill entered into his eight-week journey with a full plan, made space in his life, and kept the four parts of his life in balance.

The key in balancing your Quadrant is staying proactive with your health. You want to set your health pace rather than reacting to it. Chapters 7 and 8 will provide you with valuable insight on how to work your program consistently into your world, and that information will provide you with additional tools to help you balance your Quadrant.

Congratulations! You have established the majority of your Body Confidence Foundation!

The final two components of your Body Confidence Plan are your nutrition and exercise plans (presented in the next two chapters). I know we covered a lot of information in this chapter, and you can look forward to more in-depth information in the next two. My goal is for you to see that this is what it takes to truly learn how to permanently work your health into your world and see how it is possible!

5

YOUR FUEL

Your body is a "refuel as it goes" machine. It
needs to be fed the right fuel if you want to take
your Body Confidence to the next level.

A good way to picture fueling your body is to think about the last time you put gas in your car. You had three choices: regular unleaded (87 octane), midgrade unleaded (89 octane), and premium unleaded (91–93 octane). All three types will provide fuel for your car. The main difference between each type is that a car with a higher-performance engine requires a higher octane level to run. This is why a Ferrari needs premium gas. Your body's "engine" requires calories as fuel, and just as the octane levels in gas vary, so does the quality of calories you consume. If you want your body to run like an efficient, fast, and powerful Ferrari, you need to feed it premium fuel. My purpose in this chapter is for you to learn *what* foods you should eat, *why* you should eat them, and *how* eating the right fuel will take your Body Confidence to the next level.

To set an efficient pace for you as you take in this information and create the best success with your meals, we have split this chapter into eight sections.

Section 1—Your Body's Fuel

Before a car can use its gasoline as fuel, the gas must go through its fuel system to provide energy for the engine. If the car's fuel system is not correctly breaking down the gasoline and getting it ready to be utilized by the engine, the engine cannot use it, and the car won't run. This is similar to how your body's digestive system works to prepare your fuel (the food you eat) to be utilized as energy. Your digestive system prepares fuel by metabolizing it, or breaking it down into its simplest forms. It converts proteins to amino acids, carbohydrates to sugar, and fats to fatty acids. This breakdown of the three key nutrients is what allows your fuel to be used for energy and your digestive system to absorb vitamins, minerals, and water. Whatever it does not want or need will be eliminated by your body.

Protein, fat, and carbohydrates are the *fuel* (energy represented by calories) found in your food. The first step in getting your body to run like a Ferrari is to understand your fuel.

Protein—Your "Muscle Fuel"

Hot scrambled eggs, creamy Greek yogurt, tangy barbecued chicken, and a juicy filet mignon are all proteins, and this short list is just a sample of the types of proteins found in your meals, presented in section 5 of this chapter.

Protein Is the Building Block of Your Body

Protein is the main factor in the growth, repair, and maintenance of your body's tissue. It is composed of chains of amino acids that contain both *essential* (your body cannot make them) and *nonessential* (your body *can* make them) amino acids. Because of the difference between essential and nonessential amino acids, there are two types of protein: *complete* and *incomplete.*

Complete protein has all the essential amino acids and can be used immediately by your body. Complete protein comes primarily from animal sources like beef, chicken, fish, and turkey, or from animal by-products like milk, cheese, and eggs. There are two vegetarian sources of complete protein: soy (a bean) and quinoa (a seed). You'll find a detailed list of complete proteins in section 7 of this chapter.

Incomplete protein lacks one or more of the essential amino acids. Incomplete protein can be found in fruits, vegetables (besides soy), nuts, and grains (besides quinoa). Incomplete protein must combine with another source of protein to become complete, such as when rice and beans are combined.

Whenever I first start working with a client, I find that they never think about the type of protein they are eating. They think that all protein is created equal . . . but this is not the case! The type of protein you eat is a deciding factor in stabilizing your blood sugar. Because incomplete protein is lacking one or more of the essential amino acids, it is inferior to complete protein.

The Three Ways Complete Protein Stabilizes Your Blood Sugar and Is Superior to Incomplete Protein

1. Complete protein can be used by your body for fuel immediately, whereas incomplete protein must first combine with another source to be utilized.

2. Complete protein causes a positive release of the hormone glucagon (the one that raises your blood sugar), which in turn counteracts the hormone insulin (the one that lowers your blood sugar), resulting in stable blood sugar as the two hormones balance each other out.

3. Complete protein is of higher quality than incomplete protein. Complete protein (with the exception of soy and quinoa) is protein that contains little to no carbohydrates. Your digestive system is designed to begin chemically metabolizing carbohydrates in your mouth.

Protein doesn't begin metabolizing until it reaches your stomach. This means that when you eat protein that contains carbohydrates (almost all incomplete protein), the carbohydrates in that food are metabolizing faster than the protein. This extra speed results in the glucose entering your bloodstream faster than the amino acids, causing a blood-sugar spike. You get a great example of this when people combine the incomplete proteins rice and beans (which, as previously explained, become complete when combined) to make a complete protein. Rice and beans combined have a large amount of carbohydrates and a very small amount of complete protein. This imbalance triggers an overrelease of insulin from the blood-sugar spike, resulting in the storage of fat.

Complete Protein Strengthens Your Body

In addition to the assistance that complete protein provides in stabilizing blood-sugar levels, it also greatly assists with cell and tissue growth because it contains nitrogen as I briefly shared in Don's story in chapter 2. There are two environments in your body. One is an anabolic environment, where your body is building tissue and developing new cells, and the other is a catabolic environment, where your body breaks down tissue and cells. The determining factor is the amount of nitrogen you take in versus the amount that leaves. Simply put, more nitrogen entering than leaving equals an anabolic environment. Less nitrogen coming in than leaving equals a catabolic environment. In order to stay anabolic, it is crucial that you consume enough complete protein (and thus enough nitrogen) per day. Think of protein, especially complete protein, as "muscle fuel."

Because complete protein greatly assists in stabilizing your blood sugar and is your best source of nitrogen, *complete protein is the only type of protein that will be listed in your meal plans, under the protein column for each food item.*

Carbohydrates—Your "Brain Fuel"

Grilled asparagus, fresh blueberries, crisp roasted red potatoes, and a warm bowl of oatmeal with brown sugar are all carbohydrates, and this short list is just a sample of the types of carbohydrates found in your meals, which are presented in section 5 of this chapter.

Carbohydrates Are Your Body's Main Source of Fuel

As we discussed, *all* carbohydrates (with the exception of fiber) are broken down through digestion into glucose. Glucose is the fuel for your central nervous system (CNS). Your CNS is your command center, and along with your brain it manages every breath, heartbeat, movement, and thought you have. So think of carbohydrates as your "brain fuel."

"Brain Fuel" Can Be Classified into Two Categories, Simple and Complex.

Simple carbohydrates are named as such because your digestive system can quickly metabolize them into glucose for use as energy. Think of a time when you ate a piece of fruit or drank some juice and then within minutes felt a rush of energy. This energy rush was caused by your body quickly metabolizing the fruit or juice into glucose, making it readily available.

Complex carbohydrates are called "complex" because they take longer to break down (metabolize) into glucose. There are two types of complex carbohydrates: *starches* and *fiber*. Starches are your heavier, denser carbohydrates, like corn, wheat, potatoes, and beans. Fiber is the nondigestible portion of the carbohydrate and cannot be used for energy.

Both simple and complex carbohydrates are important in helping stabilize your blood sugar. Simple carbohydrates get broken down faster than complex carbohydrates. Complex carbohydrates are packed with more calories than simple ones. If you eat only simple carbohydrates, you will be hungry all the time and constantly find yourself with low blood sugar. If you eat only complex carbohydrates, you will end up eating too many per meal and feel full and bloated. Just remember that your meals will have multiple combinations of simple and complex carbohydrates. Some meals will have both, and some meals will only have one. Once you dive into your meal plans, you should experiment. I'll give you direction as to what combination is best for you.

Fat—Your "Fat-Burner Fuel"

A spoonful of peanut butter, a ripe avocado, fresh olives, zesty Italian dressing, and sliced almonds are all examples of fats and are just a few of the fats that you will be eating in your meals, which are presented in section 5 of this chapter.

Fat Is Your Friend

There is something you should know about fat: it is your friend, and it is essential for your body to work correctly. Let's start with the two main types of fat, the one considered "bad" and the one considered "good." Saturated fat is your "bad fat." Unsaturated fat is your "good fat." Saturated fat is considered "bad" because it raises the level of "bad" cholesterol (LDL) in your blood and can increase your risk of heart disease. Some examples of saturated fat are beef, bacon, butter, and cheese. The reality is this: saturated fat is fine to have as long as it is consumed in moderation. Your goal is consuming less than 15 grams of saturated fat per day.

Your second type of fat is unsaturated fat, the "good" kind. This type of fat can be split into two types: *monounsaturated* and *polyunsaturated.* A few examples of monounsaturated-fat sources are avocados, olives, and canola oil. A few examples of polyunsaturated-fat sources are nuts, seeds, and soybeans. Unsaturated fats do not raise your "bad" cholesterol (LDL) and may actually help in reducing it. Since these are your "good" fats, I recommended that you use unsaturated fats as your primary fat source in each meal.

Fat benefits you in four ways:

1. **Eating fat slows down digestion.** Fat inhibits the release of stomach acid (hydrochloric acid, or HCl), which in turn slows down your digestive process. By eating fat with each meal, the digestion of your carbohydrates and protein as well as your fat is slowed, stabilizing your blood sugar more easily.

2. **Eating fat causes you to release stored body fat.** When your body recognizes that an essential nutrient's consumption is being restricted, it will do everything to protect that nutrient. This means that your body will stop releasing stored fat if it senses that none is coming in. This mechanism operates similarly to the way your body behaves when it senses imminent starvation. Since fat has over twice the energy of protein and carbohydrates, your body will always hold onto its fat in times of restriction or deprivation. The simple solution is to continuously feed yourself the correct amount of fat per meal. Your body will then continuously release your unwanted stored fat.

3. **Consuming fat is needed to absorb the fat-soluble vitamins A, D, E, and K.** Fat-soluble vitamins are essential for your body to function

optimally. Without fat, these vitamins cannot be absorbed by your body. Nonabsorption of these vitamins will create vitamin deficiencies and cause health challenges.

4. **Consuming fats can provide essential fatty acids.** I detailed all the amazing benefits of omega fatty acids in chapter 4, especially how they control the overall health of your skin, hair, and nails. These benefits are possible only when you incorporate fat into your meals.

These are the reasons why the fat that you eat is your "fat-burning fuel." Your body will release its stored fat only if you feed it the right amount of fat. *Always remember: Fat Is Your Friend!*

Section 2—Fifteen Strategies for Mastering Your Meals

The first response for most people when they begin any type of nutrition plan is to go directly to their meal plans and begin the program and, as a result, possibly becoming overwhelmed. With my approach, you have a clear picture of where you are going to gain Body Confidence. Your meal parameters and meal plans will be presented in the next sections, so it is important to first understand the fifteen strategies that will provide you with the structure to seamlessly get the best foods as fuel for your day.

Strategy 1: Don't Count on the RDA

"RDA" stands for the recommended daily allowance of nutrients for each person, based on a two-thousand-calorie diet. It recommends what the daily intake of each nutrient should be. The RDA standards are good for vitamins and minerals; unfortunately, the standards are completely inadequate for protein, fat, and carbohydrates. The RDA for macronutrients is too broad and too high for carbohydrates and much too low for protein. The reality is that if you follow the RDA standards, your blood sugar will likely be unstable. The meal parameters you find in this book will provide you with the correct nutrient ratios and calories per meal to stabilize your blood sugar.

Strategy 2: Know the Three Core Principles of Blood-Sugar Stabilization

Think about your core principles of life. Typically, once set, these principles remain intact and unwavering. On the other hand, your preferences (choices) may continually change and evolve. This same logic can be applied to your nutrition. Your blood sugar will always remain stable if you consistently apply three core principles.

THREE CORE PRINCIPLES OF MAINTAINING STABLE BLOOD SUGAR

- Eat a balanced meal every three to four hours (*five to six meals per day*).
- Maintain balanced nutrient ratios (protein, fat, and carbohydrates) at every meal.
- Consume the correct amount of calories per meal.

These three principles are the core to your nutrition and need to remain intact and unwavering, just like the principles you follow in day-to-day life. Once your core is in place, the number of choices of foods you have is limitless. Following your core principles will maintain stable blood sugar, which then allows you to add variety to meals and experiment with different food choices.

Strategy 3: Believe in the Importance of the Quality of Food

Eating high-quality food (also called "clean" food) is a key factor in achieving your goals quickly. Your meal plans will be labeled "High Quality," "Medium Quality," or "Low Quality." Each meal is balanced correctly to match your nutrition parameters; the only difference is in the quality of food contained in the meal, which then determines the quality of the meal as a whole.

There are four factors that determine the quality of food:

1. **The number of ingredients in the food**—The more ingredients (listed on the food label) in a food, the more processed the food

is. A food item that is processed more gets digested faster and may therefore spike your blood sugar.

2. **The state in which the food is eaten (dry/liquid, coarsely/finely ground, raw/cooked)**—The closer to its natural state the food remains, the slower it is digested. This means that, for example, an apple is digested slower than apple juice. Slower digestion yields better blood-sugar stability.

3. **The amount of fiber in the food**—Since fiber cannot be digested, it slows down the rate of digestion. This assists with maximum blood-sugar stabilization.

IMPORTANT NOTE

Your goal is to consume at least 25 to 35 grams of fiber per day. Higher quality foods will provide a good amount of fiber. If you find yourself lacking in fiber you may choose to add a fiber supplement that contains psyllium husk. This supplement can be in a powder or capsule form. Psyllium husk is a natural fiber, and each teaspoon has 5 grams of fiber. You can get psyllium husk powder in any grocery or health-food store.

---

4. **The amount of sodium (salt) in the food**—Sodium is an excellent preservative, and the amount of salt in a food greatly enhances its taste. Unfortunately, every gram (1,000 mg) of sodium holds on to water molecules. This causes your body to become bloated and swollen and has a negative effect on how your digestive system processes food. The lower the sodium content of a food item, the higher its quality. Your goal is to limit your sodium intake to 1,500–2,000 mg per day.

IMPORTANT NOTE

For fast and optimal results, your best choice is to opt for your highest-quality meals, and what matters most is to stay consistent with your meal plans. For this reason you may want to experiment (after the ten-day Jump Start Phase) with high-, medium-, and low-quality meal plans to ensure variety and prevent burnout. Remember the Kaizen method: steady and incremental progress.

Quality of Food

Highest Quality
Least Processed and Least Refined

PROTEIN	CARBOHYDRATES	FATS
Beef	Beans, fresh	Avocado
Chicken	Brown rice	Flaxseed oil
Egg whites	Fruit	Natural nut butter
Eggs, whole	Hot cereals	Nuts
Fish	Sweet potatoes	Olive oil
Pork	Vegetables	Olives
Soy beans	Yams	
Turkey breast		
(All Other Fresh or Frozen Meat)		

Medium Quality
Medium Processed and Medium Refined

PROTEIN	CARBOHYDRATES	FATS
Canned meat	Bread - (at least 2 grams of fiber)	Canola oil
Garden burgers	Canned beans	Guacamole
Prepackaged meats	Canned fruit	Processed nut butters
Protein powder - whey, egg, and soy	Canned vegetables	Vegetable oil
Sandwich meats	Cold cereals	
Soy products, packaged	Crackers	
Dairy	Pasta	
- Cheese	Potatoes, red and white	
- Cottage cheese	Pretzels	
- Milk		
- Yogurt		

Low Quality
Most Processed and Most Refined

PROTEIN	CARBOHYDRATES	FATS
Protein bars	Bread - (less than 2 grams of fiber)	Butter
Ready-to-drink protein drinks	Ice cream (NF, LF)	Creamy salad dressing
	Potato chips	Margarine
	Tortilla chips	Mayonnaise
	White rice	Sour cream

Strategy 4: Follow Your Mealtime Guidelines

Feeding your body consistently and frequently is the key for your body to release stored fat and increase your metabolism. This is accomplished by eating several meals throughout the day.

Guidelines for mealtimes:

- **Your mealtimes each day will depend on when you wake and when you go to bed**. In general your five to six meals will follow this pattern, with the times adjusting to your schedule. (Your sample day is an excellent example of mealtimes presented in section 5 of this chapter.)

  6:30 A.M.   Meal 1: Breakfast—eat within an hour of waking. This meal can be a half meal (if you are not hungry). The bottom line is that the sooner you eat, the better for your metabolism.

  9:30 A.M.   Meal 2: Midmorning "mid" meal

  12:30 P.M.   Meal 3: Lunch

  3:30 P.M.   Meal 4: Midafternoon "mid" meal

  6:30 P.M.   Meal 5: Dinner

  9:30 P.M.   Meal 6: Bedtime—your last meal of the day should be consumed *within* an hour of going to sleep. If you are not hungry, eat a meal of only protein and fat, no carbohydrates. (Strategy 5 explains why.)

- Meals should be consumed every three to four hours throughout the day.

- If you miss a meal, simply eat one as soon as you can. Don't worry about making up the meal. Your body will naturally be hungry again before three hours are up. Make sure you eat at that time. If a long stretch of time elapsed when you missed your meal, you may be hungry in less than three hours even after your previous meal. Keep eating when you feel hungry. It's your body's way of telling you to get caught up on calories. By the second or third meal (after the meal you missed), your body will have regained its blood-sugar balance, and your hunger cycle will shift back to every three to four hours.

- The goal is to be ready to eat when it is time to eat and satisfied after each meal.

- If you are very hungry at mealtime, you waited too long to eat, and if you are full after the meal, you ate too much. If it has been four hours since your last meal and you find that you are still not hungry, cut the meal in half and eat. If the half meal made you full instead of satisfied, cut the meal into a quarter of a meal the next time this happens.

IMPORTANT NOTE

Many times your initial hunger will depend on your past nutrition habits. Your feeding drives will quickly awaken when you implement these guidelines. It is critical that you are *never* full (unless it follows your "off" plan meal, explained in strategy 14). If it is time to eat and you are not hungry, cut the meal in half; this is extremely important in order for you to achieve your Body Confidence goals. Once your appetite awakens (this could take as long as two weeks), you can eat whole meals as long as you are not full afterward.

Strategy 5: Eat Before Bed

I was talking to a dieter, and she told me how people are not supposed to eat past sundown. I followed up by asking, "Well, what happens in the fall when daylight savings hits? It gets dark at 5 P.M. That would mean everyone would go twelve to fourteen hours without food." She followed up with: "That is how our bodies are meant to be fed." I then asked, "Why?" There was a long pause before she finally responded, "I don't know why. I just know you get fat if you eat past sundown." My last response was: "Well, I am not fat, and neither are the thousands of clients I have worked with. We all eat right before bed, after sundown. Based on your theory, how is this possible?" There was another long pause, and she finally replied, with a look of hope, "I don't know . . . can you really eat before bed?" I replied, "Of course," and proceeded to explain why. I have had this conversation countless times. For some reason, people think that if they eat before bed their bodies will store fat. This assertion has no validity; it is just what people hear and in turn believe to be fact.

It's important to remember that if your blood sugar is stable, you cannot store fat. If you eat a balanced meal before bed, your blood sugar will stay stable, you will not store fat, and you will actually increase your metabolism. Digestion takes energy, and the more times your body must create energy to metabolize food, the more fat you burn. In addition, your body is designed to last six to eight hours without food—during sleep. That is why it is important to eat upon waking and within an hour of bedtime; it minimizes the chance of creating any caloric deficits.

Of course, if you eat a meal that contains a lot of carbohydrates and fat before bed, you will spike your blood-sugar levels and most likely store fat. If you eat one of your prescribed meal plans instead, you will not.

Here are the three guidelines to follow when eating your meal before bed:

1. **If you are hungry at bedtime, feel free to eat a full meal.** In section 5 you'll find meals to choose from that have simple and less dense carbohydrates, like fruits and vegetables.

2. **Avoid eating complex carbohydrates, like bread, oatmeal, rice, and pasta.** Because complex carbohydrates take longer to digest, they can feel heavy in your stomach late at night and cause bloating.

3. **If you aren't hungry and it's time to eat, eat a half meal of just protein and fat—no carbohydrates.** As your hunger cycle awakens, you will eventually become hungry at this mealtime and can then have carbohydrates.

Strategy 6: Focus Only on Complete Protein as Your Protein Source in Your Meals

Earlier in this chapter, you discovered the difference between complete and incomplete protein and how *only* complete protein (protein that has all the essential amino acids) is counted as the protein source in your meal plans. Composing each meal by first picking a complete protein source is key to keeping your blood sugar stable. Many times people think peanut butter is a good source of protein, but this is not the case. Peanut butter, as well as all nuts and nut butters, contain only incomplete protein. (They lack one or more of the essential amino acids.) Peanut butter is an excellent source of fat (as long as you are not allergic to it), and its grams of protein are not counted. This is why you will see a zero listed in our charts in the "Protein" column for all food sources that contain only incomplete protein. It's crucial that you understand this strategy as you review your meal plans and begin to exchange your food items. Your complete proteins are listed in your "Quality of Food" chart (strategy 3) and in your food exchange system (section 6 of this chapter).

Important Note: Individuals who currently or have previously experienced digestive challenges may experience temporary constipation from an increased intake of daily protein. This possible constipation is caused because your digestive system is not conditioned to metabolize the new amount of protein. Please know your body will quickly adapt. In the meantime, I recommend making these adjustments:

- Make sure to get the recommended 25–35 grams of fiber per day. If you find it hard to get fiber solely from your food, you can supplement with psyllium husk (explained in strategy 3).

- Remember to drink your water! Water will greatly assist in metabolizing your food and keep your digestive system flowing.

- Take digestive enzymes. Many people lack the necessary enzymes to digest certain foods. A quality digestive enzyme supplement will help your body effectively metabolize your food. Your local health food store will have a good selection of digestive enzymes. I suggest asking for assistance to ensure you choose the best enzymes for your body.

- Start probiotics. Probiotics are live bacteria that assist with optimal intestinal health. Your local health food store will have a good selection of probiotics. I suggest asking for assistance to ensure you choose the best probiotic for your body.

- Eat easily digestible high-quality protein sources, like egg whites and fish. Your next best choice would be chicken or turkey. Be careful of eating too much beef, as it is difficult for your system to digest.

- Cut your recommended grams of protein per meal in half for one week. In the second week start eating three quarters of your grams of protein per meal. Starting the third week eat the full grams of protein per meal. This type of pacing will provide your digestive system with the necessary time to adapt to the new protein intake.

You may choose to implement all of these recommendations or just a few. What matters most is that you quickly solve all constipation challenges. Remember . . . You are what you metabolize.

Strategy 7: Realize That Meals and Snacks Are the Same

The meals you will find in this book are labeled as breakfast, lunch, dinner, and meal replacements. Your meals and quick "mid" meals are each designed to match your nutrition parameters (calories and nutrient ratios per meal). Since each meal is correctly balanced, all of your meals, regardless of how they are labeled, can be eaten at any time. Your meals are labeled the way they are as suggestions, due only to the fact that many of us are accustomed to eating the foods used in each meal at particular times in the day. For example, eggs are a typical breakfast option. However, if you love eggs, feel free to eat an egg meal at any mealtime. Also, chicken is a typical lunch and dinner option, yet you can eat a chicken meal as a "mid" meal or even as breakfast. Obviously all of this depends on *your* food preferences. What matters most is that you have options and freedom with your meal plan.

You will notice that your meal replacements and "mid" meals are designed as quick and efficient balanced meals. They are excellent "on the go" meals and can also be used as half meals when you need them.

Strategy 8: Optimize Your Meal Order

Since your digestive system's sole purpose is to break down your food into its simplest form, understanding how this process works will assist you in maximizing the stability of your blood sugar.

As I mentioned earlier, each protein, fat, and carbohydrate is chemically broken down at a different pace. By consuming your nutrients in a particular order, you will slow digestion of carbohydrates and keep your blood sugar stable.

Here is the order I recommend:

- **Eat your protein first.** Protein begins its chemical breakdown in the stomach.

- **Eat your fat second.** Fat slows down the release of hydrochloric acid (HCl), the acid of the stomach. The breakdown of all nutrients is slowed by having a smaller amount of HCl in the stomach.

- **Eat your carbohydrates last.** Carbohydrates begin chemical breakdown immediately, in the mouth. (Since your body needs glucose and glucose comes from carbohydrates, this is the way your body is programmed.) Eating carbohydrates last allows the other nutrients (protein and fat) to begin their digestion process first. This enables a more effectively timed release of all nutrients into the blood and prevents a blood-sugar spike.

IMPORTANT NOTE

Although eating nutrients in this order is an effective Body Confidence strategy, if you want to eat a meal that has all three nutrients combined, like a salad, go ahead and eat them all together. This suggestion is designed more for a meal like turkey slices, almonds, and a banana. For a meal like this, you would eat the turkey (protein) first (with a condiment like mustard if you want), then the almonds (fat), and then the banana (carbohydrate).

Strategy 9: Learn How to Order in Restaurants

The kiss of death for any restaurant is to have a reputation for dry and boring food. Eating at a restaurant is an experience, and most of us want to feel like the food we are eating is not something we could have made at home. For this reason, restaurant food is typically loaded with fat, sodium, a lot of complex (dense) carbohydrates, and tons of calories. This is why you may feel sluggish (blood-sugar spike from excess carbs and calories) and bloated (water retention from carbs and sodium) after eating in a restaurant.

The good news is that you *can* follow your program and eat correctly in restaurants by following a few simple guidelines:

1. **Decide whether you want to eat "on plan" in the restaurant.** I suggest that each week you have an "off plan" meal (explained in strategy 14). I have made the mistake of going into a restaurant with the thought of eating "on plan" and then ending up having my "off plan" meal instead. Because I made an impulsive decision, I felt guilty and did not enjoy my meal. To make matters worse, I still craved another "off plan" meal. The adjustment I made was to mentally prepare myself for the meal and to choose beforehand whether I was going to eat correctly or have it be my "off plan" meal. Once I make a choice, I follow through with it, and now at every meal I eat in a restaurant, I eat guilt free!

2. **Make sure your blood sugar is stable when you get to the restaurant.** Have you ever gone to eat at a restaurant starving? The first thing you do is reach for the bread basket and keep on reaching until your hunger dissipates. This is your body craving sugar in an effort to stabilize itself. The simple way to prevent this is to time your meals so that you go to the restaurant ready to eat, not starving. For example, let's say you have a lunch appointment at 1 P.M. and your last meal took place at 9 A.M. You will need to eat again no later than at 1 P.M. (since you need to eat every three to four hours). The problem is that with restaurants, you need to be prepared for a thirty-minute cushion at least: the kitchen may be slow, or the waiters might be overworked. The way you can keep your blood sugar stable and prevent yourself from reaching for the bread is by eating a half meal at 11 A.M. Doing this will keep your blood sugar stable without filling you up for lunch. By the time your food arrives, you will be ready to eat a balanced meal.

3. **Request all sauce and salad dressing on the side.** Sauces and salad dressings are loaded with sodium and fat. Restaurants have the habit of using too much. Think about a house salad and the amount of dressing that comes with it. Each tablespoon of dressing has about 12 grams of fat. That means you are getting 108 calories per tablespoon (12 grams × 9 calories/gram = 108 calories). A typical salad has an average of 3 tablespoons of dressing, meaning 36 grams of fat and 324 calories!

4. **Request that all food items be prepared without oil or butter.** Fat does enhance the taste of food, which is why most food items are almost always prepared with some fat source.

5. **Know each meal will have more fat than expected (even when you request no oil or butter).** Be cautious about consuming heavy carbohydrates (brown rice, potatoes, pasta, and bread), since each meal will contain more fat than your meal parameters recommend. Cutting back on your starchy carbohydrates will assist in maintaining stable blood sugar. Eating a meal that is calorie packed with complex carbohydrates and fat will spike your blood sugar, causing you to store body fat. If you feel that the meal has too much fat, cut your starchy carbohydrates in half, or replace them completely with vegetables.

6. **Enjoy your meal, and eat at a slow pace.** The goal is to finish the meal satisfied and content. We have all felt what it's like to be full after a meal. This is a clear sign of high blood sugar and fat storage. Eating your food slowly allows you to tell when you're satisfied and thus prevent overeating.

Strategy 10: Design Your Mobile Readiness Food Kit (MRFK)

Years ago, my friend Scott introduced me to the concept of the mobile readiness food kit (MRFK). He had just started the program when he pulled up in his car. He was all fired up and said, "Mark, come on over here. I have the coolest thing to show you." I walked over to his car, and he opened the trunk. Scott had created a complete mobile food kit. I said, "This is really cool. What made you think of doing it?" Scott replied, "You know that I drive all over Los Angeles. And traffic is so unpredictable, I was tired of being unprepared with my food. So I took the easiest food options and stocked up on them so I'm always prepared. I call it my MRFK."

From that point on, I have taken Scott's concept and fine-tuned it for each client. Because life is so unpredictable, we each need our own version of an MRFK. The main reason for blood-sugar crashes is missing meals. Your MRFK will ensure that you do not miss any meals. Your meal plans are filled with quick meals.

Based on those meal plans, here are some examples of what you can keep in your MRFK:

- String cheese and apple

- Protein bars

- Beef or turkey jerky with nuts and fruit

- Ready-to-drink protein shakes

- Greek yogurt

- Cottage cheese, or lean low-sodium deli meats with nuts and fruit

- Edamame

- Hard-boiled eggs with fruit

Your MRFK can simply be protein bars in your purse, or ready-to-drink protein shakes in your briefcase. Or you can have a cooler in your car with a greater variety of food. You can even go full out, like Scott, and create a deluxe MRFK. All that matters is that you make sure you are prepared with quick food options when life throws you a curveball.

Strategy 11: Rethink How to Drink Coffee, Tea, Soda, and Alcohol

When you begin a nutrition plan, you might be inclined to eliminate everything that is considered bad for you. This is the typical "all or nothing" mind-set. The reality is that coffee, tea, soda, and alcohol can all be worked into your program. The key word in this case is *moderation*. Before I give you the run-down on each, let's discuss the effects of caffeine on your body.

Caffeine is a stimulant, a drug that causes your adrenal gland (your battery) to release the hormones adrenaline and cortisol (explained in the stress section of chapter 4), providing you with a burst of energy. Caffeine also causes your appetite to be suppressed. This is why if you drink coffee in the morning you will not be hungry . . . until the caffeine leaves your system. Then you will become very hungry. Taking caffeine in moderation is fine; just be cautious about overconsumption. Since caffeine causes an energy burst, its intake will be followed by an energy crash. (Always the case when a hormone is overreleased. Remember: what goes up must come down.) This crash is the reason you crave another caffeinated beverage. This happens because your adrenal gland begins to rely on the caffeine as a stimulant to assist with your energy production. The point to remember is that consuming caffeine in moderation is fine; just limit it to one or two servings per day. This will prevent your body from becoming completely reliant on caffeine and ensure the proper health of your adrenal glands.

In addition, caffeine is acidic, which means it causes an increase of acid in your stomach. This can cause digestive disturbances like burping, a "sour" stomach, and acid reflux (stomach acid splashing into your esophagus). Remember: since caffeine causes the release of adrenaline and cortisol, it can trigger the same negative side effects as stress: rapid heart rate, jittery feelings, and possibly diarrhea.

Here are the guidelines on how to successfully work coffee, tea, soda, and alcohol into your program.

Coffee and Tea

- Drink coffee or tea with a meal. Since the caffeine in both will suppress your appetite and increase the acid in your stomach, eating a balanced meal with a cup of coffee or tea will keep your blood sugar stable and absorb the additional stomach acid.

- Choose low-calorie coffee and tea drinks. A high-calorie coffee drink (any drink with more than 100 calories) can be consumed once a week. The rest of the week, please choose a low-calorie coffee drink (less than 100 calories).

- If a high-calorie coffee drink is a daily treat, you should count the calories as well as the protein, fat, and carbohydrate totals for the drink and take this information into account to keep your meal balanced.

- Limit drinking coffee (caffeine or decaf) to the morning and early afternoon. Late afternoon or evening coffee consumption can cause sleep irregularities.

Soda

When I eat pizza, I love to drink Diet Coke! To me, pizza just does not taste the same without Diet Coke. I know soda gets a bad rap, and honestly, it is not the best thing for you. That being said, drinking an occasional diet soda (one to three per week) is fine.

Here are the guidelines for drinking soda:

- Drink only diet soda. Drinking regular soda is like drinking liquid sugar. It will go right through your digestive system and spike your blood sugar before you can blink. Definitely stay away from regular soda, and if you don't like the taste of diet, water is always your best choice anyway.

- Caffeine-free soda is your best choice for evening or nighttime consumption.

- Be prepared for possible gas and bloating from soda, for two reasons: the carbonation, and sugar alcohols (sweeteners). Carbonation means that it contains gas bubbles. These gas bubbles are why a burp typically follows a long swig of soda. Sugar alcohols are the fake sugar created to give diet soda its sweet taste. These fake sugars cannot be digested by your body; therefore, when you consume too much, the result is gas and bloating. People with digestive challenges are more prone to the negative effects of sugar alcohols; therefore, if you experience stomach or intestinal challenges, you should avoid soda.

Alcohol

I used to base my alcohol recommendations on a certain number of glasses per week—until Abbi and I attended our close friend Pam's birthday party for her daughter. Pam had lived the program for many years and was in great shape. A couple of months before the party, she told me she wanted to take her body to a higher level. I designed a program for her, and she began implementing the strategies. Her only vice was that she drank a glass of wine three times a week. I told her it was no problem and should not affect anything.

By the time the party rolled around, she had progressed, but not at the level we both expected. I was puzzled. The effort and consistency she put in should have gotten her where she wanted to go. Then halfway through the birthday party, Pam and I realized what had happened. Abbi and I were sitting outside talking to Pam, and I saw her wine glass. It was literally the biggest wine glass I had ever seen. I looked at Pam and asked, "Pam, is this wine glass the one you use for your three glasses each week?" She looked at me and said yes. I followed up by asking, "How many ounces of wine do you think that glass holds?" She replied, "About ten ounces." I thought to myself, *She cannot be serious. That glass holds at least twenty-four ounces.* (A typical glass of wine is six ounces and has 130 calories.) I then asked Pam, "Can we go inside and measure your glass? I think you have at least twenty-four ounces of wine in that thing!"

We walked into her kitchen, took out a liquid measuring device, poured the wine in it, and—guess what—the glass had twenty-four ounces of red wine in it! Pam had a shocked look on her face, and Abbi and I could not stop laughing. We found out why Pam was holding on to her last few pounds of body fat. She was drinking an additional 390 calories of red wine three times a week. Pam made the proper adjustments, and within a few weeks she achieved her goal. The lesson I learned from this experience was never to measure alcoholic drinks by the glass, because glasses come in all shapes and sizes.

Alcohol, like caffeine, is considered a drug. When taken in moderation it has little negative impact on the body; when taken in abundance it can seriously affect your liver as well as how your body metabolizes food.

Alcohol has 7 calories per gram and, unfortunately, is void of nutrients. This means you still need to eat your recommended amounts of protein, fat, and carbohydrates to get the nutrients your body needs to function at optimal efficiency. Alcohol is typically metabolized by your body before any other nutrients. This means that the other nutrients you consume along with it will primarily be stored instead of digested as your liver handles the alcohol. I know what you might be thinking. . . . That means I can just drink alcohol and not eat, right? Well, hold on a second. Since alcohol is void of nutrients, your body still needs to get its fuel somehow. That means if you drink alcohol without eating, your body will need to consume itself (primarily muscle) to provide the necessary fuel. This, of course, will negatively impact your metabolism.

For this reason, it is important to follow the following alcohol guidelines when drinking. They will ensure that you limit the negative effects of alcohol.

- Limit alcohol consumption to a maximum of two to three drinks per week. Four examples of a drink are the following:

  1 ounce (a shot) of hard liquor—for example, vodka or scotch (60–80 calories depending on type of hard liquor)

  6 ounces of red or white wine (130 calories)

  12 ounces of typical regular beer (140–150 calories)

  12 ounces of typical light beer (100 calories)

- Avoid drinking sugary drinks, like daiquiris. These are loaded with sugar and calories.

- Eat food when you drink. This will help in maintaining stable blood-sugar levels. To prevent overconsumption of calories in a meal where you are also drinking alcohol, replace the heavy carbohydrates with lighter carbs such as fruits and vegetables. An example would be a piece of salmon (protein and fat), vegetables, and a glass of wine.

- Avoid drinking alcohol at bedtime (it can cause an imbalance between your REM and non-REM sleep).

Strategy 12: Use Protein Powder, Bars, and Ready-to-Drink Shakes

As shown in the "Quality of Food" chart on page 106, real food is always better than protein powder and meal-replacement supplements. That being said, we all live busy lives, and we need to get in at least five meals with the correct amount of protein each day. For this reason, protein powder and meal replacements definitely come in handy. Whether you choose to use them is completely up to you; all that matters is that you do not miss meals. This is why I recommend using protein powder and meal replacements on occasion.

Here are the guidelines to follow when using these supplements:

- Whether you choose protein powder, protein bars, or ready-to-drink shakes, you should keep to one to two servings at a maximum per day. This will ensure that you get in at least three "real food" meals per day.

- Find a protein bar and a ready-to-drink shake that match your nutrition parameters, and make sure you like their taste as well. The nutrition information of each product can be found on its food label. In your meal plans I recommend a variety of protein bars and ready-to-drink shakes. Each of them falls into the correct nutrition parameters. Bars and ready-to-drink shakes are loaded with ingredients and some have sugar alcohols; however, they are extremely portable and are fantastic emergency meals. Even if you don't want to eat them, it would be smart to have one or two with you . . . just in case.

- Choose a protein powder with the highest-quality protein. Think of the different quality levels of turkey breast (the all-white-meat portion of the turkey). You have the homecooked high-quality turkey breast you eat at Thanksgiving and you also have the heavily processed lower quality prepackaged turkey meat you get in the refrigerated section at the grocery store. Which do you prefer? Which will provide you with higher quality protein? The differences between the two types of turkey are huge. Let me explain: one ounce of freshly roasted Thanksgiving turkey breast has approximately 8 grams of protein, while one ounce of processed turkey breast has around 5 grams. The two turkey slices are the same weight, yet the Thanksgiving turkey meat provides 3 more grams of protein per ounce than the prepackaged turkey. This vast difference is due to the amount of preservatives and water added to the prepackaged turkey. These preservatives make the prepackaged turkey harder for your body to digest as well as a much lower quality food item than the Thanksgiving turkey breast. Your choices of protein powder are just like your choices of turkey breast. They may look similar on the surface, but when you dig deeper you will find out that their qualities can vary drastically.

To ensure you are choosing the highest quality protein powder, please follow these four simple guidelines:

1. Decide which type of protein powder you want: egg white, soy, or whey. Whey protein is the most common and comes from dairy. There are now many lactose-free whey powders. This means that even if you are lactose intolerant, you can have whey protein. Soy protein powder does not provide the same quality of protein that egg white and whey do: it has less nitrogen per gram of protein. Egg white powder, though it has the same quality of protein as whey, becomes an acquired taste. Taking all of this into consideration, the most preferred choice of protein powder is whey.

2. If you choose whey protein, the best-quality powder is hydrolyzed whey protein (I use a hydrolyzed powder called Proto Whey). Hydrolyzed whey protein has been broken down into smaller molecules for optimal protein absorption by your digestive system. Hydrolyzed whey is the Thanksgiving turkey breast of protein powders. The next best choice of protein powder type is whey isolate. Isolate is a medium-quality protein powder. Whey isolate can be compared to the higher-quality turkey breast that can be purchased at the grocery store deli counter (Boar's Head brand, for example). The lowest-quality protein powder type is whey concentrate. Whey concentrate and whey isolate are both equally absorbed by your digestive system, but whey concentrate has less protein per gram than whey isolate.

This is why whey concentrate can be compared to the prepackaged turkey breast found in the refrigerated section. The best way to determine the type of whey protein powder in a product is by looking at the nutrition label on a tub of protein powder. Avoid all powders that list whey concentrate as the first ingredient (the ingredients in a food item are listed in order from the highest quantity to the lowest quantity). The specific type of protein within the powder is why you will see such a price difference among the protein powders. Trust me, you get what you pay for. If you are going to use whey protein powder, choose hydrolyzed whey or whey isolate, preferably hydrolyzed whey, as this will ensure your body is absorbing the most amount of protein per serving.

3. Choose a powder that contains mostly protein. There are many protein powders out there that have fat and carbohydrates in them as well as protein. These are more like meal replacements. Finding a good protein that has minimal amounts of fat and carbohydrates will allow you to add it to your meal as the protein source. For example, in your meal plans you have a breakfast called "Protein Power Oatmeal." This is a quick meal that has oatmeal, peanut butter, and protein powder mixed together. Making a meal like this will allow you to eat two high-quality food items and one medium-quality food item rather than a lower quality meal-replacement shake.

4. Be aware of sugar sweeteners in protein powders. All protein powders have sugar sweeteners, usually sucralose (Splenda). There are a few powders out there that use the natural sweetener Stevia. As with protein bars and meal replacements, it is important to find the brand that works best for you and your digestive system.

Strategy 13: Initially Measure and Journal Your Food

The dieting world has turned measuring and journaling food into a hated task. Most people think that once you start doing it, you have to do it for the rest of your life. Seriously, who wants to journal and measure their food for the rest of their life? I definitely do not, and I will not ask you to do it, either. However, I do suggest that you measure and journal your food for your first three to four weeks on the program. Think about these two questions: First, if you never measure your food portions, how will you know if you are eating the correct amount of food? Second, how will you create food awareness without journaling?

The simple fact is that for you to become an expert on your nutrition, you need to roll up your sleeves and learn about food, and then learn how to incorporate your program into your day. Measuring your food will educate you on portion sizes. Think about it: once you know what a 4-ounce portion of chicken breast looks like, you never need to measure it again; you can eyeball it. However, if you never measured 4 ounces of chicken, how would you know what your portion size was supposed to look like?

Here are three guidelines to measuring your food:

1. **Buy a food scale.** (They are sold online and at many local cooking stores.)

2. **Measure every food item you eat at least once.** This will provide you with the ability to recognize the appropriate portion size for the rest of your life.

3. **All the food in your meal plans should be measured** *precooked* unless the plan indicates that the food is already cooked. Typically, depending on how long you cook meat, it can lose up to an ounce of water weight while you cook. Meaning if your meal plans say 4 ounces of ground turkey, it will be around 3 ounces cooked. For accuracy, I suggest measuring each meat source one time before you cook it and then again after you cook it. From that point on you will know the meat's post-cooking weight.

Your main objective during your first four weeks on the program is to create a health rhythm. Journaling allows you to see where you are doing well throughout your day and where you may be late for a meal or consistently experiencing a craving. This information will provide the baseline for you to make a quick adjustment. Within four weeks you will have a solid nutrition structure for each day.

There is a sample of a full-size nutrition journal on page 123. Feel free to follow this format, or get a small notebook and carry it around with you, writing down the times you eat and what you eat. Don't worry about counting the calories or protein, fat, and carbohydrate amounts. You will be following your meal plans, so you know they will already be balanced.

A Sample Nutrition Journal

Nutrition Journal KEY
Energy — L: Low   M: Medium   H: High
Hunger Before Meal — NH: not hungry   H: hungry   VH: very hungry
Hunger After Meal — SH: still hungry   S: satisfied   F: full

Meals (time am/pm)	Cal.	Fat	Carbs	Protein	Water	Energy Before	Energy After	Hunger Before	Hunger After
		grams	grams	grams	oz or L	L, M, H	L, M, H	NH, H, VH	SH, S, F
Meal 1					Notes:				
Meal Total									
Meal 2					Notes:				
Meal Total									
Meal 3					Notes:				
Meal Total									
Meal 4					Notes:				
Meal Total									
Meal 5					Notes:				
Meal Total									
Meal 6					Notes:				
Meal Total									
Daily Total									
SLEEP HOURS:									
MULTIVITAMIN & OMEGA FATTY ACIDS:									

Strategy 14: Enjoy Your Weekly "Off Plan" (aka Cheat) Meal

When I was fitness-modeling and dieting, I would live for my cheat day. It was the only thing that kept me going and, sadly, the only thing I found joy in. I would do everything to make the day last, and I dreaded my last bite of that day's food, knowing I would suffer in calorie deprivation and carbohydrate restriction for six straight days afterward. I would get depressed for three days after my cheat day. Then, by the time I made it to my fourth day, I would feel closer to my next cheat day, so I would be pulled out of my depressed state, ignited by my obsession with the food I was going to eat. I would go to the grocery store and walk down each aisle, dreaming about the different foods, lifting up my favorite foods just to smell them. The most special time I spent was in the bakery section. I love baked goods, especially doughnuts, and the smell of all the fresh bakery items would get my mouth watering! Looking back at those times, I can only laugh at myself and be thankful that I am years beyond that food prison I was living in.

Now I still love food, and I love a great "off plan" meal; it's just that this meal is no longer my be-all and end-all. This is why you must enjoy your daily meal plans and expand your food preferences. You do not want the example I shared to become you. Your weekly "off plan" meal should, of course, be something you look forward to—just not so enticing that you feel you are escaping from your normal meal plans. Finding the proper balance between your "on plan" meals and your weekly "off plan" meal will determine the level of consistency with your eating, which will determine the pace at which your Body Confidence goals are achieved.

There is one quick item I want to discuss. The standard term that people use when they have an "off plan" meal is *cheat meal*. "Cheating" makes it sound like you are doing something wrong. In the Venice Nutrition program, this is not the case. This is why I do not call any meals "cheat meals." You should have a once-a-week "off plan" meal. This just means you are eating a meal outside your nutrition parameters. Since this weekly "off plan" meal is part of your program, there is no cheating involved.

Here are four guidelines that will help you find this balance and make the most of your "off plan" meal with minimal damage (fat gain):

1. **Eat consistently throughout the day before your "off plan" meal.**
   The dieting mind-set is to starve yourself before your "off plan"

meal. This leads to saving your calories and using them all up at the "off plan" meal. As you know, this mind-set only makes you burn muscle and store fat. Your "off plan" meal is just another meal in your day. Keep eating at normal meal intervals (every three to four hours) up until your "off plan" meal. This meal frequency will keep your metabolism going, which will allow your body to burn more of the excess calories from your "off plan" meal after you eat it.

2. **Make the most of your "off plan" meal.** My "off plan" meal needs to be an experience. I used to try eating only pizza or ice cream. The problem was that I always felt it was incomplete. Abbi is the type of person who can have one slice of pizza or a piece of chocolate and feel content. I am not that kind of person. When I eat "off plan," I want to enjoy my food and make the experience last. My suggestion is to go for it. Get the appetizer, the salad, the main course, and the dessert. Enjoy your favorite foods, and make sure you feel content after the meal, because if you don't, you may still crave an "off plan" meal. Use your weekly "off plan" meal to get it all out of your system; this approach will make it much easier to jump right back "on plan" afterward.

3. **Eat a meal within four hours after your "off plan" meal.** We have discussed how your metabolism burns more energy the more meals you eat. This also applies to eating after an "off plan" meal. By eating a half meal four hours afterward, your body will work at a faster pace to metabolize your "off plan" meal, minimizing any possible fat storage. An example would be 4 ounces of cottage cheese and 5 almonds, or 1 scoop of protein powder with ½ tablespoon of peanut butter—basically, any of your meal plans but with the protein and fat amounts cut in half and the carbohydrates completely removed.

4. **Stay guilt free after your "off plan" meal.** Guilt is a feeling associated with diets. We feel guilty because the action (an "off plan" meal) was something we were not supposed to do or something that we felt we should not have done in the first place. If you eat five meals a day, that means you are eating thirty-five meals per week. If one of those meals is "off plan," you are eating thirty-four out of thirty-five "on plan" meals per week. That is 97 percent compliance! Ninety-seven

percent is fantastic in my book! My point is, you need to give yourself some slack. Enjoy your "off plan" meal, and get back on track afterward. If for some reason you have a couple of "off plan" meals in a week, just let it go; guilt will get you nowhere. Becoming an expert on your nutrition means accepting that you may fall off, and remembering that you have the education to jump right back on.

Strategy 15: Adjusting Your Plan as a Vegetarian or Vegan

Having my first nutrition center in Venice, California, provided me with great insight into vegetarian and vegan lifestyles. Venice is one of the most vegetarian/vegan-friendly places in the world. Through the years, many vegetarians and vegans have come to me for nutritional advice. Each of them seems to have similar challenges: *low energy, intense sugar cravings, low muscle tone, and high body fat*. This list made sense to me, since their nutrition was composed primarily of carbohydrates, with some fat and very little complete protein. Their blood sugar was very unstable.

Getting their blood sugar back in line was straightforward; they just implemented two actions:

Action 1 Get the correct amount of complete protein. Vegetarians will typically eat edamame, tofu, dairy, soy; whey or egg protein powder or bars; eggs; and fish. These are each great sources of complete protein. Vegans typically avoid all animal protein and eat only soy or quinoa, and take liquid amino acids. Whether you are a vegetarian or vegan, all that matters is that you get the amount of complete protein per meal that matches your nutrition parameters. This will ensure that your blood sugar remains stable.

Action 2 Avoid processed vegetarian food. Most vegetarian foods are meat imitations that are extremely processed. This type of vegetarian food is full of ingredients, very high in sodium, and because it is made from soy, contains a lower quality complete protein than found in animal protein (*based on nitrogen content per gram of protein*). Because of these reasons, eating processed vegetarian food makes it very difficult to stabilize your blood-sugar levels.

These fifteen strategies are great reference points as you go through your nutrition plan. Once you feel comfortable with each strategy, you are ready for section 3, "Choosing Your Nutrition Parameters."

Section 3—Choosing Your Nutrition Parameters

In the introduction I explained how and why I created the Venice Nutrition blood-sugar formula. Originally, there was no solution that truly seemed to stabilize someone's blood-sugar levels. The Venice Nutrition blood-sugar formula takes many factors about your health into account and, based on that information, prescribes your optimal nutrition parameters. Your nutrition parameters are your calories per meal and nutrient ratios (percentages or grams of protein, fat, and carbohydrates) based on your goal type and gender. Of course, this is simple with the power of software (which is why we created Venice Nutrition Online), but what about in a book? There are way too many calculations to use the same formula in a book. Additionally, the whole idea is to keep things relatively simple while still delivering powerful information. Because of this I decided that the best solution for determining your nutrition parameters was to prescribe the most commonly recommended nutrition parameters through my years of coaching Venice Nutrition clients. These are what I consider to be the "gold standard" nutrition parameters. These parameters make up the core of your nutrition plan. By understanding them you will learn how to make any food work in your program.

Your parameters are presented according to gender and goal type. Choose the parameters that match your gender and goal type. All of your meal plans will be designed around your parameters.

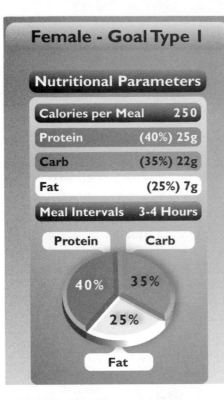

Female - Goal Type 1

Nutritional Parameters

Calories per Meal	250
Protein	(40%) 25g
Carb	(35%) 22g
Fat	(25%) 7g
Meal Intervals	3-4 Hours

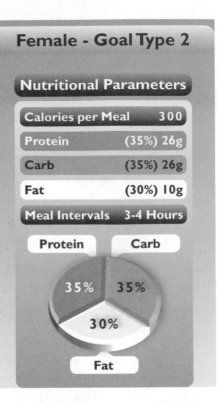

Female - Goal Type 2

Nutritional Parameters

Calories per Meal	300
Protein	(35%) 26g
Carb	(35%) 26g
Fat	(30%) 10g
Meal Intervals	3-4 Hours

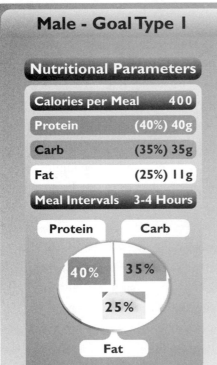

Male - Goal Type 1

Nutritional Parameters

Calories per Meal	400
Protein	(40%) 40g
Carb	(35%) 35g
Fat	(25%) 11g
Meal Intervals	3-4 Hours

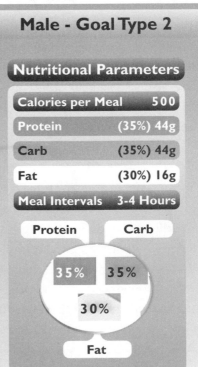

Male - Goal Type 2

Nutritional Parameters

Calories per Meal	500
Protein	(35%) 44g
Carb	(35%) 44g
Fat	(30%) 16g
Meal Intervals	3-4 Hours

Your meal parameters do not need to be exact. The standard wiggle room is this:

Calories per meal: plus or minus 20 calories per meal

You will notice that some meals are half or three-quarter meals; they are cut across the board, so the calories per meal and nutrient ratios match your parameters.

Nutrient ratios per meal: plus or minus 5%, or 3 grams, for protein, fat, and carbohydrates

It is important first that your protein matches, then your fat. Let carbohydrates make up the rest of the meal. For amounts of protein, fat, and carbohydrates per meal, you can focus either on percentages or on grams. They are essentially the same, so do what is easiest for you. For your percentages, you simply convert the recommend grams of protein, fat, and carbohydrates per meal to calories, and then divide that figure by your total recommend calories per meal. For example, female Goal Type 1 should eat 250 calories per meal. Here is how the nutrient ratios (percentages) are determined:

Protein per meal: 25 grams. Each gram of protein has 4 calories. So, 25 grams × 4 calories/gram = 100 calories. Then, 100 calories ÷ 250 calories = 0.4, or 40 percent. This means 40 percent of your meal will be protein. Here is a recap: 25 × 4 = 100; 100 ÷ 250 = 0.4 = 40%

Fat grams per meal: 7 grams. Each gram of fat has 9 calories. So, 7 grams × 9 calories/gram = 63 calories. Then, 63 calories ÷ 250 calories = 0.25, or 25 percent. This means 25 percent of your meal will be fat. Here is a recap: 7 × 9 = 63; 63 ÷ 250 = 0.25 = 25%

Carbohydrate grams per meal: 22 grams. Each gram of carbohydrates has 4 calories. So, 22 grams × 4 calories/gram = 88 calories. Then, 88 calories ÷ 250 calories = 0.35, or 35 percent. This means 35 percent of your meal will be carbohydrates. Here is a recap: 22 × 4 = 88; 88 ÷ 250 = 35%

Section 4—Simplifying Your Meals

When I first began coaching clients, I could always feel them becoming overwhelmed as I presented their meal plans to them. They would have a look that said, "Oh man, how am I going to do this? This program is hard!" I totally got it, too. It is not easy to make your health a priority in an already full life. I realized that in order to counter my clients' feelings of being overwhelmed, I needed to create a system that would simplify their meal plans and eliminate this sense of difficulty. With that goal in mind, I took a step back, thought of what I had done to simplify my nutrition, and realized I'd followed five basic steps with every meal. My method made meal plans, grocery shopping, eating in restaurants, and traveling simple. If you think about it, your meal plans are always just a combination of a protein, a fat, and a carbohydrate. Once you know the types of foods that are in each category, you simply choose one of the foods you enjoy in each category and *voila!*—you have a meal. The moment I began teaching my meal-plan method to clients, they got it. They understood that once they learned their nutrition parameters, the food categories, and their portion sizes, eating correctly was easy. Instantly, they had complete control over their nutrition.

In the next section (section 5), I introduce your Jump Start Phase and your meal plans. There is a good amount of information in these sections, so I'd like to help pace the delivery of this information by first presenting the five steps for keeping your meals simple. Implementing these five steps will show you how simple your meal plans actually are.

Here are the five steps for simplifying your nutrition plan:

Step 1: Know your recommended meal parameters (calories per meal and nutrient ratios).

Step 2: Review the meal plans that fall within your parameters.

Step 3: List at least five of your favorite proteins, fats, and carbohydrates (as shown in the "Simplify Your Meals" illustration on page 131).

Step 4: Choose a protein, fat, and carbohydrate, or a meal replacement, for each meal. (The only exception to this occurs if you choose a nonlean protein. In that case, you should avoid adding a fat choice, since a nonlean protein has both protein and fat.)

Step 5: As you become more comfortable with combining different meals, begin to add more of the food choices you enjoy to each category.

An Example of How to Simplify Your Nutrition

After reviewing your meal plans, simply follow this example and write your own food choices out on paper. This will initially narrow down the meal plans you want to follow and streamline your grocery-shopping list. Then, as you and your program evolve together, you can continue adding to your five-step method while maintaining a sense of simplicity.

Simplifying Your Meals

Protein		Fats	Carbohydrates		
Choose 1 type of Protein		**Choose 1 Fat**	**Choose 1 or 2 Carbs**		
Lean Protein	Non-Lean Protein	ONLY With Lean Protein	Grain	Fruit	Vegetables
✓ Chicken	✓ Ground beef	✓ Almonds	✓ Brown rice	✓ Apple	✓ Asparagus
✓ Low-fat cottage cheese	✓ Ground turkey	✓ Avocados	✓ Oatmeal	✓ Banana	✓ Broccoli
✓ Tuna	✓ Filet mignon	✓ Cashew	✓ Potatoes	✓ Blueberries	✓ Carrots
✓ Protein powder	✓ Pork tenderloin	✓ Peanut butter	✓ Quinoa	✓ Orange	✓ Corn
✓ Low-fat Greek yogurt	✓ Salmon	✓ Oil vinaigrette	✓ Wheat bread	✓ Strawberries	✓ Garbanzo beans
etc...	etc...	Salad dressing	etc...	etc...	etc...
		etc...			

OR

Meal Replacements
Choose 1 for a Whole Meal

✓ Edamame

✓ Protein bar (your 2 favorites)

✓ Ready-to-drink protein shake (your 2 favorites)

etc...

Section 5—Jump-Starting Your Meals

Your ten-day Jump Start Phase is designed to jump-start your metabolism and provide you with fast results via a simplified approach. After your Jump Start, you can either dive into the rest of your meal plans and add variety or choose to stay in this phase. The only difference between Jump Start meal plans and additional meal plans is quality of food. The calories, protein, fat, and carbohydrates are all based on your meal parameters. The goal in the Jump Start Phase is to eat only the highest-quality foods, since this will yield the fastest internal and external results.

There are three parts to your meal plans:

Part 1—Your Jump Start sample day

Part 2—Your Jump Start meal plans

Part 3—Your additional meal plans—for after your ten-day Jump Start Phase

There is a great chance you are above your set point. This means that by focusing only on your Jump Start meals, your initial results will be fast. Your Jump Start meals are high-quality meals (see "Quality of Food" chart on page 106).

There are three types of foods in particular that cause difficult digestion, bloating, and slower results. I recommend avoiding them during your Jump Start Phase. They are:

All bread products and cereals (except oatmeal)—These foods are heavily processed, and the majority of them contain gluten. (Oats are good because they are unprocessed and contain only a little gluten.) Gluten is a special type of protein that is found primarily in wheat, rye, and barley. Gluten is what gives bread its elasticity. It is also a complex protein that is difficult to digest. This is why most people retain water after they eat bread products or processed cereals: their digestive system struggles with breaking down gluten. The presence of gluten along with processed carbohydrates makes these foods medium quality at best. After your Jump Start program, you can eat bread products and cereals. I suggest choosing products that say "gluten free" on the label. These foods are higher quality, easier to digest, and better at stabilizing your blood sugar.

Dairy—Dairy products contain the sugar lactose. Your body makes a digestive enzyme called *lactase* to digest lactose. Many people have a degree of deficiency in lactase levels. Some people are even lactose intolerant, which means their body cannot digest lactose at all. When lactose cannot be digested, the result is gas and intestinal pressure. In addition, dairy is highly processed. For these reasons, dairy should be avoided during your Jump Start Phase. Many people love dairy, and it is the staple protein of choice for many quick and balanced meals. After your Jump Start Phase, if you love dairy, I suggest experimenting with dairy in your meals and seeing how much of it you can eat without feeling bloated.

Soy—Soybeans contain organic compounds called *isoflavones*. These compounds trigger your body to produce the female hormone estrogen. (Men have small amounts of estrogen, just as women have small amounts of testosterone.) Estrogen is a water-retaining and fat-storing hormone. For this reason, soy should be avoided during your Jump Start Phase. If you enjoy soy, I suggest eating soy in moderation after your Jump Start Phase.

Because of dairy and bread products' high level of processing as well as the digestion challenges they present, and because of the estrogen properties of soy, the majority of your Jump Start meals do not contain these food items. I also know that needing to prepare five to six meals a day can be unrealistic. This is why I have included quick "mid"-meal options for your midmorning and midafternoon meals—the most difficult ones to get in. These quick options are lower in quality, though they will still provide you with the ability to jump-start your metabolism. Also, if you want to exchange foods in your Jump Start meal plans, make sure you exchange only high-quality foods.

Fourteen Things You Need to Know About Your Meal Plans and Sample Day

1. **All of your meal plans are designed like templates.** This means that any lean protein can be exchanged for any other lean protein, any fat for any other fat, and any carbohydrate for any other carbohydrate. This truly provides you with thousands of exchange options.

2. **Your sample day is exactly that—a "sample day."** Your sample day is an example of how quickly and efficiently you can work your meals into your day, focusing primarily on the meals that work *best* at each time in a typical day (breakfast, midmorning meal, lunch, midafternoon meal, dinner, bedtime meal). You can choose to follow the sample day as provided, or use it as a reference point to design your meal structure for each day. Whichever you prefer, make sure you map out your meals and get at least five meals a day. Also, there are notes that come with each meal. These notes will provide you with additional meal ideas that you can incorporate at that time of day.

    You will also notice that with Goal Type 1 (for both male and female), your sample day may have half or three-quarter meals at your midmorning and midafternoon mealtimes. Your sample day is designed like this because most people have not established a pattern of eating consistently at those times. Therefore, their bodies are not used to metabolizing food in the midmorning and midafternoon. The adjustment is to eat half or three-quarter meals for the first ten to fourteen days, and then, as your appetite grows in the midmorning and midafternoon (*and it definitely will*), you can shift to eating a full meal at those mealtimes. Basically, if you are hungry, you should eat a full meal. If you are not hungry, eat half or three-quarters of a meal.

    If you are already eating consistently at midmorning and midafternoon, you may want to eat full meals at those times. Just choose a full meal from your Jump Start meal plans and plug it into those mealtimes. Make sure you always base your full- or half-meal size decision on your hunger.

3. **Every meal description contains notes and recommendations.** Each meal description will have tips on how to create more variety within the meal as well as add additional flavor. The notes will also share what adjustments you can make to optimally work the meal into your day.

4. **Remember that only complete protein is counted in your meal plans.** All incomplete protein will be listed as 0 grams of protein in every meal. The overall calories for the food item is accounted for.

5. **Understand that many of your meal percentages *will not* add up to 100 percent.** There are two reasons for this. First, all manufacturers and nutrition databases that provide food nutrient labels round their numbers. Some food labels may be up to 20 to 25 calories off their true total (due to the rounding of grams of protein, fat, and carbs). This leads to the nutrient percentages being off from 1 to 5 percent compared to total calories in the food item itself. Second, since incomplete protein is not counted (on the Venice Nutrition Program), this will affect the nutrient percentages per meal compared to total calories. Please know that these percentage discrepancies have no effect on your nutrition plan. It is just important to know that sometimes the math will not add up.

6. **Discover which carbohydrates work best for your body.** Every meal is centered on complete protein, then fat. The remaining available calories per meal are filled by carbohydrates. You need carbohydrates at each meal (except possibly at bedtime and after your "off plan" meal, which are both explained in the "fifteen strategies" section). You want to find out what meals satisfy you the most. This factor changes depending on who you are. You know that high-quality carbohydrates are your best choice. But you need to take it beyond that. Discover which carbohydrates work best for your body. Find out which meals bloat you a bit and which ones leave you feeling energized. Every meal in this book is balanced correctly. Your body, on the other hand, will digest each food in each meal differently. This is another reason that journaling is so helpful during the first thirty days on the program. When possible, I also recommend choosing meals that contain a high-quality simple and complex carbohydrate. As I briefly shared in section 1, fruits and vegetables are simple carbohydrates and grains (oatmeal, rice, sweet potato, beans, etc.) are complex carbohydrates. A meal that contains a high-quality simple and complex carbohydrate along with a high-quality protein and fat is a powerful combination for optimizing blood-sugar levels. Once you are aware of which carbs work best for you, you will have that knowledge forever. This knowledge will be an essential asset in your quest to permanently achieve your Body Confidence goals.

7. **All your meals are labeled as "High Quality," "Medium Quality," or "Low Quality"** (as shared earlier in section 2, strategy 3). Regardless of the quality, each meal is balanced and will stabilize your blood sugar. High-quality meals just stabilize your blood sugar more efficiently and for a longer time than medium- and low-quality meals.

8. **Certain meals are labeled "Quick Meals."** A Quick Meal is a meal that can be prepared in five minutes or less. Most medium- and low-quality meals are Quick Meals. Many high-quality meals can be made into Quick Meals by cooking your protein source in advance.

9. **All "free foods" are optional.** Your meal plans will list "free foods" to enhance the taste of the meal. These recommendations are optional. They have either zero or few calories and add only bonus flavors to each meal. If you prefer keeping your meals as simple as possible, you can skip the "free food" recommendations.

10. **You *can* eat your additional meal plans during your Jump Start Phase.** I do recommend eating only your Jump Start meals during your first ten days on the program, since they will accelerate your metabolism and yield faster results. Still, it is important to remember the ultimate goal—achieving permanent health results. If you want to ease into the program, then by all means immediately start eating the additional meal plans. The only point I want to make is that you need to understand that your initial results may come a bit slower. They will still come—just possibly not as fast. Enjoying the program from day one is very important, so by all means do what you feel will allow you to most enjoy the program.

11. **Remember your fifteen strategies to mastering your meals.** Your fifteen strategies, explained earlier in this chapter, are your guide to successfully working these meal plans into your lifestyle. Continue to read the ones that apply most to you, since they will make your meal plan process much easier.

12. **All sugar cravings will be gone and your energy will be high within two days.** It typically takes about two days for your body to detoxify itself. After that, your blood sugar will be stable. The result is high energy and no sugar cravings.

13. **Eat more meals rather than bigger meals.** Many times people think the meals will be too small and they will be ravenous the entire day. This is not the case. The frequency of meals, along with the correct calories and nutrient ratios, will keep your body consistently fed and feeling good. Now, there may be times (the longer you are on the program) when you get hungry sooner than three hours after a meal. If this is the case, go ahead and eat your next meal before the three-hour mark rather than increasing the size of your meal. As your metabolism rate increases, your body will naturally crave more food. This additional meal will give your body the calories it wants while keeping your metabolism running efficiently.

14. **Your recipes and the food-exchange system are in sections 6 and 7 of this chapter.** The quantities of the non–"free foods" ingredients are listed within your meal plans. The recipe section will teach you how to make the meal.

To view your Jump Start sample day, Jump Start meal, and additional meal plans, go to the nutrition plan that is based on your *gender* and your *goal type*.

FEMALE GOAL TYPE 1 (250-CALORIE MEAL PLANS)

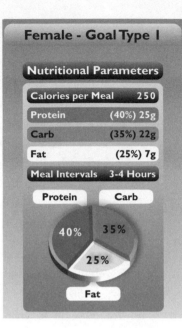

Female - Goal Type I

Nutritional Parameters

Calories per Meal	250
Protein	(40%) 25g
Carb	(35%) 22g
Fat	(25%) 7g
Meal Intervals	3-4 Hours

Protein 40% · Carb 35% · Fat 25%

Jump Start Sample Day

Remember to drink at least 8 ounces of water with every meal, and 8 ounces of water between each meal.

6:30 am

Quick Meal!

Scrambled Eggs and Side of Oatmeal (with optional flavorings)

¾ Meal (High Quality)

(Quick Meal if eggs are hardboiled)

You can increase your metabolism and jump-start the fat-burning process by eating a balanced breakfast, like eggs and oatmeal, one hour within waking. Add flavor to unsweetened oatmeal with "free foods" like Stevia, cinnamon, and vanilla extract. If you're pressed for time, the Protein Power Oatmeal breakfast is a faster option.

FOODS	CALORIES	PROTEIN(G)	CARB(G)	FAT(G)
3 egg whites	51	10.5	0.0	0.0
1 egg (whole)	80	6.4	0.5	5.6
¾ ounces oatmeal (unsweetened)	75	0.0	14.5	1.5
Totals:	**206**	**16.9 (33%)**	**15.0 (29%)**	**7.1 (31%)**

9:30 am

Quick Meal!

Protein Bar

(Low Quality)

A midmorning meal can initially be challenging to fit into your schedule. A balanced protein bar is the perfect solution. The brand of protein bar is your choice. What matters most is to find a bar that comes close to matching your caloric and nutrient ratio parameters. Cottage cheese and Greek yogurt meals are also quick midmorning options after you complete the Jump Start Phase.

FOODS	CALORIES	PROTEIN(G)	CARB(G)	FAT(G)
1 serving Think Thin, any flavor	230	20.0	24.0	8.0
Totals:	**230**	**20.0 (35%)**	**24.0 (41%)**	**8.0 (31%)**

12:30 pm

Quick Meal!

Grilled Chicken Salad

(High Quality)

(Quick Meal if chicken is prepared in advance)

A grilled chicken salad can be made and brought from home or ordered at any restaurant. If you're dining out for lunch, request that your salad dressing be served on the side. If you dislike light dressing, you can substitute it with 1 tablespoon of regular balsamic vinaigrette. You can also exchange chicken for any other high-quality lean protein like grilled shrimp.

FOODS	CALORIES	PROTEIN(G)	CARB(G)	FAT(G)
4 ounces chicken breast (boneless/skinless)	124	26.0	0.0	1.2
3 tablespoons low-fat balsamic vinaigrette salad dressing	66	0.0	3.0	6.0
2 cups garden salad (lettuce and vegetables)	70	0.0	18.0	0.0
Totals:	**260**	**26.0 (40%)**	**21.0 (32%)**	**7.2 (25%)**

3:30 pm

Quick Turkey Roll-Up with Fruit and Nuts

¾ Meal (Medium Quality)

This is a quick midafternoon meal. Dip turkey slices into mustard or any other "free food" for extra flavor. Finding the time to eat midafternoon can be challenging at first. If you need a faster, "ready to eat" meal at this time, then your Ready-to-Drink shake meal is a fantastic choice. Whether it is a shake, bar, or higher-quality meal, getting a balanced meal in during your Jump Start Phase is what matters most.

Important note: if you are still hungry after this meal, next time make it a full meal.

FOODS	CALORIES	PROTEIN(G)	CARB(G)	FAT(G)
3 ounces turkey breast, Boar's Head, low sodium	75	18.0	0.0	0.4
⅓ ounce cashews (raw)	48	0.0	2.8	4.0
3 ounces apple	51	0.0	12.9	0.3
Totals:	**174**	**18.0 (41%)**	**15.7 (36%)**	**4.7 (24%)**

6:30 pm

Salmon with Brown Rice and Asparagus

(High Quality)

This meal is both tasty and extremely high quality, due to the salmon, which is naturally high in omega-3 fatty acids (the heart-healthy, good fat). Enhance the flavor of salmon with fresh-squeezed lemon juice, herbs, and spices. You may want to occasionally substitute a filet mignon for salmon if you are in the mood for beef.

FOODS	CALORIES	PROTEIN(G)	CARB(G)	FAT(G)
4 ounces salmon	160	22.4	0.0	8.0
¼ cup brown rice (cooked)	50	0.0	11.0	0.0
4 ounces asparagus	24	0.0	4.0	0.5
Totals:	**234**	**22.4 (38%)**	**15 (26%)**	**8.5 (33%)**

9:30 pm

Protein Smoothie Without Milk (can add water and ice) ¾ Meal (Medium Quality)

A protein shake makes for a delicious and balanced dessert before bed. It will also help to keep your metabolism humming all night long. If you choose to have a meal in place of a protein shake at this time, limit the amount of starchy carbs/grains to accelerate the fat-burning process.

FOODS	CALORIES	PROTEIN(G)	CARB(G)	FAT(G)
1 scoop whey protein powder, any flavor	102	20.0	1.0	1.5
½ tablespoon natural peanut butter	50	0.0	1.6	4.0
3 ounces strawberries	27	0.0	6.0	0.3
Totals:	**179**	**20.0 (45%)**	**8.6 (19%)**	**5.8 (29%)**

Day Totals:	1283	123.3 (38%)	99.3 (31%)	41.3 (29%)

JUMP START MEALS

Breakfast

High Quality

Scrambled Eggs and Side of Oatmeal (with optional flavorings) ¾ Meal

(Quick Meal if eggs are hardboiled)

An eggs and oatmeal breakfast combo is simple to make (use instant oatmeal for easy prep) and incredibly satisfying. Give plain cooked oatmeal a boost of flavor without extra calories by stirring in "free foods" like Stevia (or any calorie-free sugar substitute), cinnamon, and vanilla extract.

FOODS	CALORIES	PROTEIN(G)	CARB(G)	FAT(G)
3 egg whites	51	10.5	0.0	0.0
1 egg (whole)	80	6.4	0.5	5.6
¾ ounce oatmeal (unsweetened)	75	0.0	14.5	1.5
Totals:	**206**	**16.9 (33%)**	**15.0 (29%)**	**7.1 (31%)**

Veggie and Egg Scramble

An egg scramble is the perfect way to sneak in extra veggies you have on hand. Add a spoonful of your favorite salsa for extra spice.

FOODS	CALORIES	PROTEIN(G)	CARB(G)	FAT(G)
3 egg whites	51	10.5	0.0	0.0
1 egg (whole)	80	6.4	0.5	5.6
½ cup spinach (cooked)	25	0.0	5.0	0.0
2 ounces broccoli	16	0.0	3.0	0.3
½ cup mushrooms	14	0.0	2.6	0.3
⅓ cup tomato	12	0.0	2.6	0.2
Totals:	**198**	**16.9 (34%)**	**13.7 (28%)**	**6.4 (29%)**

Medium Quality

Quick Meal!

Berry Banana Protein Smoothie Without Milk (add water and ice)

A protein and fruit smoothie is a sweet and refreshing way to stabilize your blood sugar fast. Try blending your favorite vanilla or chocolate protein powder with a variety of fresh or frozen fruit. Adjust the amount of water and ice to your desired consistency.

FOODS	CALORIES	PROTEIN(G)	CARB(G)	FAT(G)
1¼ scoops whey protein powder, any flavor	128	25.0	1.3	1.9
½ tablespoon natural peanut butter	50	0.0	1.6	4.0
2 ounces banana	52	0.0	13.6	0.0
2 ounces strawberries	18	0.0	4.0	0.2
Totals:	**248**	**25.0 (40%)**	**20.5 (33%)**	**6.1 (22%)**

Quick Meal!

Protein Power Oatmeal

Recipe

Protein Power Oatmeal is warm, creamy, and guaranteed to fuel your busy mornings. You can substitute the whey protein powder for soy or egg white powder. For a change of pace, swap nuts, peanut butter, or ground flax seeds for the almond butter. *For the full recipe, please see page 234.*

FOODS	CALORIES	PROTEIN(G)	CARB(G)	FAT(G)
1¼ scoops whey protein powder, any flavor	128	25.0	1.3	1.9
½ tablespoon almond butter	43	0.0	2.0	3.5
¾ ounce oatmeal (unsweetened)	75	0.0	14.5	1.5
Totals:	**246**	**25.0 (41%)**	**17.8 (29%)**	**6.9 (25%)**

Lunch

High Quality

Quick Meal!

Grilled Chicken Salad

(Quick Meal if chicken is prepared in advance)

Whether it's lunch at home or at a restaurant, grilled chicken salad is a balanced and high-quality option. You can exchange the chicken for any other lean protein like grilled white fish or shrimp and top the salad with your favorite vegetables.

FOODS	CALORIES(G)	PROTEIN(G)	CARB(G)	FAT(G)
4 ounces chicken breast (boneless/skinless)	124	26.0	0.0	1.2
3 tablespoons low-fat balsamic vinaigrette salad dressing	66	0.0	3.0	6.0
2 cups garden salad (lettuce and vegetables)	70	0.0	18.0	0.0
Totals:	**260**	**26.0 (40%)**	**21.0 (32%)**	**7.2 (25%)**

Quick Meal!

Ground Turkey Vegetable Stir-Fry

(Quick Meal if stir-fry is prepared in advance)

A stir-fry is perfect to make in bulk for grab 'n' go meals during the week. Choose your favorite veggies and season your stir-fry with garlic, fresh herbs, and spices to enhance the flavor without additional fat or calories. (See "Condiments, Seasonings, and Spices" in your Food Exchange List for a full list of "free foods.")

FOODS	CALORIES	PROTEIN(G)	CARB(G)	FAT(G)
3½ ounces ground turkey (99% fat free)	105	24.9	0.0	0.7
½ tablespoon olive oil	60	0.0	0.0	7.0
1 cup mixed vegetables	80	0.0	14.0	0.0
Totals:	**245**	**24.9 (41%)**	**14.0 (23%)**	**7.7 (28%)**

Quick Meal!

Italian Tuna Salad with Side of Fruit

Recipe

Italian Tuna Salad is made up of common pantry items (canned tuna, low-fat balsamic dressing) and any vegetable you choose. Try making this recipe in bulk and storing it in the fridge for easy meals throughout the week. If desired, substitute any other lean protein for the tuna. *For the full recipe, please see page 237.*

FOODS	CALORIES	PROTEIN(G)	CARB(G)	FAT(G)
3½ ounces albacore tuna (packed in water and drained)	105	24.5	0.0	1.8
½ ounce black olives (pitted)	19	0.0	0.4	1.9
1½ tablespoons low-fat balsamic vinaigrette salad dressing	33	0.0	1.5	3.0
½ cup bell peppers, green or red	13	0.0	3.2	0.3
⅓ cup cherry tomato	12	0.0	2.6	0.2
⅛ cup onion	6	0.0	1.3	0.0
4 ounces orange	52	0.0	13.2	0.4
Totals:	**240**	**24.5 (41%)**	**22.2 (37%)**	**7.6 (28%)**

Quick Meal!

Chicken, Fruit, and Nuts

(Quick Meal if chicken is prepared in advance)

It may seem like an odd combination, but this meal is one of our go-to staples when we're in a hurry. Try preparing grilled or baked chicken in bulk for the week so you always have a high-quality protein on hand. Then pair it with your favorite fresh fruit and unsalted nuts and you've got a quality meal that takes only minutes to make.

FOODS	CALORIES	PROTEIN(G)	CARB(G)	FAT(G)
3½ ounces chicken breast (boneless/skinless)	109	22.8	0.0	1.1
½ ounce cashews (raw)	80	0.0	4.6	6.6
4 ounces apple	68	0.0	17.2	0.4
Totals:	257	22.8 (35%)	21.8 (34%)	8.1 (28%)

Dinner

High Quality

Quick Meal!

Grilled Chicken with Spinach Bean Salad

(Quick Meal if chicken is prepared in advance)

Garbanzo beans (or any beans) add a boost of flavor and texture to a spinach salad. You can swap out the spinach for your favorite leafy greens and the chicken breast for any lean protein.

FOODS	CALORIES	PROTEIN(G)	CARB(G)	FAT(G)
4 ounces chicken breast (boneless/skinless)	124	26.0	0.0	1.2
2 tablespoons low-fat balsamic vinaigrette salad dressing	44	0.0	2.0	4.0
2 cups spinach leaves (uncooked)	14	0.0	2.0	0.0
¾ ounce garbanzo beans	77	0.0	13.5	1.5
Totals:	259	26.0 (40%)	17.5 (27%)	6.7 (23%)

Restaurant-Worthy Steak with Sweet Potato and Steamed Cauliflower

Recipe

A filet mignon is one of the leanest, tastiest cuts of beef, and that is why we recommend it. Pair your filet with delicious sweet potatoes and any steamed vegetable for a satisfying meal. *For the full recipe, please see page 239.*

FOODS	CALORIES	PROTEIN(G)	CARB(G)	FAT(G)
3 ounces filet mignon	150	24.0	0.0	7.5
2 ounces sweet potato	60	0.0	14.0	0.0
4 ounces cauliflower	28	0.0	5.7	0.0
Totals:	**238**	**24.0 (40%)**	**19.7 (33%)**	**7.5 (28%)**

Seared Scallops with Brown Rice and Spinach

Recipe

Seared scallops take only minutes to make and are a great source of high-quality protein. You can swap out the scallops for any lean protein like chicken breast, pork tenderloin, or shrimp. The spinach can also be substituted with any leafy greens. *For the full recipe, please see page 241.*

FOODS	CALORIES	PROTEIN(G)	CARB(G)	FAT(G)
5 ounces scallops	125	25.0	0.0	1.3
1 teaspoon olive oil	40	0.0	0.0	4.6
⅓ cup brown rice (cooked)	66	0.0	14.5	0.0
3½ cups spinach leaves (uncooked)	25	0.0	3.5	0.0
Totals:	**256**	**25.0 (39%)**	**18 (28%)**	**5.9 (21%)**

Salmon with Brown Rice and Asparagus

Salmon is loaded in omega-3 essential fats and should be eaten once or twice a week if possible. Enhance the flavor of salmon with fresh-squeezed lemon juice, herbs, and spices. Serve leftover salmon over a crisp salad for a satisfying lunch the next day.

FOODS	CALORIES	PROTEIN(G)	CARB(G)	FAT(G)
4 ounces salmon	160	22.4	0.0	8.0
¼ cup brown rice (cooked)	50	0.0	11.0	0.0
4 ounces asparagus	24	0.0	4.0	0.5
Totals:	234	22.4 (38%)	15.0 (26%)	8.5 (33%)

MEAL REPLACEMENTS AND QUICK "MID" MEALS

Medium Quality

Quick Meal!

Quick Turkey Roll-Up with Fruit and Nuts

¾ Meal

Having lean, low-sodium deli meat on hand is a great way to ensure you've got a fast source of protein available. Ask your local deli for the highest-quality, least-processed brand they have (like Boar's Head). Pair it with fresh fruit and unsalted nuts of your choice for a quick and balanced meal. Dip turkey slices into mustard or any other "free food" for extra flavor.

FOODS	CALORIES	PROTEIN(G)	CARB(G)	FAT(G)
3 ounces turkey breast, Boar's Head, low sodium	75	18.0	0.0	0.4
⅓ ounce cashews (raw)	48	0.0	2.8	4.0
3 ounces apple	51	0.0	12.9	0.3
Totals:	174	18.0 (41%)	15.7 (36%)	4.7 (24%)

Low Quality

Quick Meal!

Protein Bar

Protein bars are a convenient option for those times when you are too busy for an actual meal (like when you are on the go or in a meeting at work). The goal is to choose a bar that matches your nutritional parameters. For a complete list of recommended protein bars, see "Meal Replacements" in your Food Exchange List.

FOODS	CALORIES	PROTEIN(G)	CARB(G)	FAT(G)
1 serving Think Thin, any flavor	230	20.0	24.0	8.0
Totals:	**230**	**20.0 (35%)**	**24.0 (41%)**	**8.0 (31%)**

Quick Meal!

Ready-to-Drink Shake and Fruit

¾ Meal

A ready-made protein drink paired with fresh fruit is an ideal option while at work or even while traveling. For a complete list of recommended protein drinks, see "Meal Replacements" in your Food Exchange List.

FOODS	CALORIES	PROTEIN(G)	CARB(G)	FAT(G)
1 bottle (14 ounces) Muscle Milk, Light, any flavor	160	20	10	4.5
2 ounces apple	34	0.0	8.6	0.2
Totals:	**194**	**20.0 (41%)**	**18.6 (38%)**	**4.7 (22%)**

ADDITIONAL MEALS—AFTER JUMP START PHASE

Breakfast

Medium Quality

Quick Meal!

Cereal to Go with Protein Powder

By adding protein powder and nuts to cereal, you end up with a hearty breakfast that stabilizes your blood sugar and keeps you full all morning long. Simply shake protein powder and milk together in a shake cup with a lid until blended and pour over any low-sugar, high-fiber cereal. Top with nuts and enjoy. If the milk mixture is too sweet, try using only half of the protein powder together with the milk. Mix the remaining protein powder with water on the side for a quick shake.

FOODS	CALORIES	PROTEIN(G)	CARB(G)	FAT(G)
1 scoop whey protein powder, any flavor	102	20.0	1.0	1.5
5 ounces milk (low fat)	55	5.6	7.5	0.6
½ ounce bran flakes cereal	45	0.0	11.0	0.0
¼ ounce almonds (raw)	43	0.0	1.5	4.0
Totals:	**245**	**25.6 (42%)**	**21.0 (34%)**	**6.1 (22%)**

Quick Meal!

Cottage Cheese with Fruit

Cottage cheese mixed with fruit is a sweet and creamy combo that takes less than a minute to make. Fresh pineapple, blueberries, and peaches taste delicious too. Try prepping fruit in bulk for a few days so it's always ready to eat.

FOODS	CALORIES	PROTEIN(G)	CARB(G)	FAT(G)
7 ounces cottage cheese (low fat)	175	24.5	7.0	4.2
4 ounces strawberries	27	0.0	6.0	0.3
2 ounces blueberries	37	0.0	9.3	0.3
Totals:	**239**	**24.5 (41%)**	**22.3 (37%)**	**4.8 (18%)**

Protein Smoothie with Milk (can also add water and ice)

Milk adds a dose of calcium and a creamier texture to this protein smoothie. If you'd prefer, substitute the milk with low-fat Lactaid or soy milk. Almond butter or even flax seed oil can be substituted for the peanut butter.

FOODS	CALORIES	PROTEIN(G)	CARB(G)	FAT(G)
1 scoop whey protein powder, any flavor	102	20.0	1.0	1.5
2 ounces banana	52	0.0	13.6	0.0
½ tablespoon natural peanut butter	50	0.0	1.6	4.0
4 ounces milk (low fat)	60	4.0	6.0	2.5
Totals:	**264**	**24.0 (36%)**	**22.2 (34%)**	**8.0 (27%)**

Bacon, Egg, and Cheese Burrito

Recipe

A bacon, egg, and cheese burrito makes a tasty and fast breakfast, lunch, or dinner. Egg whites can easily be substituted for Egg Beaters. *For the full recipe, see page 235.*

FOODS	CALORIES	PROTEIN(G)	CARB(G)	FAT(G)
⅔ cup Egg Beaters	66	13.2	2.6	0.0
½ ounce cheddar cheese (low fat)	25	3.4	0.2	1.0
1 ounce Canadian bacon	44	6.0	0.5	2.0
1 whole-grain, low-carb wrap	110	0.0	17.0	3.0
1 ounce tomato (about 2 thin slices)	6	0.0	1.3	0.1
Totals:	**251**	**22.6 (36%)**	**21.6 (34%)**	**6.1 (22%)**

Greek Yogurt Parfait

Recipe

Unlike traditional yogurt, Greek yogurt is high in protein and low in sugar. It's best sweetened and served with your favorite fruit and nuts. For an additional boost of flavor add "free foods" like Stevia and vanilla extract. This recipe can be made in bulk for the week and is perfect for breakfast, dessert, or a snack. *For the full recipe, see page 233.*

FOODS	CALORIES	PROTEIN(G)	CARB(G)	FAT(G)
10 ounces Greek yogurt, fat free	150	25.0	11.3	0.0
1½ ounces blueberries	28	0.0	6.9	0.2
½ ounce almonds (raw)	85	0.0	3.0	8.0
Totals:	**263**	**25.0 (38%)**	**21.2 (32%)**	**8.2 (28%)**

Western-Style Omelet with Side of Fruit

Recipe

This omelet is a perfect way to use any leftover veggies you have on hand. You can even double the recipe and gently reheat the other half of the omelet in the microwave for dinner that night or breakfast the next morning. Serve with your favorite fresh fruit. *For the full recipe, see page 233.*

FOODS	CALORIES	PROTEIN(G)	CARB(G)	FAT(G)
⅔ cup Egg Beaters	66	13.2	2.6	0.0
1½ ounces ham, Boar's Head, low sodium	45	7.5	1.5	0.8
⅔ ounce cheddar cheese	73	4.6	0.7	5.9
2 tablespoons chopped tomato	6	0.0	1.3	0.1
2 tablespoons chopped onion	6	0.0	1.3	0.0
¼ cup bell peppers, green or red	7	0.0	1.6	0.1
4 ounces cantaloupe	40	0.0	9.6	0.5
Totals:	**243**	**25.3 (42%)**	**18.6 (31%)**	**7.4 (27%)**

Lunch

Medium Quality

Quick Meal!

Boca Burger with Fruit (can add lettuce, tomato, and onion)

A Boca burger is a great source of soy protein and takes only moments to prepare. You can top your burger with a small amount of ketchup or mustard. Serve with fresh fruit of your choice for a complete meal.

FOODS	CALORIES	PROTEIN(G)	CARB(G)	FAT(G)
1 Boca Burger, original	100	19.0	8.0	1
¾ ounce cheddar cheese	83	5.3	0.8	6.8
5 ounces strawberries	45	0.0	10.0	0.6
Totals:	**228**	**24.3 (43%)**	**18.8 (33%)**	**8.4 (33%)**

Quick Meal!

Chicken and Cheese Burrito

(Quick Meal if chicken is prepared in advance)

This meal is made of several staples we recommend you always have on hand: chicken breast, whole-grain/low-carb wraps, and fresh or frozen veggies (choose your favorite veggies). You can substitute the chicken for deli turkey or even grilled shrimp for a change of pace. This meal is also delicious as a grilled quesadilla. Add salsa for a boost of flavor.

FOODS	CALORIES	PROTEIN(G)	CARB(G)	FAT(G)
3 ounces chicken breast (boneless/skinless)	93	19.5	0.0	0.9
⅓ ounce cheddar cheese	36	2.3	0.3	3.0
1 whole-grain, low-carb wrap	110	0.0	17.0	3.0
¼ cup mixed vegetables	20	0.0	3.5	0.0
Totals:	**259**	**21.8 (34%)**	**20.8 (32%)**	**6.9 (24%)**

Quick Meal!

Chicken Fajita (can add tomato, lettuce, and onion)

(Quick Meal if chicken is prepared in advance)

Chicken (or shrimp) fajitas can be made at home or enjoyed at any Mexican restaurant. If dining out, request that your meal is prepared in very little oil, and use guacamole as your fat (or choose a small amount of sour cream or cheese). Skip the rice and beans and load up on bell peppers and onions. Add salsa or pico de gallo for extra flavor.

FOODS	CALORIES	PROTEIN(G)	CARB(G)	FAT(G)
3 ounces chicken breast (boneless/skinless)	109	22.8	0.0	1.1
1 tablespoon guacamole	40	0.0	0.4	4.0
2 ounces corn tortillas	100	0.0	18.4	2.0
¼ cup bell peppers, green or red	7	0.0	1.6	0.1
Totals:	**256**	**22.8 (36%)**	**20.4 (32%)**	**7.2 (25%)**

Quick Meal!

Smoked Salmon and Cream Cheese Toasts

Recipe

Smoked salmon toasts are a fun way to load up on your omega-3 essential fat. Ak-Mak crackers, a whole-grain flat-bread snack, can be found at any grocery store. This meal is also delicious served for breakfast. *For the full recipe, see page 238.*

FOODS	CALORIES	PROTEIN(G)	CARB(G)	FAT(G)
4 ounces smoked salmon	132	20.8	0.0	4.8
2 Ak-Mak crackers	46	0.0	8.0	0.8
1 tablespoon light cream cheese	35	1.0	1.0	2.5
½ small tomato, sliced	12	0.0	2.6	0.2
1 slice of red onion	12	0.0	1.3	0.0
¼ cucumber, sliced	8	0.0	1.5	0.2
Totals:	**245**	**21.8 (36%)**	**14.4 (24%)**	**8.5 (31%)**

153

Spicy Turkey Club Wrap

Recipe

A turkey club can be healthy when it's made with low-fat mayonnaise, turkey bacon, and a whole-grain wrap. You can swap out the turkey for chicken breast if you'd prefer. *For the full recipe, see page 237.*

FOODS	CALORIES	PROTEIN(G)	CARB(G)	FAT(G)
3½ ounces turkey breast, Boar's Head, low sodium	87.5	21.0	0.0	0.5
1 slice turkey bacon	33	2.5	0.0	2.5
½ tablespoon light mayonnaise	25	0.0	0.5	2.5
1 whole-grain, low-carb wrap	110	0.0	17.0	3.0
romaine lettuce leaves	1	0.0	0.2	0.0
2 slices of tomato	6	0.0	1.3	0.1
4 slices of cucumber	4	0.0	0.8	0.1
Totals:	**266.5**	**23.5 (35%)**	**19.8 (30%)**	**8.7 (29%)**

Sushi Meal (can add wasabi and ginger)

When ordering sushi, aim for sashimi (slices of fish that can be served on top of or alongside rice). Some sushi restaurants even offer brown rice in place of white rice, which is a better choice for stable blood sugar due to the increased fiber. Add soy sauce for a boost of flavor.

FOODS	CALORIES	PROTEIN(G)	CARB(G)	FAT(G)
2 ounces sashimi, tuna (albacore)	98	14.4	0.0	4.2
2 ounces sashimi, salmon	80	11.2	0.0	4.0
1 piece vegetable roll	31	0.0	5.6	0.6
¼ cup brown rice (cooked)	50	0.0	11.0	0.0
Totals:	**259**	**25.6 (40%)**	**16.6 (26%)**	**8.8 (31%)**

Quick Meal!

Cranberry Chicken Salad Wrap

Recipe

(Quick Meal if chicken is prepared in advance)

This creamy chicken salad can be served in a wrap, on top of a salad, or with a side of fruit. Try making the chicken salad mixture in bulk for grab 'n' go meals for the week. *For the full recipe, see page 236.*

FOODS	CALORIES	PROTEIN(G)	CARB(G)	FAT(G)
3 ounces chicken breast (boneless/skinless)	109	22.8	0.0	1.1
1 tablespoon Greek yogurt (fat free)	8	1.3	0.6	0.0
½ tablespoon light mayonnaise	25	0.0	0.5	2.5
1 whole-grain, low-carb wrap	110	0.0	17.0	3.0
½ cup spinach leaves (uncooked)	4	0.0	0.5	0.0
2 slices of tomato	6	0.0	1.3	0.1
½ tablespoon dried cranberries	16	0.0	4.0	0.0
Totals:	**278**	**24.1(35%)**	**23.9 (34%)**	**6.7 (22%)**

Quick Meal!

Tuna Wrap (can add lettuce, tomato, and onion)

A tuna wrap is a fast and easy meal to pack for work. To boost the flavor, add celery, onion, lettuce, tomato, and even fresh herbs like parsley. Season to taste with salt and pepper.

FOODS	CALORIES	PROTEIN(G)	CARB(G)	FAT(G)
3 ounces albacore tuna (in water)	90	21.0	0.0	1.5
¾ tablespoon light mayonnaise	38	0.0	0.8	3.8
1 whole-grain, low-carb wrap	110	0.0	17.0	3.0
Totals:	**238**	**21.0 (35%)**	**17.8 (30%)**	**8.3 (31%)**

Dinner

High Quality

Greek Brown Rice Salad with Chicken

Recipe

This recipe can easily be prepared in bulk for quick meals all week long. You can also substitute the chicken for lean chopped pork tenderloin or grilled shrimp. *For the full recipe, see page 240.*

FOODS	CALORIES	PROTEIN(G)	CARB(G)	FAT(G)
4 ounces chicken breast (boneless/skinless)	124	26.0	0.0	1.2
1½ tablespoons low-fat balsamic vinaigrette salad dressing	33	0.0	1.5	3.0
½ ounce black olives (pitted)	19	0.0	0.4	1.9
⅓ cup brown rice (cooked)	66	0.0	14.5	0.0
½ cup arugula (raw)	4	0.0	0.5	0.1
2 tablespoons chopped tomato	6	0.0	1.3	0.1
¼ cup cucumber	4	0.0	0.8	0.1
Totals:	**256**	**26.0 (41%)**	**19.0 (30%)**	**6.4 (23%)**

Orange Honey Mustard Pork Tenderloin with Asparagus

Recipe

A juicy glaze adds plenty of flavor to plain old pork. Use leftovers in stir-frys, salads, or wraps the rest of the week. You can also substitute the asparagus for another vegetable if you'd prefer. *For the full recipe, see page 242.*

FOODS	CALORIES	PROTEIN(G)	CARB(G)	FAT(G)
4 ounces pork tenderloin	136	24.0	0.0	4.0
1 teaspoon olive oil	40	0.0	0.0	4.6
5 ounces asparagus	30	0.0	5.0	0.6
1 tablespoon Orange Honey Mustard Glaze (see recipe)	40	0.0	10.0	0.0
Totals:	**246**	**24.0 (39%)**	**15.0 (24%)**	**9.2 (34%)**

Shrimp, Rice, and Vegetable Stir-Fry

A rice and vegetable stir-fry goes well with any lean protein like shrimp, chicken, lean ground turkey, or pork tenderloin. Olive oil can be swapped out for peanut oil or sesame oil. To further enhance the flavor, you can add soy sauce, garlic, herbs, and spices. For a full list of "free foods" see "Condiments, Seasonings, and Spices" in your Food Exchange List.

FOODS	CALORIES	PROTEIN(G)	CARB(G)	FAT(G)
4 ounces shrimp	112	24.0	0.0	1.0
½ tablespoon olive oil	60	0.0	0.0	7.0
¼ cup brown rice (cooked)	50	0.0	11.0	0.0
4 ounces broccoli	32	0.0	6.0	0.6
Totals:	**254**	**24.0 (38%)**	**17.0 (27%)**	**8.6 (30%)**

Medium Quality

Quick Meal!

BBQ Chicken and Salad

(Quick Meal if chicken is prepared in advance)

BBQ Chicken (or shrimp or pork tenderloin) can be grilled or baked in the oven. You can substitute any low-fat dressing with roughly the same amount of fat for the balsamic vinaigrette. A side salad or your favorite vegetable completes the meal.

FOODS	CALORIES	PROTEIN(G)	CARB(G)	FAT(G)
4 ounces chicken breast (boneless/skinless)	124	26.0	0.0	1.2
2 tablespoons low-fat balsamic vinaigrette salad dressing	44	0.0	2.0	4.0
1½ cups garden salad (lettuce and vegetables)	53	0.0	13.5	0.0
1 tablespoon BBQ sauce	30	0.0	7.0	0.0
Totals:	**251**	**26.0 (41%)**	**22.5 (36%)**	**5.2 (19%)**

Lean Turkey Burger (can add lettuce, tomato, and onion)

To boost the flavor, lean ground turkey can be seasoned with garlic, herbs, and spices (see "Condiments, Seasonings, and Spices" in your Food Exchange List). On occasion, you can also substitute 99% fat-free ground beef for the turkey (because even lean ground beef has fat, omit the avocado to keep the fat content down).

FOODS	CALORIES	PROTEIN(G)	CARB(G)	FAT(G)
3 ounces ground turkey (99% fat free)	90	21.3	0.0	0.6
¾ ounce avocado	38	0.0	1.5	3.8
1 wheat bun	130	0.0	20.0	3.0
Totals:	**258**	**21.3 (33%)**	**21.5 (33%)**	**7.4 (26%)**

Turkey Meat Sauce with Pasta and Veggies

Try making this meal in bulk for the week. For added flavor, sauté onion and garlic with ground turkey. Add tomato sauce and fresh basil and season with salt and pepper.

FOODS	CALORIES	PROTEIN(G)	CARB(G)	FAT(G)
3½ ounces ground turkey (93% fat free)	155	23.8	0.0	7.4
2 ounces pasta (cooked)	74	0.0	16.0	1.0
¼ cup tomato sauce	15	0.0	3.0	0.0
2 ounces broccoli	16	0.0	3.0	0.3
Totals:	**260**	**23.8 (37%)**	**22.0 (34%)**	**8.7 (30%)**

Salmon with Red Potatoes, Vegetable, and Dessert

A filet mignon or orange roughy can easily be substituted for the salmon. Try chopping the potatoes, spraying them with fat-free cooking spray, and seasoning them with garlic, herbs, and spices before roasting. Or, if you'd like, substitute brown rice, sweet potatoes, or extra veggies in place of them. You can also add fresh-squeezed lemon juice to enhance the taste of the salmon.

FOODS	CALORIES	PROTEIN(G)	CARB(G)	FAT(G)
4 ounces salmon	160	22.4	0.0	8.0
2 ounces red potatoes	50	0.0	10.0	0.0
2 ounces snow peas	24	0.0	4.0	0.0
1 cup Jello (sugar free)	20	0.0	4.0	0.0
Totals:	**254**	**22.4 (35%)**	**18.0 (28%)**	**8.0 (28%)**

MEAL REPLACEMENTS AND QUICK "MID" MEALS

Medium Quality

Quick Meal!

Edamame
¾ **Meal**

Edamame is the perfect snack food. Not only is edamame the ideal balance of complete protein (from soy), carbohydrates, and fat, it's also loaded with vitamins and antioxidants. Buy it fresh or frozen in your local supermarket and boil until tender. Salt lightly and enjoy.

FOODS	CALORIES	PROTEIN(G)	CARB(G)	FAT(G)
1 cup edamame	200	16.0	18.0	6.0
Totals:	**200**	**16.0 (32%)**	**18.0 (36%)**	**6.0 (27%)**

Quick Meal!

Turkey, String Cheese, and Fruit

1/2 Meal

Sliced turkey, string cheese, and fruit is a fast and portable snack perfect for any time of day. Substitute the apple with any of your favorite fruits.

FOODS	CALORIES	PROTEIN(G)	CARB(G)	FAT(G)
1 ounce turkey breast, Boar's Head, low sodium	25	6.0	0.0	0.1
1 ounce mozzarella string cheese	80	8.0	1.0	5.0
2 ounces apple	34	0.0	8.6	0.2
Totals:	**139**	**14.0 (40%)**	**9.6 (27%)**	**5.3 (34%)**

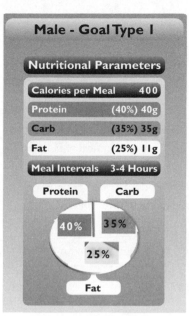

Male - Goal Type 1

Nutritional Parameters

Calories per Meal	400
Protein	(40%) 40g
Carb	(35%) 35g
Fat	(25%) 11g
Meal Intervals	3-4 Hours

Protein 40%
Carb 35%
Fat 25%

Jump Start Sample Day

Remember to drink at least 12 ounces of water with every meal, and 12 ounces of water between each meal.

6:30 am

Quick Meal!

Scrambled Eggs and Side of Oatmeal (with optional flavorings)

¾ Meal (High Quality)

(Quick Meal if eggs are hardboiled)

You can increase your metabolism and jump-start the fat-burning process by eating a balanced breakfast, like eggs and oatmeal, one hour within waking. Add flavor to unsweetened oatmeal with "free foods" like Stevia, cinnamon, and vanilla extract. If you're pressed for time, the Protein Power Oatmeal breakfast is a faster option.

FOODS	CALORIES	PROTEIN(G)	CARB(G)	FAT(G)
6 egg whites	102	21.0	0.0	0.0
1 egg (whole)	80	6.4	0.5	5.6
1 ounce oatmeal (unsweetened)	100	0.0	19.3	2.0
1½ ounces blueberries	28	0.0	6.9	0.2
Totals:	**310**	**27.4 (35%)**	**26.7 (34%)**	**7.8 (23%)**

9:30 am

Protein Bar

¾ Meal (Low Quality)

A midmorning meal can initially be challenging to fit into your schedule. A balanced protein bar is the perfect solution. The brand of protein bar is your choice. What matters most is to find a bar that comes close to matching your caloric and nutrient ratio parameters. Cottage cheese and Greek yogurt meals are also quick midmorning options after you complete the Jump Start Phase.

Important note: if you are still hungry after this meal, next time make it a full meal.

FOODS	CALORIES	PROTEIN(G)	CARB(G)	FAT(G)
1 serving Pure protein bar, any flavor	310	31.0	25.0	10.0
Totals:	**310**	**31.0 (40%)**	**25.0 (32%)**	**10.0 (29%)**

12:30 pm

Grilled Chicken Salad

(High Quality)

(Quick Meal if chicken is prepared in advance)

A grilled chicken salad can be made and brought from home or ordered at any restaurant. If you're dining out for lunch, request that your salad dressing be served on the side. You can also use a couple of tablespoons of low-fat balsamic vinaigrette in place of the oil and vinegar. The chicken can be exchanged for any other high-quality, lean protein like grilled shrimp.

FOODS	CALORIES	PROTEIN(G)	CARB(G)	FAT(G)
6 ounces chicken breast (boneless/skinless)	187	39.0	0.0	1.8
1½ tablespoons salad dressing, oil/vinegar	105	0.0	1.5	12.0
3 cups garden salad (lettuce and vegetables)	105	0.0	27.0	0.0
Totals:	**397**	**39.0 (39%)**	**28.5 (29%)**	**13.8 (31%)**

3:30 pm

Quick Meal!

Quick Turkey Roll-Up with Fruit and Nuts

¾ Meal (Medium Quality)

This is a quick midafternoon meal. Dip turkey slices into mustard or any other "free food" for extra flavor. Finding the time to eat midafternoon can be challenging at first. If you need a faster, "ready to eat" meal at this time, then your Ready-to-Drink shake meal is a fantastic choice. Whether it is a shake, bar, or higher-quality meal, getting a balanced meal in during your Jump Start Phase is what matters most.

Important note: if you are still hungry after this meal, next time make it a full meal.

FOODS	CALORIES	PROTEIN(G)	CARB(G)	FAT(G)
4½ ounces turkey breast, Boar's Head, low sodium	125	27.0	0.0	0.6
½ ounce cashews (raw)	80	0.0	4.6	6.6
5 ounces pear	85	0.0	21.5	0.6
Totals:	**290**	**27.0 (37%)**	**26.1 (36%)**	**7.8 (24%)**

6:30 pm

Salmon with Sweet Potato and Asparagus

(High Quality)

This meal is both tasty and extremely high quality due to the salmon, which is naturally high in omega-3 fatty acids (the heart-healthy, good fat). Enhance the flavor of salmon with fresh-squeezed lemon juice, herbs, and spices. You may want to occasionally substitute a filet mignon for salmon if you are in the mood for beef.

FOODS	CALORIES	PROTEIN(G)	CARB(G)	FAT(G)
6 ounces salmon	240	33.6	0.0	12.0
4 ounces sweet potato	120	0.0	28.0	0.0
3 ounces asparagus	18	0.0	3.0	0.4
Totals:	**378**	**33.6 (36%)**	**31.0 (33%)**	**12.4 (30%)**

9:30 pm

Quick Meal!

Protein Smoothie Without Milk (add water and ice)   ½ Meal (Medium Quality)

A protein shake makes for a delicious and balanced dessert before bed. It will also help to keep your metabolism humming all night long. If you chose to have a meal in place of a protein shake at this time, limit the amount of starchy carbs/grains and make it a half meal like this protein shake for enhanced fat burning and improved nighttime digestion.

FOODS	CALORIES	PROTEIN(G)	CARB(G)	FAT(G)
1 scoop whey protein powder, any flavor	102	20.0	1.0	1.5
½ tablespoon natural peanut butter	50	0.0	1.6	4.0
2 ounces banana	52	0.0	13.6	0.0
Totals:	**204**	**20.0 (39%)**	**16.2 (32%)**	**5.5 (24%)**
Day Totals:	**1889**	**178 (38%)**	**153.5 (33%)**	**57.3 (27%)**

JUMP START MEALS

Breakfast

High Quality

Quick Meal!

Scrambled Eggs, Side of Oatmeal and Fruit (with optional flavorings)

¾ Meal

(Quick Meal if eggs are hardboiled)

An eggs and oatmeal breakfast combo is simple to make (use instant oatmeal for easy prep) and incredibly satisfying. Give plain cooked oatmeal a boost of flavor without extra calories by stirring in "free foods" like Stevia (or any calorie-free sugar substitute), cinnamon, and vanilla extract.

FOODS	CALORIES	PROTEIN(G)	CARB(G)	FAT(G)
6 egg whites	102	21.0	0.0	0.0
1 egg (whole)	80	6.4	0.5	5.6
1 ounce oatmeal (unsweetened)	100	0.0	19.3	2.0
1½ ounces blueberries	28	0.0	6.9	0.2
Totals:	**310**	**27.4 (35%)**	**26.7 (34%)**	**7.8 (23%)**

Veggie and Egg Scramble with Side of Fruit

¾ Meal

An egg scramble is the perfect way to sneak in extra veggies you have on hand. Add a spoonful of your favorite salsa for extra spice.

FOODS	CALORIES	PROTEIN(G)	CARB(G)	FAT(G)
5 egg whites	85	17.5	0.0	0.0
2 eggs (whole)	160	12.8	1.0	11.2
½ cup spinach (cooked)	25	0.0	5.0	0.0
2 ounces broccoli	16	0.0	3.0	0.3
½ cup mushrooms	14	0.0	2.6	0.3
⅓ cup tomato	12	0.0	2.6	0.2
3 ounces strawberries	27	0.0	6.0	0.3
Totals:	**339**	**30.3 (36%)**	**20.2 (24%)**	**12.3 (33%)**

Medium Quality

Quick Meal!

Berry Banana Protein Smoothie Without Milk (add water and ice)

A protein and fruit smoothie is a sweet and refreshing way to stabilize your blood sugar fast. Try blending your favorite vanilla or chocolate protein powder with a variety of fresh or frozen fruit. Adjust the amount of water and ice to your desired consistency.

FOODS	CALORIES	PROTEIN(G)	CARB(G)	FAT(G)
2 scoops whey protein powder, any flavor	204	40.0	2.0	3.0
1 tablespoon natural peanut butter	100	0.0	3.2	8.0
5 ounces strawberries	45	0.0	10.0	0.6
2 ounces banana	52	0.0	13.6	0.0
Totals:	**401**	**40.0 (40%)**	**28.8 (29%)**	**11.6 (26%)**

Quick Meal!

Protein Power Oatmeal

Recipe

Protein Power Oatmeal is warm, creamy, and guaranteed to fuel your busy mornings. You can substitute the whey protein powder for soy or egg white powder. For a change of pace, swap nuts, peanut butter, or ground flax seeds for the almond butter. *For the full recipe, see page 234.*

FOODS	CALORIES	PROTEIN(G)	CARB(G)	FAT(G)
2 scoops whey protein powder, any flavor	204	40.0	2.0	3.0
¾ tablespoon almond butter	64	0.0	3.0	5.3
1½ ounces oatmeal (unsweetened)	150	0.0	29.0	3.0
Totals:	**418**	**40.0 (38%)**	**34.0 (33%)**	**11.3 (24%)**

Lunch

High Quality

Quick Meal!

Grilled Chicken Salad

(Quick Meal if chicken is prepared in advance)

Whether it's lunch at home or at a restaurant, Grilled Chicken Salad is a balanced and high-quality option. You can exchange the chicken for any other lean protein like grilled white fish or shrimp and top the salad with your favorite vegetables.

FOODS	CALORIES	PROTEIN(G)	CARB(G)	FAT(G)
6 ounces chicken breast (boneless/skinless)	187	39.0	0.0	1.8
1½ tablespoons oil and vinegar salad dressing	105	0.0	1.5	12.0
3 cups garden salad (lettuce and vegetables)	105	0.0	27.0	0.0
Totals:	**397**	**39.0 (39%)**	**28.5 (29%)**	**13.8 (31%)**

Quick Meal!

Ground Turkey, Rice and Broccoli Stir-Fry

(Quick Meal if stir-fry is prepared in advance)

A stir-fry is perfect to make in bulk for grab 'n' go meals during the week. Season your stir-fry with garlic, fresh herbs, and spices to enhance the flavor without additional fat or calories. (See "Condiments, Seasonings, and Spices" in your Food Exchange List for a full list of "free foods.")

FOODS	CALORIES	PROTEIN(G)	CARB(G)	FAT(G)
5 ounces ground turkey (99% fat free)	150	35.5	0.0	1.0
¾ tablespoon olive oil	90	0.0	0.0	10.5
½ cup brown rice (cooked)	100	0.0	22.0	0.0
4 ounces broccoli	32	0.0	6.0	0.6
Totals:	**372**	**35.5 (38%)**	**28.0 (30%)**	**12.1 (29%)**

Quick Meal!

Italian Tuna Salad with Side of Fruit
Recipe

Italian Tuna Salad is made up of common pantry items (canned tuna, low-fat balsamic dressing) and any vegetable you choose. Try making this recipe in bulk and storing it in the fridge for easy meals all week long. If desired, substitute any other lean protein for the tuna. *For the full recipe, see page 237.*

FOODS	CALORIES	PROTEIN(G)	CARB(G)	FAT(G)
6 ounces albacore tuna (in water)	180	42.0	0.0	3.0
½ tablespoon olive oil	60	0.0	0.0	7.0
¼ ounce black olives (pitted)	9	0.0	0.2	1.0
½ cup bell peppers, green or red	13	0.0	3.2	0.3
⅓ cup cherry tomato	12	0.0	2.6	0.2
⅛ cup onion	6	0.0	1.3	0.0
8 ounces orange slices	104	0.0	26.4	0.7
Totals:	**384**	**42.0 (43%)**	**33.7 (35%)**	**12.2 (28%)**

Quick Meal!

Chicken, Fruit, and Nuts

(Quick Meal if chicken is prepared in advance)

It may seem like an odd combination, but this meal is one of our go-to staples when we're in a hurry. Try preparing grilled or baked chicken in bulk for the week so you always have a high-quality protein on hand. Then pair it with your favorite fresh fruit and unsalted nuts and you've got a quality meal that takes only minutes to make.

FOODS	CALORIES	PROTEIN(G)	CARB(G)	FAT(G)
5½ ounces chicken breast (boneless/skinless)	171	35.8	0.0	1.7
¾ ounce cashews (raw)	120	0.0	6.9	9.9
6 ounces apple	102	0.0	25.8	0.6
Totals:	**393**	**35.8 (36%)**	**32.7 (33%)**	**12.2 (28%)**

Dinner

High Quality

Restaurant-Worthy Steak with Sweet Potato and Steamed Cauliflower

Recipe

A filet mignon is one of the leanest, tastiest cuts of beef, and that is why we recommend it. Pair your filet with delicious sweet potatoes and any steamed vegetable for a satisfying meal. *For the full recipe, see page 239.*

FOODS	CALORIES	PROTEIN(G)	CARB(G)	FAT(G)
5 ounces filet mignon	250	40.0	0.0	12.5
4 ounces sweet potato	120	0.0	28.0	0.0
4 ounces cauliflower	28	0.0	5.7	0.0
Totals:	**398**	**40.0 (40%)**	**33.7 (34%)**	**12.5 (28%)**

Quick Meal!

Grilled Chicken with Spinach Bean Salad and Fruit

(Quick Meal if chicken is prepared in advance)

Garbanzo beans (or any beans) add a boost of flavor and texture to a spinach salad. You can swap the spinach for your favorite leafy greens and the chicken breast for any lean protein. Top off the meal with your favorite fruit as dessert.

FOODS	CALORIES	PROTEIN(G)	CARB(G)	FAT(G)
5 ounces chicken breast (boneless/skinless)	156	32.5	0.0	1.5
1 tablespoon oil and vinegar salad dressing	70	0.0	1.0	8.0
2 cups spinach leaves (uncooked)	14	0.0	2.0	0.0
¾ ounce garbanzo beans	77	0.0	13.5	1.5
8 ounces watermelon	72	0.0	16.0	0.9
Totals:	**389**	**32.5 (33%)**	**32.5 (33%)**	**11.9 (28%)**

Seared Scallops with Brown Rice and Spinach   Recipe

Seared scallops take only minutes to make and are a great source of high-quality protein. You can swap out the scallops for any lean protein like chicken breast, pork tenderloin, or shrimp. The spinach can also be substituted with any other leafy greens. *For the full recipe, see page 241.*

FOODS	CALORIES	PROTEIN(G)	CARB(G)	FAT(G)
7½ ounces scallops	188	37.5	0.0	1.9
½ tablespoon olive oil	60	0.0	0.0	7.0
⅔ cup brown rice (cooked)	132	0.0	29.0	0.0
4 cups spinach leaves (uncooked)	28	0.0	4.0	0.0
Totals:	**408**	**37.5 (37%)**	**33.0 (32%)**	**8.9 (20%)**

Salmon with Brown Rice and Asparagus

Salmon is loaded in heart-healthy, omega-3 essential fats and should be eaten once or twice a week if possible. Enhance the flavor of salmon with fresh-squeezed lemon juice, herbs, and spices. Serve leftover salmon over a crisp salad for a satisfying lunch the next day.

FOODS	CALORIES	PROTEIN(G)	CARB(G)	FAT(G)
6 ounces salmon	240	33.6	0.0	12.0
½ cup brown rice (cooked)	100	0.0	22.0	0.0
5 ounces asparagus	30	0.0	5.0	0.6
Totals:	**370**	**33.6 (36%)**	**27.0 (29%)**	**12.6 (31%)**

MEAL REPLACEMENTS AND QUICK "MID" MEALS

Medium Quality

Quick Meal!

Quick Turkey Roll-Up with Fruit and Nuts

¾ Meal

Having lean, low-sodium deli meat on hand is a great way to ensure you've got a fast source of protein available. Ask your local deli for the highest-quality, least-processed brand they have (like Boar's Head). Pair it with fresh fruit and unsalted nuts of your choice for a quick and balanced meal. Dip turkey slices into mustard or any other "free food" for extra flavor.

FOODS	CALORIES	PROTEIN(G)	CARB(G)	FAT(G)
4 ounces turkey breast, Boar's Head, low sodium	100	24.0	0.0	0.5
½ ounce cashews (raw)	80	0.0	4.6	6.6
5 ounces pear	85	0.0	21.5	0.6
Totals:	**265**	**24.0 (36%)**	**26.1 (39%)**	**7.7 (26%)**

Low Quality

Protein Bar
¾ Meal

Protein bars are a convenient option for those times when you are too busy for an actual meal (like when you're on the go or in a meeting at work). The goal is to choose a bar that matches your nutritional parameters. For a complete list of recommended protein bars, see "Meal Replacements" in your Food Exchange List.

FOODS	CALORIES	PROTEIN(G)	CARB(G)	FAT(G)
1 serving Pure protein bar, any flavor	310	32.0	24.0	10.0
Totals:	**310**	**32.0 (41%)**	**24.0 (31%)**	**10.0 (29%)**

Ready-to-Drink Shake
¾ Meal

An all-in-one protein shake is another fast and convenient option for those times when you're on the go. Choose any ready-to-drink shake that is close to your nutritional parameters.

FOODS	CALORIES	PROTEIN(G)	CARB(G)	FAT(G)
1 serving Myoplex (EAS) Ready-to-Drink Shake (17 ounces), any flavor	310	43.0	20.0	7.0
Totals:	**310**	**43.0 (55%)**	**20.0 (26%)**	**7.0 (20%)**

ADDITIONAL MEALS—AFTER JUMP START PHASE

Breakfast

Medium Quality

Quick Meal!

Cereal with Protein Powder

By adding protein powder and nuts to cereal, you end up with a hearty breakfast that stabilizes your blood sugar and keeps you full all morning long. Simply shake half of the protein powder and milk together in a shake cup with a lid until blended and pour over any low-sugar, high-fiber cereal. Top with nuts and enjoy. Mix the remaining protein powder with water on the side for a quick shake.

FOODS	CALORIES	PROTEIN(G)	CARB(G)	FAT(G)
1½ scoops whey protein powder, any flavor	153	30	1.5	2.3
6 ounces milk (low fat)	90	6.0	9.0	3.8
¼ ounce almonds (raw)	43	0.0	1.5	4.0
1¼ ounces bran flakes cereal	113	0.0	27.5	0.0
Totals:	**399**	**36.0 (36%)**	**39.5 (40%)**	**10.1 (23%)**

Quick Meal!

Cottage Cheese with Fruit and Nuts

Cottage cheese mixed with fruit is a sweet and creamy combo that takes less than a minute to make. Fresh pineapple, raspberries, and peaches taste delicious too. Try prepping fruit in bulk for a few days so it's always ready to eat.

FOODS	CALORIES	PROTEIN(G)	CARB(G)	FAT(G)
10 ounces cottage cheese (low fat)	250	35.0	10.0	6.0
¼ ounce almonds (raw)	43	0.0	1.5	4.0
4 ounces strawberries	36	0.0	8.0	0.4
3 ounces blueberries	56	0.0	13.9	0.4
Totals:	**385**	**35.0 (36%)**	**33.4 (35%)**	**10.8 (25%)**

Protein Smoothie with Milk (can also add water and ice)

Milk adds a dose of calcium and a creamier texture to this protein smoothie. If you'd prefer, substitute the milk with low-fat Lactaid or soy milk. Almond butter or even flax seed oil can be substituted for the peanut butter.

FOODS	CALORIES	PROTEIN(G)	CARB(G)	FAT(G)
1½ scoops whey protein powder, any flavor	153	30.0	1.5	2.3
4 ounces milk (low fat)	60	4.0	6.0	2.5
1 tablespoon natural peanut butter	100	0.0	3.2	8.0
3 ounces banana	78	0.0	20.4	0.0
Totals:	**391**	**34.0 (35%)**	**31.1 (32%)**	**12.8 (29%)**

Bacon, Egg, and Cheese Sandwich

Recipe

A bacon, egg, and cheese sandwich makes a tasty and fast breakfast, lunch, or dinner. Egg whites can easily be substituted for Egg Beaters. *For the full recipe, see page 235.*

FOODS	CALORIES	PROTEIN(G)	CARB(G)	FAT(G)
1 cup Egg Beaters	100	20.0	4.0	0.0
¾ ounce cheddar cheese	83	5.3	0.8	6.8
2 ounces Canadian bacon	88	12.0	1.0	4.0
1 whole-wheat English muffin	130	0.0	25.6	1.6
1 ounce tomato (about 2 thin slices)	6	0.0	1.3	0.1
Totals:	**407**	**37.3 (37%)**	**32.7 (32%)**	**12.5 (28%)**

Greek Yogurt Parfait

¾ Meal; Recipe

Unlike traditional yogurt, Greek yogurt is high in protein and low in sugar. It's best sweetened and served with your favorite fruit and nuts. This recipe can be made in bulk for the week and is perfect for breakfast, dessert or a snack. *For the full recipe, see page 233.*

FOODS	CALORIES	PROTEIN(G)	CARB(G)	FAT(G)
12 ounces Greek yogurt (low fat)	222	29.1	13.8	6.9
¼ ounce almonds (raw)	43	0.0	1.5	4.0
3 ounces blueberries	56	0.0	13.9	0.4
Totals:	321	29.1 (36%)	29.2 (36%)	11.3 (32%)

Western-Style Omelet with Side of Fruit

Recipe

This omelet is a perfect way to use any leftover veggies you have on hand. You can even double the recipe and gently reheat the other half of the omelet in the microwave for dinner that night or breakfast the next morning. Serve with your favorite fresh fruit. *For the full recipe, see page 233.*

FOODS	CALORIES	PROTEIN(G)	CARB(G)	FAT(G)
1¼ cups Egg Beaters	125	25.0	5.0	0.0
1½ ounces ham, Boar's Head, low sodium	45	7.5	1.5	0.8
1 ounce cheddar cheese	110	7.0	1.0	9.0
2 tablespoons chopped tomato	6	0.0	1.3	0.1
2 tablespoons chopped onion	6	0.0	1.3	0.0
¼ cup bell peppers, green or red	7	0.0	1.6	0.1
8 ounces cantaloupe	80	0.0	19.2	1.0
Totals:	379	39.5 (42%)	30.9 (33%)	11 (26%)

Lunch

Medium Quality

Quick Meal!

Double Boca Burger with Fruit (can add lettuce, tomato, and onion)

A Boca burger is a great source of soy protein and takes only moments to prepare. You can top your burger with a small amount of ketchup or mustard. Serve with fresh fruit of your choice for a complete meal.

FOODS	CALORIES	PROTEIN(G)	CARB(G)	FAT(G)
1½ Boca Burgers, original	150	28.5	12.0	1.5
1½ ounces cheddar cheese	165	10.5	1.5	13.5
5 ounces pear	85	0.0	21.5	0.6
Totals:	**400**	**39.0 (39%)**	**35.0 (35%)**	**15.6 (35%)**

Quick Meal!

Chicken and Cheese Burrito

(Quick Meal if chicken is prepared in advance)

This meal is made of several staples we recommend you always have on hand: chicken breast, whole grain/low carb wraps, and fresh or frozen veggies (choose your favorite veggies). You can substitute the chicken for deli turkey or even grilled shrimp for a change of pace. This meal is also delicious as a grilled quesadilla. Add salsa for a boost of flavor.

FOODS	CALORIES	PROTEIN(G)	CARB(G)	FAT(G)
5 ounces chicken breast (boneless/skinless)	156	32.5	0.0	1.5
1 ounce cheddar cheese	110	7.0	1.0	9.0
1 serving whole-grain, low-carb wrap	83	0.0	12.8	2.3
⅓ cup mixed vegetables	60	0.0	10.5	0.0
Totals:	**409**	**39.5 (39%)**	**24.3 (24%)**	**12.8 (28%)**

Quick Meal!

Chicken Fajita (can add tomato, lettuce, and onion)

(Quick Meal if chicken is prepared in advance)

Chicken (or shrimp) fajitas can be made at home or enjoyed at any Mexican restaurant. If dining out, request that your meal is prepared in very little oil, and use guacamole as your fat (or choose a small amount of sour cream or cheese). Skip the rice and beans and load up on bell peppers and onions. Add salsa or pico de gallo for a boost of flavor.

FOODS	CALORIES	PROTEIN(G)	CARB(G)	FAT(G)
6 ounces chicken breast (boneless/skinless)	187	39.0	0.0	1.8
1½ tablespoons guacamole	60	0.0	0.6	6.0
3 ounces corn tortillas	125	0.0	23.0	2.5
¼ cup bell peppers, green or red	7	0.0	1.6	0.1
Totals:	**379**	**39.0 (41%)**	**25.2 (27%)**	**10.4 (25%)**

Quick Meal!

Smoked Salmon and Cream Cheese Toasts with Side of Fruit   Recipe

Smoked salmon toasts are a fun way to load up on your omega-3 essential fat. Ak-Mak crackers, a whole-grain flat-bread snack, can be found at any grocery store. This meal is also delicious served for breakfast. Serve leftover smoked salmon on the side and pair this dish with your favorite fresh fruit. *For the full recipe, see page 238.*

FOODS	CALORIES	PROTEIN(G)	CARB(G)	FAT(G)
7 ounces smoked salmon	231	36.4	0.0	8.4
1 tablespoon light cream cheese	35	1.0	1.0	2.5
3 Ak-Mak crackers	69	0.0	12.0	1.2
½ small tomato, sliced	12	0.0	2.6	0.2
¼ cucumber, sliced	8	0.0	1.5	0.2
1 thin slice of red onion	6	0.0	1.3	0.0
3 ounces apple	51	0.0	12.9	0.3
Totals:	**412**	**37.4 (36%)**	**31.3 (30%)**	**12.8 (28%)**

Spicy Turkey Club Sandwich with Side of Fruit

Recipe

A turkey club can be healthy when it's made with low-fat mayonnaise, turkey bacon, and whole-wheat bread. You can swap out the turkey for chicken breast if you'd prefer. *For the full recipe, see page 237.*

FOODS	CALORIES	PROTEIN(G)	CARB(G)	FAT(G)
6 ounces turkey breast, Boar's Head, low sodium	150	36.0	0.0	0.8
1 slice turkey bacon	33	2.5	0.0	2.5
1 tablespoon light mayonnaise	50	0.0	1.0	5.0
2 slices whole-wheat bread	140	0.0	24.0	2.0
romaine lettuce leaves	1	0.0	0.2	0.0
2 slices of tomato	6	0.0	1.3	0.1
4 slices of cucumber	4	0.0	0.8	0.1
3 ounces strawberries	27	0.0	6.0	0.3
Totals:	**411**	**38.5 (38%)**	**33.3 (32%)**	**10.8 (24%)**

Sushi Meal (can add wasabi and ginger)

When ordering sushi, aim for sashimi (slices of fish that can be served on top of or alongside rice). Some sushi restaurants even offer brown rice in place of white rice, which is a better choice for stable blood sugar due to the increased fiber. Add soy sauce for a boost of flavor.

FOODS	CALORIES	PROTEIN(G)	CARB(G)	FAT(G)
2 ounces sashimi, tuna (albacore)	98	14.4	0.0	4.2
2 ounces sashimi, yellowtail	82	13.6	0.0	3.2
1 ounce sashimi, salmon	40	5.6	0.0	2.0
4 pieces vegetable roll	124	0.0	22.4	2.4
¼ cup brown rice (cooked)	50	0.0	11.0	0.0
Totals:	**394**	**33.6 (34%)**	**33.4 (34%)**	**11.8 (27%)**

Quick Meal!

Cranberry Pecan Chicken Salad Wrap

Recipe

(Quick Meal if chicken is prepared in advance)

This creamy chicken salad can be served in a wrap, on top of a salad, or with a side of fruit. Try making the chicken salad mixture in bulk for grab 'n' go meals for the week. *For the full recipe, see page 236.*

FOODS	CALORIES	PROTEIN(G)	CARB(G)	FA(G)T
5 ounces chicken breast (boneless/skinless)	171	35.8	0.0	1.7
1 tablespoon Greek yogurt (fat free)	8	1.3	0.6	0.0
¼ ounce pecans (raw)	47	0.0	1.6	4.6
¾ tablespoon light mayonnaise	38	0.0	0.8	3.8
1 whole-grain, low-carb wrap	110	0.0	17.0	3.0
½ cup spinach leaves (uncooked)	4	0.0	0.5	0.0
2 slices of tomato	6	0.0	1.3	0.1
1 tablespoon dried cranberries	31	0.0	8.0	0.0
Totals:	**415**	**37.1 (36%)**	**29.8 (29%)**	**13.2 (29%)**

Quick Meal!

Tuna Wrap and Fruit (can add lettuce, tomato, and onion)

A tuna wrap is a great meal to pack for work. To boost the flavor, you can add relish, celery, lettuce, tomato, onion, lemon, and fresh herbs, and season with salt and pepper. Serve with your choice of fruit.

FOODS	CALORIES	PROTEIN(G)	CARB(G)	FAT(G)
5 ounces albacore tuna (in water)	150	35.0	0.0	2.5
1 tablespoon light mayonnaise	50	0.0	1	5
1 whole-grain, low-carb wrap	110	0.0	17	3
6 ounces orange slices	78	0.0	19.8	0.5
Totals:	**388**	**35.0 (36%)**	**37.8 (39%)**	**11 (26%)**

Dinner

High Quality

Greek Brown Rice Salad with Chicken

Recipe

This recipe can easily be prepared in bulk for quick meals all week long. You can also substitute the chicken for lean chopped pork tenderloin or grilled shrimp. *For the full recipe, see page 240.*

FOODS	CALORIES	PROTEIN(G)	CARB(G)	FAT(G)
5½ ounces chicken breast (boneless/skinless)	171	35.8	0.0	1.7
¾ ounces black olives (pitted)	28	0.0	0.5	2.9
2½ tablespoons light balsamic vinaigrette salad dressing	55	0.0	2.5	5.0
⅔ cup brown rice (cooked)	132	0.0	29.0	0.0
½ cup arugula lettuce leaves	4	0.0	0.5	0.1
2 tablespoons chopped tomato	6	0.0	1.3	0.1
¼ cup cucumber	4	0.0	0.8	0.1
Totals:	**400**	**35.8 (36%)**	**34.6 (35%)**	**9.9 (22%)**

Orange Honey Mustard Pork Tenderloin with Asparagus

Recipe

A juicy glaze adds plenty of flavor to plain old pork. Use leftovers in stir-frys, salads, or wraps the rest of the week. You can also substitute the asparagus for another vegetable if you'd prefer. *For the full recipe, see page 242.*

FOODS	CALORIES	PROTEIN(G)	CARB(G)	FAT(G)
6½ ounces pork tenderloin	221	39.0	0.0	6.5
1 teaspoon olive oil	40	0.0	0.0	4.6
7 ounces asparagus	42	0.0	7.0	0.9
2 tablespoons Orange Honey Mustard Glaze (see recipe)	80	0.0	22.0	0.0
Totals:	**383**	**39.0 (41%)**	**29.0 (30%)**	**12.0 (28%)**

Shrimp, Rice, and Vegetable Stir-Fry

A rice and vegetable stir-fry goes well with any lean protein like shrimp, chicken, lean ground turkey, or pork tenderloin. Olive oil can be swapped out for peanut oil or sesame oil. To further enhance the flavor, you can add soy sauce, garlic, herbs, and spices. For a full list of "free foods," see "Condiments, Seasonings, and Spices" in your Food Exchange List.

FOODS	CALORIES	PROTEIN(G)	CARB(G)	FAT(G)
6 ounces shrimp	168	36.0	0.0	1.5
¾ tablespoon olive oil	90	0.0	0.0	10.5
¼ cup brown rice (cooked)	50	0.0	11.0	0.0
1 cup mixed vegetables	80	0.0	14.0	0.0
Totals:	388	36.0 (37%)	25.0 (26%)	12.0 (28%)

Medium Quality

BBQ Chicken, Pasta, and Side Salad

BBQ chicken (or shrimp or pork tenderloin) can be grilled or baked in the oven. You can substitute any low-fat dressing with roughly the same amount of fat for the balsamic vinaigrette. A side salad or your favorite vegetable completes the meal.

FOODS	CALORIES	PROTEIN(G)	CARB(G)	FAT(G)
6 ounces chicken breast (boneless/skinless)	187	39.0	0.0	1.8
1 tablespoon oil and vinegar salad dressing	70	0.0	1.0	8.0
1 cup garden salad (lettuce and vegetables)	35	0.0	9.0	0.0
2 ounces pasta (cooked)	74	0.0	16.0	1.0
½ cup tomato sauce	30	0.0	6.0	0.0
1 tablespoon BBQ sauce	30	0.0	7.0	0.0
Totals:	426	39.0 (37%)	39.0 (37%)	10.8 (23%)

Lean Turkey Burger (can add lettuce, tomato and onion)

To boost the flavor, lean ground turkey can be seasoned with garlic, herbs, and spices (see "Condiments, Seasonings, and Spices" in your Food Exchange List). On occasion, you can also substitute 99% fat-free ground beef for the turkey (because even lean ground beef has fat, omit the avocado to keep the fat content down).

FOODS	CALORIES	PROTEIN(G)	CARB(G)	FAT(G)
6 ounces ground turkey (99% fat free)	180	42.6	0.0	1.2
2 ounces avocado	100	0.0	4.0	10.0
1 wheat bun	130	0.0	20.0	3.0
Totals:	**410**	**42.6 (42%)**	**24.0 (23%)**	**14.2 (31%)**

Turkey Meat Sauce with Pasta and Veggies

Try making this meal in bulk for the week. For added flavor, sauté onion and garlic with ground turkey. Add tomato sauce and fresh basil and season with salt and pepper.

FOODS	CALORIES	PROTEIN(G)	CARB(G)	FAT(G)
5 ounces ground turkey (93% fat free)	222	34	0.0	10.5
3 ounces pasta (cooked)	111	0.0	24.0	1.5
½ cup tomato sauce	30	0.0	6.0	0.0
3 ounces broccoli	24	0.0	4.5	.5
Totals:	**387**	**34 (35%)**	**34.5 (36%)**	**12.5 (29%)**

Salmon with Red Potatoes, Corn, and Dessert

A filet mignon or orange roughy can easily be substituted for the salmon. Try chopping the potatoes, spraying them with fat-free cooking spray, and seasoning them with garlic, herbs, and spices before roasting. Or, if you'd like, substitute brown rice, sweet potatoes, or extra veggies in place of them. You can also add fresh-squeezed lemon juice to enhance the taste of the salmon.

FOODS	CALORIES	PROTEIN(G)	CARB(G)	FAT(G)
7 ounces salmon	280	39.2	0.0	14.0
2 ounces red potatoes	50	0.0	10.0	0.0
¼ cup corn	40	0.0	10.0	0.0
1 serving Dreyers Fruit Bar	30	0.0	8.0	0.0
Totals:	**400**	**39.2 (39%)**	**28.0 (28%)**	**14.0 (31%)**

MEAL REPLACEMENTS AND QUICK "MID" MEALS

Medium Quality

Quick Meal!

Edamame

½ Meal

Edamame is the perfect snack food. Not only is edamame the ideal balance of complete protein (from soy), carbohydrates, and fat, it's also loaded with vitamins and antioxidants. Buy it fresh or frozen in your local supermarket and boil until tender. Salt lightly and enjoy.

FOODS	CALORIES	PROTEIN(G)	CARB(G)	FAT(G)
1 cup edamame	200	16.0	18.0	6.0
Totals:	**200**	**16.0 (32%)**	**18.0 (36%)**	**6.0 (27%)**

Turkey, String Cheese, and Fruit

½ Meal

Sliced turkey, string cheese, and fruit is a fast and portable snack perfect for any time of day. Substitute the apple with any of your favorite fruits.

FOODS	CALORIES	PROTEIN(G)	CARB(G)	FAT(G)
2 ounces turkey breast, Boar's Head, low sodium	50	12.0	0.0	0.3
1 ounce mozzarella string cheese	80	8.0	1.0	5.0
5 ounces apple	85	0.0	21.5	0.5
Totals:	**215**	**20.0 (37%)**	**22.5 (42%)**	**5.8 (24%)**

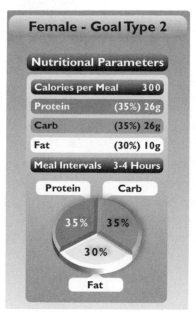

Nutritional Parameters

Calories per Meal	300
Protein	(35%) 26g
Carb	(35%) 26g
Fat	(30%) 10g
Meal Intervals	3-4 Hours

Protein 35%   Carb 35%   Fat 30%

FEMALE GOAL TYPE 2 (300-CALORIE MEAL PLANS)

Jump Start Sample Day

Remember to drink at least 8 ounces of water with every meal, and 8 ounces of water between each meal.

6:30 am

Quick Meal!

Scrambled Eggs and Side of Oatmeal (with optional flavorings)

¾ Meal (High Quality)

(Quick Meal if eggs are hardboiled)

You can increase your metabolism and maximize muscle growth by eating a balanced breakfast, like eggs and oatmeal, one hour within waking. Add flavor to unsweetened oatmeal with "free foods" like Stevia, cinnamon, and vanilla extract. If you're pressed for time, the Protein Power Oatmeal breakfast is a faster option.

FOODS	CALORIES	PROTEIN(G)	CARB(G)	FAT(G)
4 egg whites	68	14.0	0.0	0.0
1 egg (whole)	80	6.4	0.5	5.6
1 ounce oatmeal (unsweetened)	100	0.0	19.3	2.0
Totals:	**248**	**20.4 (33%)**	**19.8 (32%)**	**7.6 (28%)**

9:30 am

Protein Bar

¾ Meal (Low Quality)

A midmorning meal can initially be challenging to fit into your schedule. A balanced protein bar is the perfect solution. The brand of protein bar is your choice. What matters most is to find a bar that comes close to matching your caloric and nutrient ratio parameters. Cottage cheese and Greek yogurt meals are also quick midmorning options after you complete the Jump Start Phase.

Important Note: You are always better off eating high-quality food to maximize results, especially with weight gain as your goal. If you can replace this low-quality meal with a high-quality meal, you will quickly feel the difference in energy, meal satisfaction, and in the speed of your results.

FOODS	CALORIES	PROTEIN(G)	CARB(G)	FAT(G)
1 serving Think Thin, any flavor	230	20.0	24.0	8.0
Totals:	**230**	**20.0 (35%)**	**24.0 (41%)**	**8.0 (31%)**

12:30 pm

Grilled Chicken Salad

(High Quality)

(Quick Meal if chicken is prepared in advance)

A grilled chicken salad can be made and brought from home or ordered at any restaurant. If you're dining out for lunch, request that your salad dressing be served on the side. If you dislike light dressing, you can substitute it with 1 tablespoon of regular balsamic vinaigrette. You can also exchange chicken for any other high-quality, lean-protein like grilled shrimp.

FOODS	CALORIES	PROTEIN(G)	CARB(G)	FAT(G)
4 ounces chicken breast (boneless/skinless)	124	26.0	0.0	1.2
1 tablespoon low-fat balsamic vinaigrette salad dressing	70	0.0	1.0	8.0
3 cups garden salad (lettuce and vegetables)	105	0.0	27.0	0.0
Totals:	**299**	**26.0 (35%)**	**28.0 (37%)**	**9.2 (28%)**

3:30 pm

Quick Turkey Roll-Up with Mustard (optional), Fruit, and Nuts   (Medium Quality)

This is a quick midafternoon meal. Dip turkey slices into mustard or any other "free food" for extra flavor. Finding the time to eat midafternoon can be challenging at first. If you need a faster, "ready to eat" meal at this time, then your Ready-to-Drink shake meal is a fantastic choice. Whether it is a shake, bar, or higher-quality meal, getting a balanced meal in during your Jump Start Phase is what matters most.

Important Note: You are always better off eating high-quality food to maximize results, especially with weight gain as your goal. If you can replace this medium-quality meal with a high-quality meal, you will quickly feel the difference in energy, meal satisfaction, and in the speed of your results.

FOODS	CALORIES	PROTEIN(G)	CARB(G)	FAT(G)
4½ ounces turkey breast, Boar's Head, low sodium	113	27.0	0.0	0.6
½ ounce cashews (raw)	80	0.0	4.6	6.6
5 ounces apple	85	0.0	21.5	0.5
Totals:	**278**	**27.0 (39%)**	**26.1 (37%)**	**7.7 (25%)**

6:30 pm

Salmon with Brown Rice and Asparagus   (High Quality)

This meal is both tasty and extremely high quality due to the salmon, which is naturally high in omega-3 fatty acids (the heart-healthy, good fat). Enhance the flavor of salmon with fresh-squeezed lemon juice, herbs, and spices. You may want to occasionally substitute a filet mignon for salmon if you are in the mood for beef.

FOODS	CALORIES	PROTEIN(G)	CARB(G)	FAT(G)
4½ ounces salmon	180	25.2	0.0	9.0
½ cup brown rice (cooked)	100	0.0	22.0	0.0
3 ounces asparagus	18	0.0	3.0	0.4
Totals:	**298**	**25.2 (34%)**	**25.0 (34%)**	**9.4 (28%)**

9:30 pm

Protein Smoothie Without Milk (add water and ice)

¾ Meal (Medium Quality)

A protein shake makes for a delicious and balanced dessert before bed. It will also fuel your muscles through the night and assist you in increasing your lean body mass. If you choose to have a meal in place of a protein shake at this time, limit the amount of starchy carbs/grains to prevent possible bloating and optimize nighttime digestion.

FOODS	CALORIES	PROTEIN(G)	CARB(G)	FAT(G)
1 scoop whey protein powder, any flavor	102	20.0	1.0	1.5
¾ tablespoon natural peanut butter	75	0.0	2.4	6.0
7 ounces strawberries	63	0.0	14.0	0.8
Totals:	**240**	**20.0 (33%)**	**17.4 (29%)**	**8.3 (31%)**
Day Totals:	**1593**	**138.6 (35%)**	**140.3 (35%)**	**50.2 (29%)**

JUMP START MEALS

Breakfast

High Quality

Quick Meal!

Scrambled Eggs and Side of Oatmeal (with optional flavorings)

¾ Meal

(Quick Meal if eggs are hardboiled)

An eggs and oatmeal breakfast combo is simple to make (use instant oatmeal for easy prep) and incredibly satisfying. Give plain cooked oatmeal a boost of flavor without extra calories by stirring in "free foods" like Stevia (or any calorie-free sugar substitute), cinnamon, and vanilla extract.

FOODS	CALORIES	PROTEIN(G)	CARB(G)	FAT(G)
4 egg whites	68	14.0	0.0	0.0
1 egg (whole)	80	6.4	0.5	5.6
1 ounce oatmeal (unsweetened)	100	0.0	19.3	2.0
Totals:	**248**	**20.4 (33%)**	**19.8 (32%)**	**7.6 (28%)**

Veggie and Egg Scramble with Side of Fruit

¾ Meal

An egg scramble is the perfect way to sneak in extra veggies you have on hand. Add a spoonful of your favorite salsa for extra spice. Choose your favorite fruit as a side.

FOODS	CALORIES	PROTEIN(G)	CARB(G)	FAT(G)
4 egg whites	68	14.0	0.0	0.0
1 egg (whole)	80	6.4	0.5	5.6
½ cup spinach (cooked)	25	0.0	5.0	0.0
2 ounces broccoli	16	0.0	3.0	0.3
½ cup mushrooms	14	0.0	2.6	0.3
⅓ cup tomato	12	0.0	2.6	0.2
2 ounces blueberries	37	0.0	9.3	0.3
Totals:	**252**	**20.4 (32%)**	**23 (37%)**	**6.7 (24%)**

Medium Quality

Quick Meal!

Berry Banana Protein Smoothie Without Milk (add water and ice)

A protein and fruit smoothie is a sweet and refreshing way to stabilize your blood sugar fast. Try blending your favorite vanilla or chocolate protein powder with a variety of fresh or frozen fruit. Adjust the amount of water and ice to your desired consistency.

FOODS	CALORIES	PROTEIN(G)	CARB(G)	FAT(G)
1¼ scoops whey protein powder, any flavor	128	25.0	1.3	1.9
1 tablespoon natural peanut butter	100	0.0	3.2	8.0
2 ounces banana	52	0.0	13.6	0.0
3 ounces strawberries	27	0.0	6.0	0.3
Totals:	**307**	**25.0 (33%)**	**24.1 (31%)**	**10.2 (30%)**

Quick Meal!

Protein Power Oatmeal

Recipe

Protein Power Oatmeal is warm, creamy, and guaranteed to fuel your busy mornings. You can substitute the whey protein powder for soy or egg white powder. For a change of pace, swap nuts, peanut butter, or ground flax seeds for the almond butter. *For the full recipe, see page 234.*

FOODS	CALORIES	PROTEIN(G)	CARB(G)	FAT(G)
1¼ scoops whey protein powder, any flavor	128	25.0	1.3	1.9
1 tablespoon almond butter	85	0.0	4.0	7.0
1 ounce oatmeal (unsweetened)	100	0.0	19.3	2.0
Totals:	**313**	**25.0 (32%)**	**24.6 (31%)**	**10.9 (31%)**

Lunch

High Quality

Grilled Chicken Salad

(Quick Meal if chicken is prepared in advance)

Whether it's lunch at home or at a restaurant, Grilled Chicken Salad is a balanced and high-quality option. You can exchange the chicken for any other lean protein like grilled white fish or shrimp and top the salad with your favorite vegetables.

FOODS	CALORIES	PROTEIN(G)	CARB(G)	FAT(G)
4 ounces chicken breast (boneless/skinless)	124	26.0	0.0	1.2
1 tablespoon oil and vinegar salad dressing	70	0.0	1.0	8.0
3 cups garden salad (lettuce and vegetables)	105	0.0	27.0	0.0
Totals:	**299**	**26.0 (35%)**	**28.0 (37%)**	**9.2 (28%)**

Ground Turkey Vegetable Stir-Fry

(Quick Meal if stir-fry is prepared in advance)

A stir-fry is perfect to make in bulk for grab 'n' go meals during the week. Choose your favorite veggies and season your stir-fry with garlic, fresh herbs, and spices to enhance the flavor without additional fat or calories. (See "Condiments, Seasonings, and Spices" in your Food Exchange List for a full list of "free foods.")

FOODS	CALORIES	PROTEIN(G)	CARB(G)	FAT(G)
3½ ounces ground turkey (99% fat free)	105	24.9	0.0	0.7
2 teaspoons olive oil	79	0.0	0.0	9.2
1½ cups mixed vegetables	120	0.0	21.0	0.0
Totals:	**304**	**24.9 (33%)**	**21.0 (28%)**	**9.9 (29%)**

Quick Meal!

Italian Tuna Salad with Side of Fruit

Recipe

Italian Tuna Salad is made up of common pantry items (canned tuna, low-fat balsamic dressing) and any vegetable you choose. Try making this recipe in bulk and storing it in the fridge for easy meals throughout the week. If desired, substitute any other lean protein for the tuna. *For the full recipe, see page 237.*

FOODS	CALORIES	PROTEIN(G)	CARB(G)	FAT(G)
4 ounces albacore tuna (in water)	120	28.0	0.0	2.0
½ ounce black olives (pitted)	19	0.0	0.4	1.9
3 tablespoons low-fat balsamic vinaigrette salad dressing	66	0.0	3.0	6.0
½ cup bell peppers, green or red	13	0.0	3.2	0.3
⅓ cup cherry tomato	12	0.0	2.6	0.2
⅛ cup onion	6	0.0	1.3	0.0
5 ounces orange slices	65	0.0	16.5	0.5
Totals:	**301**	**28.0 (37%)**	**27.0 (36%)**	**10.9 (32%)**

Quick Meal!

Chicken, Fruit, and Nuts

(Quick Meal if chicken is prepared in advance)

It may seem like an odd combination, but this meal is one of our go-to staples when we're in a hurry. Try preparing grilled or baked chicken in bulk for the week so you always have a high-quality protein on hand. Then pair it with your favorite fresh fruit and unsalted nuts and you've got a quality meal that takes only minutes to make.

FOODS	CALORIES	PROTEIN(G)	CARB(G)	FAT(G)
4 ounces chicken breast (boneless/skinless)	124	26.0	0.0	1.2
⅔ ounce cashews (raw)	106	0.0	6.1	8.7
4 ounces apple	68	0.0	17.2	0.4
Totals:	**298**	**26.0 (35%)**	**23.3 (31%)**	**10.3 (31%)**

Dinner

High Quality

Quick Meal!

Grilled Chicken with Spinach Bean Salad

(Quick Meal if chicken is prepared in advance)

Garbanzo beans (or any beans) add a boost of flavor and texture to a spinach salad. You can swap the spinach for your favorite leafy greens and the chicken breast for any lean protein.

FOODS	CALORIES	PROTEIN(G)	CARB(G)	FAT(G)
4 ounces chicken breast (boneless/skinless)	124	26.0	0.0	1.2
3 tablespoons low-fat balsamic vinaigrette salad dressing	66	0.0	3.0	6.0
2 cups spinach leaves (uncooked)	14	0.0	2.0	0.0
1 ounce garbanzo beans	102	0.0	18.0	2.0
Totals:	**306**	**26.0 (34%)**	**23.0 (30%)**	**9.2 (27%)**

Restaurant-Worthy Steak with Sweet Potato and Steamed Cauliflower

Recipe

A filet mignon is one of the leanest, tastiest cuts of beef, and that is why we recommend it. Pair your filet with delicious sweet potatoes and any steamed vegetable for a satisfying meal. *For the full recipe, see page 239.*

FOODS	CALORIES	PROTEIN(G)	CARB(G)	FAT(G)
3½ ounces filet mignon	175	28.0	0.0	8.8
3 ounces sweet potato	90	0.0	21.0	0.0
5 ounces cauliflower	35	0.0	7.1	0.0
Totals:	**300**	**28.0 (37%)**	**28.1 (37%)**	**8.8 (26%)**

Seared Scallops with Brown Rice and Spinach — Recipe

Seared scallops take only minutes to make and are a great source of high-quality protein. You can swap out the scallops for any lean protein like chicken breast, pork tenderloin, or shrimp. The spinach can also be substituted with any leafy greens. *For the full recipe, see page 241.*

FOODS	CALORIES	PROTEIN(G)	CARB(G)	FAT(G)
5 ounces scallops	125	25.0	0.0	1.3
½ tablespoon olive oil	60	0.0	0.0	7.0
½ cup brown rice (cooked)	100	0.0	22.0	0.0
2 cups spinach leaves (uncooked)	14	0.0	2.0	0.0
Totals:	**299**	**25.0 (33%)**	**24.0 (32%)**	**8.3 (25%)**

Salmon with Brown Rice and Asparagus

Salmon is loaded in heart-healthy, omega-3 essential fats and should be eaten once or twice a week if possible. Add some fresh-squeezed lemon juice to enhance the taste of the salmon. Serve leftover salmon over a crisp salad for a satisfying lunch the next day.

FOODS	CALORIES	PROTEIN(G)	CARB(G)	FAT(G)
4½ ounces salmon	180	25.2	0.0	9.0
½ cup brown rice (cooked)	100	0.0	22.0	0.0
3 ounces asparagus	18	0.0	3.0	0.4
Totals:	**298**	**25.2 (34%)**	**25.0 (34%)**	**9.4 (28%)**

MEAL REPLACEMENTS AND QUICK "MID" MEALS

Medium Quality

Quick Meal!

Quick Turkey Roll-Up with Fruit and Nuts

Having lean, low-sodium deli meat on hand is a great way to ensure you've got a fast source of protein available. Ask your local deli for the highest-quality, least-processed brand they have (like Boar's Head). Pair it with fresh fruit and unsalted nuts of your choice for a quick and balanced meal. Dip turkey slices into mustard or any other "free food" for extra flavor.

FOODS	CALORIES	PROTEIN(G)	CARB(G)	FAT(G)
4½ ounces turkey breast, Boar's Head, low sodium	113	27.0	0.0	0.6
½ ounce cashews (raw)	80	0.0	4.6	6.6
5 ounces apple	85	0.0	21.5	0.5
Totals:	**278**	**27.0 (39%)**	**26.1 (38%)**	**7.7 (25%)**

Low Quality

Quick Meal!

Protein Bar

¾ **Meal**

Protein bars are a convenient option for those times when you are too busy for an actual meal (like when you are on the go or in a meeting at work). The goal is to choose a bar that matches your nutritional parameters. For a complete list of recommended protein bars, see "Meal Replacements" in your Food Exchange List.

FOODS	CALORIES	PROTEIN(G)	CARB(G)	FAT(G)
1 serving Think Thin, any flavor	230	20.0	24.0	8.0
Totals:	**230**	**20.0(35%)**	**24.0 (41%)**	**8.0 (31%)**

Quick Meal!

Ready-to-Drink Shake, Nuts, and Fruit

A ready-made protein drink paired with fresh fruit is an ideal option while at work or even while traveling. For a complete list of recommended protein drinks, see "Meal Replacements" in your Food Exchange List.

FOODS	CALORIES	PROTEIN(G)	CARB(G)	FAT(G)
1 bottle (14 ounce) of Muscle Milk, Light, any flavor	150	25.0	5.0	3.5
⅓ ounce almonds (raw)	56	0.0	2	5.3
4 ounces apple	68	0.0	17.2	0.4
Totals:	**274**	**25.0 (36%)**	**24.2 (35%)**	**9.2 (30%)**

ADDITIONAL MEALS—AFTER JUMP START PHASE

Breakfast

Medium Quality

Quick Meal!

Cereal to Go with Protein Powder

By adding protein powder and nuts to cereal, you end up with a hearty breakfast that stabilizes your blood sugar and keeps you full all morning long. Simply shake protein powder and milk together in a shake cup with a lid until blended and pour over any low-sugar, high-fiber cereal. Top with nuts and enjoy. If the milk mixture is too sweet, try using only half of the protein powder together with the milk. Mix the remaining protein powder with water on the side for a quick shake.

FOODS	CALORIES	PROTEIN(G)	CARB(G)	FAT(G)
1 scoop whey protein powder, any flavor	102	20.0	1.0	1.5
5 ounces milk (nonfat)	55	5.6	7.5	0.6
⅔ ounce bran flakes cereal	59	0.0	14.5	0.0
½ ounce almonds (raw)	85	0.0	3.0	8.0
Totals:	**301**	**25.6 (34%)**	**26.0 (35%)**	**10.1 (30%)**

Cottage Cheese with Fruit

Cottage cheese mixed with fruit is a sweet and creamy combo that takes less than a minute to make. Fresh pineapple, raspberries, and peaches taste delicious too. Try prepping fruit in bulk for a few days so it's always ready to eat.

FOODS	CALORIES	PROTEIN(G)	CARB(G)	FAT(G)
7 ounces cottage cheese (low fat)	175	24.5	7.0	4.2
⅓ ounce almonds (raw)	56	0.0	2.0	5.3
4 ounces strawberries	27	0.0	6.0	0.3
2 ounces blueberries	37	0.0	9.3	0.3
Totals:	**295**	**24.5 (33%)**	**24.3 (33%)**	**10.1 (31%)**

Protein Smoothie with Milk (can also add water and ice)

Milk adds a dose of calcium and a creamier texture to this protein smoothie. If you'd prefer, substitute the milk with low-fat Lactaid or soy milk. Almond butter or even flax seed oil can be substituted for the peanut butter.

FOODS	CALORIES	PROTEIN(G)	CARB(G)	FAT(G)
1 scoop whey protein powder, any flavor	102	20.0	1.0	1.5
2 ounces banana	52	0.0	13.6	0.0
2 teaspoons natural peanut butter	75	0.0	2.4	6.0
5 ounces milk (low fat)	75	5.0	7.5	3.1
Totals:	**304**	**25.0 (33%)**	**24.5 (32%)**	**10.6 (31%)**

Bacon, Egg, and Cheese Burrito

Recipe

A bacon, egg, and cheese burrito makes a tasty and fast breakfast, lunch, or dinner. If you'd like, you can skip the Canadian bacon and double the amount of cheese. Egg whites can also be substituted for Egg Beaters. *For the full recipe, see page 235.*

FOODS	CALORIES	PROTEIN(G)	CARB(G)	FAT(G)
⅔ cup Egg Beaters	66	13.2	2.6	0.0
½ ounce cheddar cheese (low fat)	55	3.5	0.5	4.5
1 ounce Canadian bacon	44	6.0	0.5	2.0
1 whole-grain, low-carb wrap	110	0.0	17.0	3.0
1 slice of tomato	6	0.0	1.3	0.1
Totals:	**281**	**22.7 (32%)**	**21.9 (31%)**	**9.6 (31%)**

Greek Yogurt Parfait

Recipe

Unlike traditional yogurt, Greek yogurt is high in protein and low in sugar. It's best sweetened and served with your favorite fruit and nuts. For an additional boost of flavor add "free foods" like Stevia and vanilla extract. This recipe can be made in bulk for the week and is perfect for breakfast, dessert, or a snack. *For the full recipe, see page 233.*

FOODS	CALORIES	PROTEIN(G)	CARB(G)	FAT(G)
10 ounces Greek yogurt, fat free	150	25.0	11.3	0.0
2 ounces blueberries	37	0.0	9.3	0.3
⅔ ounce almonds (raw)	112	0.0	4.0	10.6
Totals:	**299**	**25.0 (33%)**	**24.6 (33%)**	**10.9 (33%)**

Quick Meal!

Western-Style Omelet with Side of Fruit

Recipe

This omelet is a perfect way to use any leftover veggies you have on hand. You can even double the recipe and gently reheat the other half of the omelet in the microwave for dinner that night or breakfast the next morning. Serve with your favorite fresh fruit. *For the full recipe, see page 233.*

FOODS	CALORIES	PROTEIN(G)	CARB(G)	FAT(G)
⅔ cup Egg Beaters	66	13.2	2.6	0.0
1½ ounces ham, Boar's Head, low sodium	45	7.5	1.5	0.8
¾ ounce cheddar cheese	83	5.3	0.8	6.8
2 tablespoons chopped tomato	6	0.0	1.3	0.1
2 tablespoons chopped onion	6	0.0	1.3	0.0
¼ cup bell peppers, green or red	7	0.0	1.6	0.1
6 ounces cantaloupe	60	0.0	14.4	0.8
Totals:	**273**	**26.0 (38%)**	**23.5 (34%)**	**8.6 (28%)**

Lunch

Medium Quality

Quick Meal!

Boca Burger with Fruit (can add lettuce, tomato, and onion)

A Boca burger is a great source of soy protein and takes only moments to prepare. You can top your burger with a small amount of ketchup or mustard. Serve with fresh fruit of your choice for a complete meal.

FOODS	CALORIES	PROTEIN(G)	CARB(G)	FAT(G)
1 Boca Burger, original	100	19	8.0	1
1 ounce cheddar cheese	110	7	1	9
4 ounces grapes	80	0.0	20.4	1
Totals:	**290**	**26.0 (36%)**	**29.4 (40%)**	**11 (34%)**

Quick Meal!

Chicken and Cheese Burrito

(Quick Meal if chicken is prepared in advance)

This meal is made of several staples we recommend you always have on hand: chicken breast, whole-grain/low-carb wraps, and fresh or frozen veggies (choose your favorite veggies). You can substitute the chicken for deli turkey or even grilled shrimp for a change of pace. This meal is also delicious as a grilled quesadilla. Add salsa for a boost of flavor.

FOODS	CALORIES	PROTEIN(G)	CARB(G)	FAT(G)
3 ounces chicken breast (boneless/skinless)	93	19.5	0.0	0.9
½ ounce cheddar cheese	55	3.5	0.5	4.5
1 whole-grain, low-carb wrap	110	0.0	17.0	3.0
½ cup mixed vegetables	40	0.0	7.0	0.0
Totals:	**298**	**23.0 (31%)**	**24.5 (33%)**	**8.4 (25%)**

Quick Meal!

Chicken Fajita (can add tomato, lettuce, and onion)

(Quick Meal if chicken is prepared in advance)

Chicken (or shrimp) fajitas can be made at home or enjoyed at any Mexican restaurant. If dining out, request that your meal be prepared in very little oil, and use guacamole as your fat (or choose a small amount of sour cream or cheese). Skip the rice and beans and load up on bell peppers and onions. Add salsa or pico de gallo for extra flavor.

FOODS	CALORIES	PROTEIN(G)	CARB(G)	FAT(G)
3½ ounces chicken breast (boneless/skinless)	109	22.8	0.0	1.1
2 tablespoons guacamole	80	0.0	0.8	8.0
2 ounces corn tortillas	100	0.0	18.4	2.0
¼ cup bell peppers, green or red	7	0.0	1.6	0.1
Totals:	**296**	**22.8 (31%)**	**20.8 (28%)**	**11.2 (34%)**

Quick Meal!

Smoked Salmon and Cream Cheese Toasts   Recipe

Smoked salmon toasts are a fun way to load up on your omega-3 essential fat. Ak-Mak crackers, a whole-grain flat-bread snack, can be found at any grocery store. This meal is also delicious served for breakfast. *For the full recipe, see page 238.*

FOODS	CALORIES	PROTEIN(G)	CARB(G)	FAT(G)
4½ ounces smoked salmon	149	23.4	0.0	5.4
3 Ak-Mak crackers	69	0.0	12.0	1.2
½ small tomato, sliced	12	0.0	2.6	0.2
¼ cucumber, sliced	8	0.0	1.5	0.2
1 thin slice of red onion	6	0.0	1.3	0.0
1½ tablespoons cream cheese (low fat)	50	3.0	1.0	3.0
Totals:	**294**	**26.4 (36%)**	**18.4 (25%)**	**10.0 (31%)**

Quick Meal!

Spicy Turkey Club Wrap with Side of Fruit   Recipe

A turkey club can be healthy when it's made with low-fat mayonnaise, turkey bacon, and a whole-grain wrap. You can swap out the turkey for chicken breast if you'd prefer. *For the full recipe, see page 237.*

FOODS	CALORIES	PROTEIN(G)	CARB(G)	FAT(G)
3½ ounces turkey breast, Boar's Head, low sodium	87.5	21.0	0.0	0.5
1 slice turkey bacon	33	2.5	0.0	2.5
1 tablespoon light mayonnaise	50	0.0	1.0	5.0
1 whole-grain, low-carb wrap	110	0.0	17.0	3.0
romaine lettuce leaves	1	0.0	0.2	0.0
2 slices of tomato	6	0.0	1.3	0.1
4 slices of cucumber	4	0.0	0.8	0.1
2 ounces strawberries	18	0.0	4.0	0.2
Totals:	**309.5**	**23.5 (30%)**	**24.3 (31%)**	**11.4 (33%)**

Sushi Meal (can add wasabi and ginger)

When ordering sushi, aim for sashimi (slices of fish that can be served on top of or alongside rice). Some sushi restaurants even offer brown rice in place of white rice, which is a better choice for stable blood sugar due to the increased fiber. Add soy sauce for a boost of flavor.

FOODS	CALORIES	PROTEIN(G)	CARB(G)	FAT(G)
2 ounces sashimi, tuna (albacore)	98	14.4	0.0	4.2
1 ounce sashimi, salmon	40	5.6	0.0	2.0
1 ounce sashimi, yellowtail	41	6.8	0.0	1.6
3 pieces vegetable roll	93	0.0	16.8	1.8
¼ cup brown rice (cooked)	50	0.0	11.0	0.0
Totals:	**322**	**26.8 (33%)**	**27.8 (35%)**	**9.6 (27%)**

Quick Meal!

Cranberry Chicken Salad Wrap   Recipe

(Quick Meal if chicken is prepared in advance)

This creamy chicken salad can be served in a wrap, on top of a salad, or with a side of fruit. Try making the chicken salad mixture in bulk for grab 'n' go meals for the week. *For the full recipe, see page 236.*

FOODS	CALORIES	PROTEIN(G)	CARB(G)	FAT(G)
3½ ounces chicken breast (boneless/skinless)	109	22.8	0.0	1.1
1 tablespoon Greek yogurt (fat free)	8	1.3	0.6	0.0
½ tablespoon light mayonnaise	50	0.0	1.0	5.0
1 whole-grain, low-carb wrap	110	0.0	17.0	3.0
½ cup spinach leaves, (uncooked)	4	0.0	0.5	0.0
2 slices of tomato	6	0.0	1.3	0.1
½ tablespoon dried cranberries	16	0.0	4.0	0.0
Totals:	**303**	**24.1 (32%)**	**24.4 (32%)**	**9.2 (27%)**

Tuna Wrap (can add Lettuce, Tomato, and Onion) with Side of Fruit

A tuna wrap is a fast and easy meal to pack for work. To boost the flavor, add celery, onion, lettuce, tomato, and even fresh herbs like parsley. Season to taste with salt and pepper.

FOODS	CALORIES	PROTEIN(G)	CARB(G)	FAT(G)
3½ ounces albacore tuna (in water)	105	24.5	0.0	1.7
1 tablespoon light mayonnaise	50	0.0	1.0	5.0
1 whole-grain, low-carb wrap	110	0.0	17.0	3.0
3 ounces orange slices	39	0.0	9.9	0.3
Totals:	**304**	**24.5 (32%)**	**27.9 (37%)**	**10 (30%)**

Dinner

High Quality

Greek Brown Rice Salad with Chicken   Recipe

This recipe can easily be prepared in bulk for quick meals all week long. You can also substitute the chicken for lean chopped pork tenderloin or grilled shrimp. *For the full recipe, see page 240.*

FOODS	CALORIES	PROTEIN(G)	CARB(G)	FAT(G)
4 ounces chicken breast (boneless/skinless)	124	26.0	0.0	1.2
2½ tablespoons low-fat balsamic vinaigrette salad dressing	55	0.0	2.5	5.0
½ ounce black olives (pitted)	19	0.0	0.4	1.9
½ cup brown rice (cooked)	100	0.0	22.0	0.0
½ cup arugula (raw)	4	0.0	0.5	0.1
2 tablespoons chopped tomato	6	0.0	1.3	0.1
¼ cup cucumber	4	0.0	0.8	0.1
Totals:	**312**	**26.0 (33%)**	**27.5 (35%)**	**8.4 (24%)**

Orange Honey Mustard Pork Tenderloin with Asparagus   Recipe

A juicy glaze adds plenty of flavor to plain old pork. Use leftovers in stir-frys, salads, or wraps the rest of the week. You can also substitute the asparagus for another vegetable if you'd prefer. *For the full recipe, see page 242.*

FOODS	CALORIES	PROTEIN(G)	CARB(G)	FAT(G)
4 ounces pork tenderloin	136	24.0	0.0	4.0
1 teaspoon olive oil	40	0.0	0.0	4.6
5 ounces asparagus	30	0.0	5.0	0.6
2 tablespoons Orange Honey Mustard Glaze (see recipe)	80	0.0	20.0	0.0
Totals:	**286**	**24.0 (34%)**	**25.0 (35%)**	**9.2 (29%)**

Shrimp, Rice, and Vegetable Stir-Fry

A rice and vegetable stir-fry goes well with any lean protein like shrimp, chicken, lean ground turkey, or pork tenderloin. Olive oil can be swapped out for peanut oil or sesame oil. To further enhance the flavor, you can add soy sauce, garlic, herbs, and spices. For a full list of "free foods" see "Condiments, Seasonings, and Spices" in your Food Exchange List.

FOODS	CALORIES	PROTEIN(G)	CARB(G)	FAT(G)
4 ounces shrimp (raw or steamed)	112	24.0	0.0	1.0
½ tablespoon olive oil	60	0.0	0.0	7.0
⅓ cup brown rice (cooked)	66	0.0	14.5	0.0
6 ounces broccoli	48	0.0	9.0	1.0
Totals:	**286**	**24.0 (34%)**	**23.5 (33%)**	**9.0 (28%)**

Medium Quality

Quick Meal!

BBQ Chicken and Salad

(Quick Meal if chicken is prepared in advance)

BBQ chicken (or shrimp or pork tenderloin) can be grilled or baked in the oven. You can substitute any low-fat dressing with roughly the same amount of fat for the balsamic vinaigrette. A side salad or your favorite vegetable completes the meal.

FOODS	CALORIES	PROTEIN(G)	CARB(G)	FAT(G)
4 ounces chicken breast (boneless/skinless)	124	26.0	0.0	1.2
3 tablespoons low-fat balsamic vinaigrette salad dressing	66	0.0	3.0	6.0
2 cups garden salad (lettuce and vegetables)	70	0.0	18.0	0.0
1 tablespoon BBQ sauce	30	0.0	7.0	0.0
Totals:	**290**	**26.0 (36%)**	**28.0 (39%)**	**7.2 (22%)**

Lean Turkey Burger (can add lettuce, tomato, and onion)

To boost the flavor, lean ground turkey can be seasoned with garlic, herbs, and spices (see "Condiments, Seasonings, and Spices" in your Food Exchange List). On occasion, you can also substitute 99% fat-free ground beef for the turkey (because even lean ground beef has fat, omit the avocado to keep the fat content down).

FOODS	CALORIES	PROTEIN(G)	CARB(G)	FAT(G)
3½ ounces ground turkey (99% fat free)	105	24.9	0.0	0.7
1½ ounces avocado	75	0.0	3.0	7.5
1 wheat bun	130	0.0	20.0	3.0
Totals:	**310**	**24.9 (32%)**	**23.0 (30%)**	**11.2 (33%)**

Turkey Meat Sauce with Pasta and Veggies

Try making this meal in bulk for the week. For added flavor, sauté onion and garlic with ground turkey. Add tomato sauce and fresh basil, and season with salt and pepper.

FOODS	CALORIES	PROTEIN(G)	CARB(G)	FAT(G)
4 ounces ground turkey (93% fat free)	178	27.2	0.0	8.4
2 ounces pasta (cooked)	74	0.0	16.0	1.0
½ cup tomato sauce	30	0.0	6.0	0.0
2 ounces broccoli	16	0.0	3.0	0.3
Totals:	298	27.2 (37%)	25.0 (34%)	9.7 (29%)

Salmon with Red Potatoes, Vegetable, and Dessert

A filet mignon or orange roughy can easily be substituted for the salmon. Try chopping the potatoes, spraying them with fat-free cooking spray and seasoning them with garlic, herbs, and spices before roasting. Or, if you'd like, substitute brown rice, sweet potatoes, or extra veggies in place of them. Enhance the flavor of salmon with fresh-squeezed lemon juice, herbs, and spices.

FOODS	CALORIES	PROTEIN(G)	CARB(G)	FAT(G)
4½ ounces salmon	180	25.2	0.0	9.0
3 ounces red potatoes	75	0.0	15.0	0.0
2 ounces snow peas	24	0.0	4.0	0.0
1 cup Jello (sugar free)	20	0.0	4.0	0.0
Totals:	299	25.2 (34%)	23.0 (31%)	9.0 (27%)

MEAL REPLACEMENTS AND QUICK "MID" MEALS

Medium Quality

Quick Meal!

Edamame
¾ Meal

Edamame is the perfect snack food. Not only is edamame the ideal balance of complete protein (from soy), carbohydrates, and fat, it's also loaded with vitamins and antioxidants. Buy it fresh or frozen in your local supermarket and boil until tender. Salt lightly and enjoy.

FOODS	CALORIES	PROTEIN(G)	CARB(G)	FAT(G)
1¼ cups edamame	250	20.0	22.5	7.5
Totals:	**250**	**20.0 (32%)**	**22.5 (36%)**	**7.5 (27%)**

Quick Meal!

Turkey, String Cheese, and Fruit
¾ Meal

Sliced turkey, string cheese, and fruit is a fast and portable snack perfect for any time of day. Substitute the apple with any of your favorite fruits.

FOODS	CALORIES	PROTEIN(G)	CARB(G)	FAT(G)
2 ounces turkey breast, Boar's Head, low sodium	50	12.0	0.0	0.3
1 ounce mozzarella string cheese	80	8.0	1.0	5.0
5 ounces apple	85	0.0	21.5	0.5
Totals:	**215**	**20.0 (37%)**	**22.5 (42%)**	**5.8 (24%)**

MALE GOAL TYPE 2 (500-CALORIE MEAL PLANS)

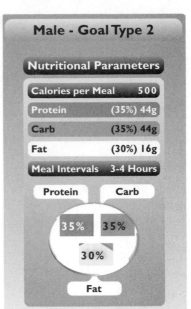

Male - Goal Type 2

Nutritional Parameters

Calories per Meal	500
Protein	(35%) 44g
Carb	(35%) 44g
Fat	(30%) 16g
Meal Intervals	3-4 Hours

Jump Start Sample Day

Remember to drink at least 12 ounces of water with every meal, and 12 ounces of water between each meal.

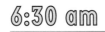 **6:30 am**

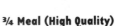 **Quick Meal!**

Scrambled Eggs and Side of Oatmeal (with optional flavorings)

¾ Meal (High Quality)

(Quick Meal if eggs are hardboiled)

You can increase your metabolism and maximize muscle growth by eating a balanced breakfast, like eggs and oatmeal, one hour within waking. Add flavor to unsweetened oatmeal with "free foods" like Stevia, cinnamon, and vanilla extract. If you're pressed for time, the Protein Power Oatmeal breakfast is a faster option.

FOODS	CALORIES	PROTEIN(G)	CARB(G)	FAT(G)
6 egg whites	102	21.0	0.0	0.0
2 eggs (whole)	160	12.8	1.0	11.2
1 ounce oatmeal (unsweetened)	100	0.0	19.3	2.0
2 ounces blueberries	37	0.0	9.3	0.3
Totals:	**399**	**33.8 (34%)**	**29.6 (30%)**	**13.5 (30%)**

9:30 am

Quick Meal!

Ready-to-Drink Shake, Almonds, and Apple

(Low Quality)

A midmorning meal can initially be challenging to fit into your schedule. A "ready to drink shake" or protein bar is a good solution. The brand you use is your choice. What matters most is to find a "ready to drink shake" or bar that comes close to matching your caloric and nutrient ratio parameters. Add your favorite unsalted nuts and fruit to complete the meal.

Important Note: You are always better off eating high-quality food to maximize results, especially with weight gain as your goal. If you can replace this low-quality meal with a high-quality meal, you will quickly feel the difference in energy, meal satisfaction, and in the speed of your results.

FOODS	CALORIES	PROTEIN(G)	CARB(G)	FAT(G)
1 serving Myoplex (EAS) Ready-to-Drink Shake (17 ounces)	310	43.0	20.0	7.0
½ ounce almonds (raw)	85	0.0	3.0	8.0
6 ounces apple	102	0.0	25.8	0.6
Totals:	**497**	**43.0 (35%)**	**48.8 (39%)**	**15.6 (28%)**

12:30 pm

Quick Meal!

Ground Turkey, Rice, and Broccoli Stir-Fry

(High Quality)

(Quick Meal if stir-fry is prepared in advance)

A stir-fry is perfect to make in bulk for grab 'n' go meals during the week. Season your stir-fry with garlic, fresh herbs, and spices to enhance the flavor without additional fat or calories. (See "Condiments, Seasonings, and Spices" in your Food Exchange List for a full list of "free foods.")

FOODS	CALORIES	PROTEIN(G)	CARB(G)	FAT(G)
6 ounces ground turkey (99% fat free)	180	42.6	0.0	1.2
1 tablespoon olive oil	120	0.0	0.0	14.0
¾ cup brown rice (cooked)	150	0.0	33.0	0.0
6 ounces broccoli	48	0.0	9.0	1.0
Totals:	**498**	**42.6 (34%)**	**42.0 (34%)**	**16.2 (29%)**

3:30 pm

Chicken, Fruit, and Nuts

(High Quality)

(Quick Meal if chicken is prepared in advance)

It may seem like an odd combination, but this meal is one of our go-to staples when we're in a hurry. Try preparing grilled or baked chicken in bulk for the week so you always have a high-quality protein on hand. Then pair it with your favorite fresh fruit and unsalted nuts and you've got a quality meal that takes only minutes to make.

FOODS	CALORIES	PROTEIN(G)	CARB(G)	FAT(G)
6½ ounces chicken breast (boneless/skinless)	202	42.3	0.0	2.0
1 ounce cashews (raw)	160	0.0	9.2	13.2
5 ounces banana	130	0.0	34.0	0.0
Totals:	**492**	**42.3 (34%)**	**43.2 (35%)**	**15.2 (28%)**

6:30 pm

Salmon with Sweet Potato and Asparagus

(High Quality)

This meal is both tasty and extremely high quality, due to the salmon, which is naturally high in omega-3 fatty acids (the heart-healthy, good fat). Enhance the flavor of salmon with fresh-squeezed lemon juice, herbs, and spices You may want to occasionally substitute a filet mignon for salmon if you are in the mood for beef.

FOODS	CALORIES	PROTEIN(G)	CARB(G)	FAT(G)
8 ounces salmon	320	44.8	0.0	16.0
5 ounces sweet potato	150	0.0	35.0	0.0
5 ounces asparagus	30	0.0	5.0	0.6
Totals:	**500**	**44.8 (36%)**	**40.0 (32%)**	**16.6 (30%)**

9:30 pm

Quick Meal!

Protein Smoothie Without Milk (add water and ice)   (Medium Quality)

A protein shake makes for a delicious and balanced dessert before bed. Use a shaker to mix the powder in water and then eat the unsalted nuts and fruit of your choice. Eating before bed will fuel your muscles through the night and assist you in increasing your lean body mass. If you choose to have a meal in place of a protein shake at this time, limit the amount of starchy carbs/grains to optimize nighttime digestion and prevent any possible bloating.

FOODS	CALORIES	PROTEIN(G)	CARB(G)	FAT(G)
2 servings whey hydrolyzed protein powder, any flavor	270	40.0	14.0	8.0
½ ounce almonds (raw)	85	0.0	3.0	8.0
7 ounces apple	119	0.0	30.1	0.7
Totals:	**474**	**40 (34%)**	**47.1 (40%)**	**16.7 (32%)**
Day Totals:	**2860**	**246.5 (34%)**	**250.7 (35%)**	**93.8 (30%)**

JUMP START MEALS

Breakfast

High Quality

Quick Meal!

Scrambled Eggs and Side of Oatmeal (with optional flavorings) ¾ Meal

(Quick Meal if eggs are hardboiled)

An eggs and oatmeal breakfast combo is simple to make (use instant oatmeal for easy prep) and incredibly satisfying. Give plain cooked oatmeal a boost of flavor without extra calories by stirring in "free foods" like Stevia (or any calorie-free sugar substitute), cinnamon, and vanilla extract.

FOODS	CALORIES	PROTEIN(G)	CARB(G)	FAT(G)
6 egg whites	102	21.0	0.0	0.0
2 eggs (whole)	160	12.8	1.0	11.2
1 ounce oatmeal (unsweetened)	100	0.0	19.3	2.0
2 ounces blueberries	37	0.0	9.3	0.3
Totals:	**399**	**33.8 (34%)**	**29.6 (30%)**	**13.5 (30%)**

Veggie and Egg Scramble with Side of Fruit

¾ Meal

An egg scramble is the perfect way to sneak in extra veggies you have on hand. Add a spoonful of your favorite salsa for extra spice. Choose your favorite fruit as a side.

FOODS	CALORIES	PROTEIN(G)	CARB(G)	FAT(G)
5 egg whites	85	17.5	0.0	0.0
2 eggs (whole)	160	12.8	1.0	11.2
½ cup spinach (cooked)	25	0.0	5.0	0.0
2 ounces broccoli	16	0.0	3.0	0.3
½ cup mushrooms	14	0.0	2.6	0.3
⅓ cup tomato	12	0.0	2.6	0.2
7 ounces grapefruit	77	0.0	18.9	0.5
Totals:	**389**	**30.3 (31%)**	**33.1 (34%)**	**12.5 (29%)**

Medium Quality

Quick Meal!

Berry Banana Protein Smoothie Without Milk (add water and ice)

A protein and fruit smoothie is a sweet and refreshing way to stabilize your blood sugar fast. Try blending your favorite vanilla or chocolate protein powder with a variety of fresh or frozen fruit. Adjust the amount of water and ice to your desired consistency.

FOODS	CALORIES	PROTEIN(G)	CARB(G)	FAT(G)
2 scoops whey protein powder, any flavor	204	40.0	2.0	3.0
1½ tablespoons natural peanut butter	150	0.0	4.8	12.0
7 ounces strawberries	63	0.0	14.0	0.8
3 ounces banana	78	0.0	20.4	0.0
Totals:	**495**	**40.0 (32%)**	**41.2 (33%)**	**15.8 (29%)**

Protein Power Oatmeal

Recipe

Protein Power Oatmeal is warm, creamy and guaranteed to fuel your busy mornings. You can substitute the whey protein powder for soy or egg white powder. For a change of pace, swap nuts, peanut butter, or ground flax seeds for the almond butter. *For the full recipe, see page 234.*

FOODS	CALORIES	PROTEIN(G)	CARB(G)	FAT(G)
2 scoops whey protein powder, any flavor	204	40.0	2.0	3.0
1½ tablespoons almond butter	128	0.0	6.0	10.5
1¾ ounces oatmeal (unsweetened)	175	0.0	33.8	3.5
Totals:	**507**	**40.0 (32%)**	**41.8 (33%)**	**17.0 (30%)**

Lunch

High Quality

Grilled Chicken Salad

(Quick Meal if chicken is prepared in advance)

Whether it's lunch at home or at a restaurant, grilled chicken salad is a balanced and high-quality option. You can exchange the chicken for any other lean protein like grilled white fish or shrimp and top the salad with your favorite vegetables.

FOODS	CALORIES	PROTEIN(G)	CARB(G)	FAT(G)
6½ ounces chicken breast (boneless/skinless)	202	42.3	0.0	2.0
2 tablespoons oil and vinegar salad dressing	140	0.0	2.0	16.0
4½ cups garden salad (lettuce and vegetables)	158	0.0	40.5	0.0
Totals:	**500**	**42.3 (34%)**	**42.5 (34%)**	**18.0 (32%)**

Ground Turkey, Rice, and Broccoli Stir-Fry

(Quick Meal if stir-fry is prepared in advance)

A stir-fry is perfect to make in bulk for grab 'n' go meals during the week. Season your stir-fry with garlic, fresh herbs, and spices to enhance the flavor without additional fat or calories. (See "Condiments, Seasonings, and Spices" in your Food Exchange List for a full list of "free foods.")

FOODS	CALORIES	PROTEIN(G)	CARB(G)	FAT(G)
6 ounces ground turkey (99% fat free)	180	42.6	0.0	1.2
1 tablespoon olive oil	120	0.0	0.0	14.0
¾ cup brown rice (cooked)	150	0.0	33.0	0.0
6 ounces broccoli	48	0.0	9.0	1.0
Totals:	**498**	**42.6 (34%)**	**42.0 (34%)**	**16.2 (29%)**

Italian Tuna Salad with Side of Fruit

Recipe

Italian Tuna Salad is made up of common pantry items (canned tuna, low-fat balsamic dressing) and any vegetable you choose. Try making this recipe in bulk and storing it in the fridge for easy meals throughout the week. If desired, substitute any other lean protein for the tuna. *For the full recipe, see page 237.*

FOODS	CALORIES	PROTEIN(G)	CARB(G)	FAT(G)
6 ounces albacore tuna (in water)	180	42.0	0.0	3.0
1 tablespoon olive oil	120	0.0	0.0	14.0
¼ ounce back olives (pitted)	9	0.0	0.2	1.0
½ cup bell peppers, green or red	13	0.0	3.2	0.3
⅓ cup cherry tomato	12	0.0	2.6	0.2
⅛ cup onion	6	0.0	1.3	0.0
10 ounces orange slices	130	0.0	33.0	0.9
Totals:	**470**	**42.0 (36%)**	**40.3 (34%)**	**19.4 (37%)**

Quick Meal!

Chicken, Fruit, and Nuts

(Quick Meal if chicken is prepared in advance)

It may seem like an odd combination, but this meal is one of our go-to staples when we're in a hurry. Try preparing grilled or baked chicken in bulk for the week so you always have a high quality protein on hand. Then pair it with your favorite fresh fruit and unsalted nuts and you've got a quality meal that takes only minutes to make.

FOODS	CALORIES	PROTEIN(G)	CARB(G)	FAT(G)
6½ ounces chicken breast (boneless/skinless)	202	42.3	0.0	2.0
1 ounce cashews (raw)	160	0.0	9.2	13.2
8 ounces apple	136	0.0	34.4	0.8
Totals:	**498**	**42.3 (34%)**	**43.6 (35%)**	**16.0 (29%)**

Dinner
High Quality

Quick Meal!

Grilled Chicken with Spinach Bean Salad and Fruit

(Quick Meal if chicken is prepared in advance)

Garbanzo beans (or any beans) add a boost of flavor and texture to a spinach salad. You can swap the spinach for your favorite leafy greens and the chicken breast for any lean protein.

FOODS	CALORIES	PROTEIN(G)	CARB(G)	FAT(G)
6½ ounces chicken breast (boneless/skinless)	202	42.3	0.0	2.0
1½ tablespoons oil and vinegar salad dressing	105	0.0	1.5	12.0
2 cups spinach leaves (uncooked)	14	0.0	2.0	0.0
1 ounce garbanzo beans	102	0.0	18.0	2.0
3½ ounces grapes	70	0.0	17.8	0.9
Totals:	**493**	**42.3 (34%)**	**39.3 (32%)**	**16.9 (31%)**

Restaurant-Worthy Steak with Sweet Potato and Steamed Cauliflower

Recipe

A filet mignon is one of the leanest, tastiest cuts of beef, and that is why we recommend it. Pair your filet with delicious sweet potatoes and any steamed vegetable for a satisfying meal. *For the full recipe, see page 239.*

FOODS	CALORIES	PROTEIN(G)	CARB(G)	FAT(G)
6 ounces filet mignon	300	48.0	0.0	15.0
6 ounces sweet potato	180	0.0	42.0	0.0
4 ounces cauliflower	28	0.0	5.7	0.0
Totals:	**508**	**48.0 (38%)**	**47.7 (38%)**	**15.0 (27%)**

Seared Scallops with Brown Rice and Spinach

Recipe

Seared scallops take only minutes to make and are a great source of high-quality protein. You can swap out the scallops for any lean protein like chicken breast, pork tenderloin, or shrimp. The spinach can also be substituted with any leafy greens. *For the full recipe, see page 241.*

FOODS	CALORIES	PROTEIN(G)	CARB(G)	FAT(G)
8 ounces scallops	200	40.0	0.0	2.0
1 tablespoon olive oil	120	0.0	0.0	14.0
¾ cup brown rice (cooked)	150	0.0	33.0	0.0
4 cups spinach leaves (uncooked)	28	0.0	4.0	0.0
Totals:	**498**	**40.0 (32%)**	**37.0 (30%)**	**16.0 (29%)**

Salmon with Brown Rice and Asparagus

Salmon is loaded in heart-healthy, omega-3 essential fats and should be eaten once or twice a week if possible. Add fresh-squeezed lemon juice to enhance the taste of the salmon. Serve left-over salmon over a crisp salad for a satisfying lunch the next day.

FOODS	CALORIES	PROTEIN(G)	CARB(G)	FAT(G)
8 ounces salmon	320	44.8	0.0	16.0
¾ cup brown rice (cooked)	150	0.0	33.0	0.0
5 ounces asparagus	30	0.0	5.0	0.6
Totals:	**500**	**44.8 (36%)**	**38.0 (30%)**	**16.6 (30%)**

MEAL REPLACEMENTS AND QUICK "MID" MEALS

Medium Quality

Quick Meal!

Quick Turkey Roll-Up with Fruit and Nuts
¾ Meal

Having lean, low-sodium deli meat on hand is a great way to ensure you've got a fast source of protein available. Ask your local deli for the highest-quality, least-processed brand they have (like Boar's Head). Pair it with fresh fruit and unsalted nuts of your choice for a quick and balanced meal. Dip turkey slices into mustard or any other "free food" for extra flavor.

FOODS	CALORIES	PROTEIN(G)	CARB(G)	FAT(G)
6 ounces turkey breast, Boar's Head, low sodium	150	36.0	0.0	0.8
¾ ounce cashews (raw)	120	0.0	6.9	9.9
7 ounces pear	119	0.0	30.1	0.8
Totals:	**389**	**36.0 (37%)**	**37.0 (38%)**	**11.5 (27%)**

Low Quality

Protein Bar

¾ Meal

Protein bars are a convenient option for those times when you are too busy for an actual meal (like when you are on the go or in a meeting at work). The goal is to choose a bar that matches your nutritional parameters. For a complete list of recommended protein bars, see "Meal Replacements" in your Food Exchange List.

FOODS	CALORIES	PROTEIN(G)	CARB(G)	FAT(G)
1 serving Pure protein bar	310	32.0	24.0	10.0
Totals:	**310**	**32.0 (41%)**	**24.0 (31%)**	**10.0 (29%)**

Ready-to-Drink Shake, Almonds, and Apple

A ready-made protein drink paired with fresh fruit is an ideal option while at work or even while traveling. For a complete list of recommended protein drinks, see "Meal Replacements" in your Food Exchange List.

FOODS	CALORIES	PROTEIN(G)	CARB(G)	FAT(G)
1 serving Myoplex (EAS) Ready-to-Drink Shake (17 ounces)	310	43.0	20.0	7.0
½ ounce almonds (raw)	85	0.0	3.0	8.0
6 ounces apple	102	0.0	25.8	0.6
Totals:	**497**	**43.0 (35%)**	**48.8 (39%)**	**15.6 (28%)**

ADDITIONAL MEALS—AFTER JUMP START PHASE

Breakfast

Medium Quality

Quick Meal!

Cereal To Go with Protein Powder

By adding protein powder and nuts to cereal, you end up with a hearty breakfast that stabilizes your blood sugar and keeps you full all morning long. Simply shake half of the protein powder and milk together in a shake cup with a lid until blended and pour over any low-sugar, high-fiber cereal. Top with nuts and enjoy. Mix the remaining protein powder with water on the side for a quick shake.

FOODS	CALORIES	PROTEIN(G)	CARB(G)	FAT(G)
2 scoops whey protein powder, any flavor	204	40.0	2.0	3.0
6 ounces milk (low fat)	90	6.0	9.0	3.8
½ ounce almonds (raw)	85	0.0	3.0	8.0
1¼ ounces bran flakes cereal	113	0.0	27.5	0.0
Totals:	**492**	**46.0 (37%)**	**41.5 (34%)**	**14.8 (27%)**

Quick Meal!

Cottage Cheese with Fruit and Nuts

Cottage cheese mixed with fruit is a sweet and creamy combo that takes less than a minute to make. Fresh pineapple, raspberries, and peaches taste delicious too. Try prepping fruit in bulk for a few days so it's always ready to eat.

FOODS	CALORIES	PROTEIN(G)	CARB(G)	FAT(G)
12 ounces cottage cheese (low fat)	300	42.0	12.0	7.2
½ ounce almonds (raw)	85	0.0	3.0	8.0
4 ounces blueberries	74	0.0	18.5	0.5
4 ounces strawberries	36	0.0	8.0	0.4
Totals:	**495**	**42.0 (34%)**	**41.5 (34%)**	**16.1 (29%)**

Protein Smoothie with Milk (can add water and ice)

Milk adds a dose of calcium and a creamier texture to this protein smoothie. If you prefer, substitute the milk with low-fat Lactaid or soy milk. Almond butter or even flax seed oil can be substituted for the peanut butter.

FOODS	CALORIES	PROTEIN(G)	CARB(G)	FAT(G)
2 scoops whey protein powder, any flavor	204	40.0	2.0	3.0
6 ounces milk (low fat)	90	6.0	9.0	3.8
1 tablespoon natural peanut butter	100	0.0	3.2	8.0
4 ounces banana	104	0.0	27.2	0.0
Totals:	**498**	**46.0 (37%)**	**41.4 (33%)**	**14.8 (27%)**

Bacon, Egg, and Cheese Sandwich   Recipe

A bacon, egg, and cheese sandwich makes a tasty and fast breakfast, lunch, or dinner. Egg whites can easily be substituted for Egg Beaters. *For the full recipe, see page 235.*

FOODS	CALORIES	PROTEIN(G)	CARB(G)	FAT(G)
1½ cups Egg Beaters	150	30.0	6.0	0.0
1 ounce cheddar cheese	110	7.0	1.0	9.0
2 ounces Canadian bacon	88	12.0	1.0	4.0
1 whole-wheat English muffin	130	0.0	25.6	1.6
1 slice of tomato	6	0.0	1.3	0.1
Totals:	**484**	**49.0 (40%)**	**34.9 (29%)**	**14.7 (27%)**

Greek Yogurt Parfait

Unlike traditional yogurt, Greek yogurt is high in protein and low in sugar. It's best sweetened and served with your favorite fruit and nuts. For an additional boost of flavor add "free foods" like Stevia and vanilla extract. This recipe can be made in bulk for the week and is perfect for breakfast, dessert or a snack. *For the full recipe, see page 233.*

FOODS	CALORIES	PROTEIN(G)	CARB(G)	FAT(G)
12 ounces Greek yogurt, (low fat)	222	29.1	13.8	6.9
½ ounce almonds (raw)	85	0.0	3.0	8.0
4 ounces blueberries	74	0.0	18.5	0.5
Totals:	**381**	**29.1 (31%)**	**35.3 (37%)**	**15.4 (36%)**

Western-Style Omelet with Side of Fruit and Toast

This omelet is a perfect way to use any leftover veggies you have on hand. You can even double the recipe and gently re-heat the other half of the omelet in the microwave for dinner that night or breakfast the next morning. Serve with your favorite fresh fruit. *For the full recipe, see page 233.*

FOODS	CALORIES	PROTEIN(G)	CARB(G)	FAT(G)
1¼ cups Egg Beaters	125	25.0	5.0	0.0
1½ ounces ham, Boar's Head, low sodium	45	7.5	1.5	0.8
1½ ounces cheddar cheese	165	10.5	1.5	13.5
2 tablespoons chopped tomato	6	0.0	1.3	0.1
2 tablespoons chopped onion	6	0.0	1.3	0.0
¼ cup bell peppers, green or red	7	0.0	1.6	0.1
10 ounces cantaloupe	100	0.0	24.0	1.3
1 slice wheat bread	70	0.0	12.0	1.0
I Can't Believe It's Not Butter spray (optional), as needed for wheat toast	0	0.0	0.0	0.0
Totals:	**524**	**43.0 (33%)**	**48.2 (37%)**	**16.8 (29%)**

Lunch

Medium Quality

Quick Meal!

Double Boca Burger with Fruit (can add lettuce, tomato, and onion)

A Boca burger is a great source of soy protein and takes only moments to prepare. You can top your burger with a small amount of ketchup or mustard. Serve with fresh fruit of your choice for a complete meal.

FOODS	CALORIES	PROTEIN(G)	CARB(G)	FAT(G)
2 Boca burgers, original	200	38.0	16.0	2
1½ ounces cheddar cheese	165	10.5	1.5	13.5
7 ounces pear	119	0.0	30.1	0.8
Totals:	**484**	**48.5 (40%)**	**47.6 (39%)**	**16.3 (30%)**

Quick Meal!

Chicken and Cheese Burrito

(Quick Meal if chicken is prepared in advance)

This meal is made of several staples we recommend you always have on hand: chicken breast, whole-grain/low-carb wraps and fresh or frozen veggies (choose your favorite veggies). You can substitute the chicken for deli turkey or even grilled shrimp for a change of pace. This meal is also delicious as a grilled quesadilla. Add salsa for a boost of flavor.

FOODS	CALORIES	PROTEIN(G)	CARB(G)	FAT(G)
5 ounces chicken breast (boneless/skinless)	156	32.5	0.0	1.5
1¼ ounces cheddar cheese	138	8.8	1.3	11.3
1 whole-grain, low-carb wrap	110	0.0	17.0	3.0
1¼ cups mixed vegetables	100	0.0	17.5	0.0
Totals:	**504**	**41.3 (33%)**	**35.8 (28%)**	**15.8 (28%)**

Chicken Fajita (can add tomato, lettuce, and onion)

(Quick Meal if chicken is prepared in advance)

Chicken (or shrimp) fajitas can be made at home or enjoyed at any Mexican restaurant. If dining out, request that your meal be prepared in very little oil, and use guacamole as your fat (or choose a small amount of sour cream or cheese). Skip the rice and beans and load up on bell peppers and onions. Add salsa or pico de gallo for a boost of flavor.

FOODS	CALORIES	PROTEIN(G)	CARB(G)	FAT(G)
6 ounces chicken breast (boneless/skinless)	187	39.0	0.0	1.8
2½ tablespoons guacamole	100	0.0	1.0	10.0
4 ounces corn tortillas	200	0.0	36.8	4.0
¼ cup bell peppers, green or red	7	0.0	1.6	0.1
Totals:	**494**	**39.0 (32%)**	**39.4 (32%)**	**15.9 (29%)**

Smoked Salmon and Cream Cheese Toasts with Side of Fruit   Recipe

Smoked salmon toasts are a fun way to load up on your omega-3 essential-fat. Ak-Mak crackers, a whole-grain flat-bread snack, can be found at any grocery store. This meal is also delicious served for breakfast. *For the full recipe, see page 238.*

FOODS	CALORIES	PROTEIN(G)	CARB(G)	FAT(G)
7 ounces smoked salmon	231	36.4	0.0	8.4
3 tablespoons light cream cheese	105	3.0	3.0	7.5
4 Ak-Mak crackers	92	0.0	16.8	1.6
½ small tomato, sliced	12	0.0	2.6	0.2
¼ cucumber, sliced	8	0.0	1.5	0.2
1 thin slice of red onion	6	0.0	1.3	0.0
3 ounces apple	51	0.0	12.9	0.3
Totals:	**505**	**39.4 (31%)**	**38.1 (30%)**	**18.2 (32%)**

Quick Meal!

Spicy Turkey Club Sandwich with Side of Fruit   Recipe

A turkey club can be healthy when it's made with low-fat mayonnaise, turkey bacon, and whole-wheat bread. You can swap out the turkey for chicken breast if you prefer. *For the full recipe, see page 237.*

FOODS	CALORIES	PROTEIN(G)	CARB(G)	FAT(G)
6 ounces turkey breast, Boar's Head, low sodium	150	36.0	0.0	0.8
2 slices turkey bacon	67	5.0	0.0	5.0
1½ tablespoons light mayonnaise	75	0.0	1.5	7.5
2 slices whole-wheat bread	140	0.0	24.0	2.0
Romaine lettuce leaves	1	0.0	0.2	0.0
2 slices of tomato	6	0.0	1.3	0.1
4 slices of cucumber	4	0.0	0.8	0.1
6 ounces strawberries	54	0.0	12.0	0.7
Totals:	**497**	**41.0 (33%)**	**39.8 (32%)**	**16.2 (30%)**

Sushi Meal (can add wasabi and ginger)

When ordering sushi, aim for sashimi (slices of fish that can be served on top of or alongside rice). Some sushi restaurants even offer brown rice in place of white rice, which is a better choice for stable blood sugar due to the increased fiber. Add soy sauce for a boost of flavor.

FOODS	CALORIES	PROTEIN(G)	CARB(G)	FAT(G)
2 ounces sashimi, tuna (albacore)	98	14.4	0.0	4.2
2 ounces sashimi, yellowtail	82	13.6	0.0	3.2
2 ounces sashimi, salmon	80	11.2	0.0	4.0
4 pieces vegetable roll	124	0.0	22.4	2.4
½ cup brown rice (cooked)	100	0.0	22.0	0.0
Totals:	**484**	**39.2 (32%)**	**44.4 (37%)**	**13.8 (26%)**

Quick Meal!

Cranberry Pecan Chicken Salad Wrap

Recipe

(Quick Meal if chicken is prepared in advance)

This creamy chicken salad can be served in a wrap, on top of a salad, or with a side of fruit. Try making the chicken salad mixture in bulk for grab 'n' go meals for the week. *For the full recipe, see page 236.*

FOODS	CALORIES	PROTEIN(G)	CARB(G)	FAT(G)
6 ounces chicken breast (boneless/skinless)	187	39.0	0.0	1.8
1 tablespoon Greek yogurt (fat free)	8	1.3	0.6	0.0
⅓ ounce pecans (raw)	62	0.0	2.1	6.1
1 tablespoon light mayonnaise	50	0.0	1.0	5.0
1 whole-grain, low-carb wrap	110	0.0	17.0	3.0
½ cup spinach leaves (uncooked)	4	0.0	0.5	0.0
2 slices of tomato	6	0.0	1.3	0.1
2½ tablespoons dried cranberries	78	0.0	20.0	0.0
Totals:	**505**	**40.3 (32%)**	**42.5 (34%)**	**16.0 (29%)**

Quick Meal!

Tuna Wrap and Fruit (can add lettuce, tomato, and onion)

A tuna wrap is a fast and easy meal to pack for work. To boost the flavor, add celery, onion, lettuce, tomato, and even fresh herbs like parsley. Season to taste with salt and pepper.

FOODS	CALORIES	PROTEIN(G)	CARB(G)	FAT(G)
6 ounces albacore tuna (in water)	180	42.0	0.0	3.0
2 tablespoons light mayonnaise	100	0.0	2.0	10.0
1 whole-grain, low-carb wrap	110	0.0	17.0	3.0
8 ounces orange slices	104	0.0	26.4	0.7
Totals:	**494**	**42.0 (34%)**	**45.4 (37%)**	**16.7 (30%)**

Dinner

High Quality

Greek Brown Rice Salad with Chicken   **Recipe**

This recipe can easily be prepared in bulk for quick meals all week long. You can also substitute the chicken for lean chopped pork tenderloin or grilled shrimp. *For the full recipe, see page 240.*

FOODS	CALORIES	PROTEIN(G)	CARB(G)	FAT(G)
6 ounces chicken breast (boneless/skinless)	187	39.0	0.0	1.8
½ ounce cheese, feta	80	4.2	0.0	6.3
¾ ounce black olives (pitted)	28	0.0	0.5	2.9
2 tablespoons light balsamic vinaigrette salad dressing	44	0.0	2.0	4.0
¾ cup brown rice (cooked)	150	0.0	33.0	0.0
2 tablespoons chopped tomato	6	0.0	1.3	0.1
½ cup arugula lettuce leaves	4	0.0	0.5	0.1
¼ cup cucumber	4	0.0	0.8	0.1
Totals:	**503**	**43.2 (35%)**	**38.1 (30%)**	**15.3 (27%)**

Orange Honey Mustard Pork Tenderloin with Asparagus   **Recipe**

A juicy glaze adds plenty of flavor to plain old pork. Use leftovers in stir-frys, salads, or wraps the rest of the week. You can also substitute the asparagus for another vegetable. *For the full recipe, see page 242.*

FOODS	CALORIES	PROTEIN(G)	CARB(G)	FAT(G)
7 ounces pork tenderloin	238	42.0	0.0	7.0
½ tablespoon olive oil	60	0.0	0.0	7.0
10 ounces asparagus	60	0.0	10.0	1.3
3 tablespoons Orange Honey Mustard Glaze (see recipe)	120	0.0	30.0	0.0
Totals:	**478**	**42.0 (35%)**	**40.0 (33%)**	**15.3 (29%)**

Shrimp, Rice, and Vegetable Stir-Fry

A rice and vegetable stir-fry goes well with any lean protein like shrimp, chicken, lean ground turkey, or pork tenderloin. Olive oil can be swapped out for peanut oil or sesame oil. To further enhance the flavor, add soy sauce, garlic, herbs, and spices. For a full list of "free foods," see "Condiments, Seasonings, and Spices" in your Food Exchange List.

FOODS	CALORIES	PROTEIN(G)	CARB(G)	FAT(G)
7 ounces shrimp (raw or steamed)	196	42.0	0.0	1.8
1 tablespoon olive oil	120	0.0	0.0	14.0
½ cup brown rice (cooked)	100	0.0	22.0	0.0
1 cup mixed vegetables	80	0.0	14.0	0.0
Totals:	**496**	**42.0 (34%)**	**36.0 (29%)**	**15.8 (29%)**

Medium Quality

BBQ Chicken, Pasta, and Side Salad

BBQ chicken (or shrimp or pork tenderloin) can be grilled or baked in the oven. You can substitute any low-fat dressing with roughly the same amount of fat for the balsamic vinaigrette. A side salad or your favorite vegetable completes the meal.

FOODS	CALORIES	PROTEIN(G)	CARB(G)	FAT(G)
7 ounces chicken breast (boneless/skinless)	218	45.5	0.0	2.1
1½ tablespoons oil and vinegar salad dressing	105	0.0	1.5	12.0
1 cup garden salad (lettuce and vegetables)	35	0.0	9.0	0.0
3 ounces pasta (cooked)	111	0.0	24.0	1.5
¼ cup tomato sauce	15	0.0	3.0	0.0
1 tablespoon BBQ sauce	30	0.0	7.0	0.0
Totals:	**514**	**45.5 (35%)**	**44.5 (35%)**	**15.6 (27%)**

Lean Turkey Burger (can add lettuce, tomato, and onion) and Fruit

To boost the flavor, lean ground turkey can be seasoned with garlic, herbs, and spices (see "Condiments, Seasonings, and Spices" in your Food Exchange List). On occasion, you can also substitute 99% fat-free ground beef for the turkey (because even lean ground beef has fat, omit the avocado to keep the fat content down).

FOODS	CALORIES	PROTEIN(G)	CARB(G)	FAT(G)
6 ounces ground turkey (99% fat free)	180	42.6	0.0	1.2
1½ ounces avocado	75	0.0	3.0	7.5
1 wheat bun	130	0.0	20.0	3.0
7 ounces nectarine	98	0.0	23.1	0.7
Totals:	**483**	**42.6 (35%)**	**46.1 (38%)**	**12.4 (23%)**

Turkey Meat Sauce with Pasta and Veggies

Try making this meal in bulk for the week. For added flavor, sauté onion and garlic with ground turkey. Add tomato sauce and fresh basil, and season with salt and pepper.

FOODS	CALORIES	PROTEIN(G)	CARB(G)	FAT(G)
6 ounces ground turkey (93% fat free)	266	40.8	0.0	12.6
4 ounces pasta (cooked)	148	0.0	32.0	2.0
½ cup tomato sauce	30	0.0	6.0	0.0
4 ounces broccoli	32	0.0	6.0	0.6
Totals:	**476**	**40.8 (34%)**	**44.0 (37%)**	**15.2 (29%)**

Salmon with Red Potatoes, Corn, and Dessert

A filet mignon or orange roughy can easily be substituted for the salmon. Try chopping the potatoes, spraying them with fat-free cooking spray, and seasoning them with garlic, herbs, and spices before roasting. Or, if you'd like, substitute brown rice, sweet potatoes, or extra veggies in place of them. Enhance the flavor of salmon with fresh-squeezed lemon juice, herbs, and spices.

FOODS	CALORIES	PROTEIN(G)	CARB(G)	FAT(G)
8 ounces salmon	320	44.8	0.0	16.0
2½ ounces red potatoes	63	0.0	12.5	0.0
½ cup corn	80	0.0	20.0	0.0
1 serving Dreyers Fruit Bar	30	0.0	8.0	0.0
Totals:	**493**	**44.8 (36%)**	**40.5 (33%)**	**16.0 (29%)**

MEAL REPLACEMENTS AND QUICK "MID" MEALS

Medium Quality

Quick Meal!

Edamame

½ Meal

Edamame is the perfect snack food. Not only is edamame the ideal balance of complete protein (from soy), carbohydrates, and fat, it's also loaded with vitamins and antioxidants. Buy it fresh or frozen in your local supermarket and boil until tender. Salt lightly and enjoy.

FOODS	CALORIES	PROTEIN(G)	CARB(G)	FAT(G)
1¼ cups edamame	250	20.0	22.5	7.5
Totals:	**250**	**20.0 (32%)**	**22.5 (36%)**	**7.5 (27%)**

Quick Meal!

Turkey, String Cheese, Nuts, and Fruit

½ Meal

Sliced turkey, string cheese, nuts, and fruit is a fast and portable snack perfect for any time of day. Substitute the apple with any of your favorite fruits.

FOODS	CALORIES	PROTEIN(G)	CARB(G)	FAT(G)
3 ounces turkey breast, Boar's Head, low sodium	75	18.0	0.0	0.4
1 ounce mozzarella string cheese	80	8.0	1.0	5.0
¼ ounce almonds (raw)	43	0.0	1.5	4.0
6 ounces apple	102	0.0	25.8	0.6
Totals:	**300**	**26.0 (35%)**	**28.3 (38%)**	**10.0 (30%)**

Section 6—Diving into Tasty Recipes

At Venice Nutrition, we know how important it is to have fast, fun, and simple meals you can count on to work seamlessly into your lifestyle. The following recipes will show you how to easily create flavorful and delicious meals from basic, everyday foods. You'll learn how to whip up a balanced breakfast, grill a steak to tender perfection, and make plain old poultry sing. You'll also learn how to use ingredients like fresh veggies and herbs, capers, Greek yogurt, lemon, and vanilla to elevate the flavor and texture of even the simplest dishes. Most important, you'll discover that eating well can be quite enjoyable!

SPECIAL NOTE

You will notice that many of the ingredients in the recipes lack a quantity. This is because the recipes are customized to your personal nutrition parameters. Please refer to the actual meal in your meal plan that goes with the recipe for your specific amounts of these ingredients. Also, please take note of any special recommendations for particular nutrition guidelines in some of the meals.

BREAKFAST

Greek Yogurt Parfait

Creamy, vanilla-sweetened Greek yogurt (a high-protein, low-sugar yogurt found in specialty markets and many grocery stores) is layered between fresh berries and nuts in this mouth-watering parfait.

> Greek yogurt, plain, low fat (*for 250- and 300-calorie meal plans, use fat-free Greek yogurt*)
> ½ teaspoon vanilla extract
> Splenda or Stevia to taste
> blueberries, rinsed and dried
> almonds, slivered or chopped

Stir together Greek yogurt, Splenda or Stevia, and vanilla extract. Layer the mixture in a glass with the berries and nuts. If you are in a hurry, simply mix all ingredients together until combined. Enjoy.

- Great for on-the-go.
- Also a delicious and fast snack or dessert.

Western-Style Omelet with Side of Fruit

Chopped ham, melted cheddar cheese, fresh vegetables, and salsa come together for a hearty omelet that's sure to fill you up without filling you out.

> fat-free cooking spray, as needed
> chopped tomato
> chopped onion
> chopped bell pepper, red or green
> deli ham, lean, low sodium, chopped
> Egg beaters
> cheddar cheese
> 2 tablespoons salsa (optional)
> cantaloupe, sliced or cut into chunks
> 1 slice of wheat bread (*add slice of wheat toast for 500-calorie meal plan only*)
> I Can't Believe It's Not Butter spray (optional), as needed for wheat toast (*for 500-calorie meal plan only*)

Heat a nonstick frying pan (use a small frying pan for 250- and 300-calorie meal plans, use a medium-size frying pan for 400- and 500-calorie meal plans) over medium heat and coat generously with fat-free cooking spray. Sauté vegetables until tender. Add chopped ham and sauté until hot. Remove veggies and ham from pan and set aside. Clean pan to prevent Egg Beaters from sticking. Reduce heat on pan to medium low and coat with cooking spray. Once pan is hot, add eggs. As eggs begin to cook on the edges, use a spatula to gently push edges to the center of the pan. Tilt pan as needed to let eggs cook evenly all around. Once eggs are almost set, top with vegetables, ham, and cheese. Fold omelet over and heat until cheese is melted and eggs are done. Remove from pan and top with salsa, if desired. Serve omelet with fruit and enjoy. *For 500-calorie meal plans,* toast wheat bread and spray with I Can't Believe It's Not Butter spray (optional). Serve toast with omelet and fruit.

- Great way to use leftover veggies.

Protein Power Oatmeal

If you're short on time in the morning and are in need of a fast and hearty breakfast, Protein Power Oatmeal is the perfect choice. Warm, creamy oats are combined with chocolate or vanilla protein powder and natural nut butter for a fat-burning, metabolism-boosting meal.

instant oatmeal, dry, unsweetened
whey or soy protein powder, vanilla or chocolate flavored
natural almond butter or natural peanut butter
Splenda or Stevia to taste (optional)

Stir oats and water (for correct amount of water, see oatmeal package) in a bowl, and microwave on high according to package directions. Very slowly, stir in protein powder a little at a time until the mixture is smooth and creamy. Add natural almond butter or peanut butter and Splenda or Stevia, if desired, and mix well. Enjoy.

- Great for on-the-go.

- High in fiber.

- Helps to lower cholesterol.

Bacon, Egg, and Cheese Sandwich/Burrito

Our breakfast sandwich is a fun and healthy twist on a classic favorite. Egg Beaters, Canadian bacon, and sharp cheddar cheese provide muscle-building protein, while a whole-grain English muffin or wrap adds a hearty dose of filling fiber.

> fat-free cooking spray, as needed
> Canadian bacon
> Egg Beaters
> sharp cheddar cheese (*for 250- and 300-calorie meal plans,*
> *use low-fat cheddar cheese*)
> whole-wheat English muffin (*for 250- and 300-calorie meal plans,*
> *use a low carbohydrate, whole-grain wrap*)
> I Can't Believe It's Not Butter spray (optional) (*exclude for 250- and*
> *300-calorie meal plans*)
> 2 slices tomato (optional)

Heat a small frying pan over medium heat and coat with fat-free cooking spray. Once pan is hot, add slice of Canadian bacon. Cook until lightly browned on both sides and set aside. Wipe pan clean with a paper towel. Coat pan lightly with fat-free cooking spray and return to medium/low heat. Add eggs and gently scramble. Melt cheddar cheese on top. In the meantime, toast the English muffin and spray with I Can't Believe It's Not Butter spray, if desired (*exclude this step for 250- and 300-calorie meal plans*). Fill English muffin with eggs, cheese, bacon, and tomato (optional). Enjoy any leftover eggs on the side. For 250- and 300-calorie meal plans, place egg, cheese, and bacon inside of whole-grain wrap. Roll up and enjoy.

- Great for on-the-go if using a whole-grain wrap (250- and 300-calorie meal plans).

LUNCH

Cranberry Pecan Chicken Salad Wrap

A combination of low-fat mayonnaise and plain Greek yogurt is the key to our creamy, low-fat chicken salad. Sweetened, dried cranberries, crunchy pecans (*exclude pecans for 250- and 300-calorie meal plans*), and fresh tarragon add a touch of unexpected flavor and texture to this tasty wrap.

boneless, skinless chicken breast, cooked, and chopped or shredded
    (for best results, make sure chicken is tender, not dry)
light mayonnaise
1 to 2 tablespoons fat-free, plain Greek yogurt, depending on
    desired creaminess
dried cranberries
pecans, chopped (*exclude pecans for 250- and 300-calorie meal plans*)
fresh tarragon, chopped (*for 250- and 300-calorie meal plans,*
    use 2 teaspoons of tarragon; for 400- and 500-calorie meal plans,
    use 1 tablespoon tarragon)
kosher or sea salt, to taste
fresh ground black pepper, to taste
2 slices tomato (optional)
½ cup baby spinach leaves or lettuce
whole-grain, low-carbohydrate wrap

Mix the first six ingredients (chicken through tarragon) in a small bowl until well combined. Season to taste with salt and pepper. Place chicken salad mixture in wrap along with spinach leaves and sliced tomato, if desired. Roll up and enjoy.

- Great for on-the-go.

- Excellent way to use leftover chicken.

Italian Tuna Salad with Side of Fruit

Flaky, white tuna is tossed with Italian-style vegetables and dressed in tangy vinaigrette. Fresh basil is the perfect garnish for this simple yet elegant salad.

albacore tuna in water, drained and flaked
⅓ cup cherry tomatoes, cut in half
⅛ cup onion, chopped
½ cup bell pepper, green or red, chopped
Good-quality black kalamata olives, pitted and chopped
extra-virgin olive oil (*for 250- and 300-calorie meal plans, use low-fat balsamic vinaigrette dressing instead of olive oil and lemon juice; we like Newman's Own Lighten Up balsamic vinaigrette*)
2 tablespoons fresh lemon juice (*exclude from 250- and 300-calorie meal plans*)
fresh ground black pepper, to taste
1 tablespoon capers, drained
1 tablespoon chopped fresh basil
orange slices

Combine flaked tuna, vegetables, and olives in a bowl. Whisk together extra-virgin olive oil and fresh lemon juice, and drizzle over tuna mixture (*for 250- and 300-calorie meal plans, toss tuna mixture with low-fat balsamic vinaigrette*). Season to taste with black pepper, and toss gently. Top with fresh basil and capers. Serve with fruit and enjoy.

- Great way to use leftover veggies.

Spicy Turkey Club Sandwich/Wrap

If you're tired of eating the *same old* turkey sandwich day after day, try our turkey club version with a twist. Lean, low-sodium turkey is stacked high and layered between crisp turkey bacon, lettuce, tomato, cucumber, and our special hot and spicy pepper mayonnaise.

fat-free cooking spray, as needed
turkey bacon
2 slices whole-wheat bread (*for 250- and 300-calorie meal plans, use low-carb whole-wheat wrap*)
light mayonnaise
Sriracha sauce (a hot chili sauce found in the international aisle at your favorite supermarket), to taste
deli turkey breast, lean, low sodium

romaine lettuce leaves
2 slices tomato
4 slices cucumber
strawberries, rinsed and dried (*exclude strawberries for 250-calorie meal plan*)

Heat a small frying pan over medium heat. Coat pan with cooking spray and cook turkey bacon until crisp. Drain cooked bacon on a paper towel. In the meantime, toast wheat bread. Combine low-fat mayonnaise with enough Sriracha sauce to achieve desired heat (because Sriracha sauce is *very* spicy, it's best to add only a drop or two at a time). Spread spicy mayo on both slices of toasted wheat bread (*for 250- and 300-calorie meal plans, spread spicy mayo on whole-wheat wrap*). Add turkey, turkey bacon, lettuce, tomato, and cucumber slices. Serve with fruit (*exclude fruit for 250-calorie meal plan*) and enjoy.

Smoked Salmon and Cream Cheese Toasts

Instead of traditional lox and cream cheese on a bagel, lighten up with our Smoked Salmon and Cream Cheese Toasts. Whole-grain crackers are topped with low-fat cream cheese and then stacked with smoked salmon, red onion, and sliced cucumber for a vibrant and flavorful lunch.

Ak-Mak whole-grain crackers
low-fat cream cheese
smoked salmon
½ small tomato, sliced
¼ cucumber, thinly sliced
1 thin slice of red onion
fresh ground black pepper, to taste (optional)
apple (*exclude apple for 250- and 300-calorie meal plans*)

Spread approximately 1 teaspoon of cream cheese on each cracker. Top with desired amount of smoked salmon, tomato, cucumber, and onion. Season with fresh ground black pepper (optional). Enjoy any leftover smoked salmon on the side. Serve with fruit (*exclude fruit for 250- and 300-calorie meal plans*).

• Makes a great breakfast or snack, too.

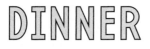

DINNER

Restaurant-Worthy Steak with Sweet Potato and Steamed Cauliflower

If you've ever gone out to eat and indulged in a perfectly juicy steak but have struggled to cook it just right at home, this recipe is for you. A flavorful, tender steak is easy to make with the right cut of beef and our simple preparation!

sweet potato
cauliflower florets
grilling cooking spray, fat free, as needed
filet mignon
kosher salt
fresh ground black pepper

For the sweet potato: Wash, scrub, and dry the sweet potato. Stab with a fork, place on a sheet pan in a 400-degree oven, and roast for approximately one hour, or until fork tender.

For the cauliflower: To steam cauliflower on stove top, bring a pot with approximately one inch of water to a boil. Place a metal steamer filled with the cauliflower florets inside the pot and place a lid on top. Steam cauliflower until tender and drain. To steam cauliflower in the microwave, place the cauliflower florets in a microwave-safe bowl with a small amount of water. Cover with plastic wrap, leaving one corner open to vent. Microwave on high until tender. Carefully remove plastic wrap, to avoid steam burn, and drain.

For the steak: Remove steak from refrigerator and let it come to room temperature (takes about 30 to 40 minutes). Spray gas grill with grilling cooking spray. Preheat the grill over medium-high heat. Five minutes before placing steak on the grill, turn heat down to medium. Season steak generously on both sides with salt and pepper. Place steak directly over flame on the grill. For medium-rare steak, cook approximately 4 to 7 minutes per side depending on size and thickness (an 8-ounce, 1¼-inch-thick filet will take about 6 minutes per side). Remove steak from grill, cover loosely with foil, and allow the meat to rest for 5 minutes to seal in juices before slicing. Serve steak with sweet potato and cauliflower and enjoy.

Indoor/Alternate Cooking Method: Remove steak from refrigerator and let it come to room temperature (takes about 30 to 40 minutes). Heat a heavy frying pan over medium heat and spray generously with regular fat-free cooking spray. Season steak generously on both sides with salt and pepper. Once pan is very hot, place steak in pan (it should sizzle). For medium-rare steak, cook approximately 5 to 7 minutes per side depending on size and thickness (an 8-ounce, 1¼-inch-thick filet will take about 6 to 7 minutes per side). Remove steak from heat, cover loosely with foil, and allow the meat to rest for 5 minutes to seal in juices.

Tips for a perfect steak:

- Season well with salt and pepper (it brings out the flavor of the meat).
- Flip steak only once and handle as little as possible.
- Cooking times will vary. To check for doneness, make a very small ¼-inch slit on the top of the steak and take a peek. If it's too rare on top, keep cooking (remember, the middle of the steak will be the rarest portion of the meat).
- Always rest steak after cooking (it will be a lot juicier).
- Practice makes perfect . . . the more you cook steak, the better you'll be at it!

Greek Brown Rice Salad with Chicken

Brown rice takes a creative turn with Greek-inspired flavors in this dish. Fresh cucumber, black olives, tomato, grilled chicken breast, and balsamic vinaigrette come together for a tasty explosion in our robust Greek Brown Rice Salad.

boneless, skinless chicken breast, cooked, and chopped or shredded (for best results, make sure chicken is tender, not dry)
brown rice, cooked
2 tablespoons chopped tomato
¼ cup chopped cucumber
½ cup arugula leaves, rough chopped
good-quality black kalamata olives, pitted and chopped
1 tablespoon chopped fresh parsley
light balsamic vinaigrette (*we like Newman's Own Lighten Up balsamic vinaigrette*)
kosher salt, to taste
fresh ground black pepper, to taste

pinch of garlic powder (optional)
pinch of oregano (optional)
Feta cheese, crumbled (*for 500-calorie meal plan only*)

Combine first 7 ingredients (chicken through the parsley) in a bowl. Add balsamic vinaigrette and toss. Season to taste with salt, pepper, garlic powder, and oregano. Top with feta cheese (*500-calorie meal plan only*). Serve at room temperature or chilled. Enjoy.

• Makes a great lunch the next day.

Seared Scallops with Brown Rice and Spinach

Perfectly caramelized, juicy sea scallops require only simple preparation and very few ingredients. Pair sautéed spinach and brown rice with our sweet and succulent scallops for an elegant meal you won't forget.

For the scallops
sea scallops
kosher salt, to taste
fresh ground black pepper, to taste
fat-free cooking spray, as needed
extra-virgin olive oil

For the spinach and brown rice
fat-free cooking spray, as needed
spinach leaves, raw
2 tablespoons chicken stock or water
kosher or sea salt, to taste
fresh ground black pepper, to taste
pinch of garlic powder
1 tablespoon fresh lemon juice
brown rice, cooked

For the scallops: Lightly rinse scallops with water and gently pat completely dry with a paper towel. Remove the beard (rough edge) of the scallop with your hands. Season scallops with salt and pepper. Heat a frying pan coated with fat-free cooking spray over medium-high heat. Brush the pan with olive oil. Once pan is hot, gently add scallops one at a time (scallops should sizzle once hitting the pan). Allow scallops to caramelize (get a golden-brown exterior) without touching or flipping them for approximately 2 to 3 minutes. Repeat on the other side. Gently remove scallops from pan.

For the spinach: Spray the same pan with fat-free cooking spray. Add spinach and chicken stock or water to pan, stir and cover. Cook approximately 2 to 3 minutes or until spinach is wilted. Season with salt, pepper, and garlic powder, and stir to combine. Squeeze fresh lemon over spinach. Serve scallops with prepared brown rice and spinach. Enjoy.

Orange Honey Mustard Pork Tenderloin with Asparagus

Our sweet and salty Orange Honey Mustard Sauce makes the perfect glaze for lean pork tenderloin. Serve sliced pork tenderloin dripping in our sticky glaze, with roasted asparagus on the side, for a simple yet sophisticated meal.

For the pork
1 pound pork tenderloin
kosher or sea salt, as needed
fresh ground black pepper, as needed
garlic powder, as needed
fat-free cooking spray, as needed

For the glaze
½ cup orange marmalade
2 tablespoons honey
1 tablespoon plus 1 teaspoon low-sodium soy sauce
1½ tablespoons mustard

For the asparagus
asparagus spears, tough ends removed
fat-free cooking spray, as needed
extra-virgin olive oil
kosher or sea salt
fresh ground black pepper

For the pork: Preheat oven to 350 degrees. Place pork on a foil-lined baking sheet and season lightly with salt, pepper, and a pinch of garlic powder. In a small saucepot, combine orange marmalade, honey, soy sauce, and mustard. Pour approximately one-quarter of the glaze in a small bowl and brush over pork tenderloin. Place pork in oven for 15 minutes. Turn pork over once and brush any leftover glaze on sheet pan back onto the pork. Continue cooking pork for approximately 17 to 22 minutes (oven times will vary) until pork is just firm and cooked throughout (pork should be just slightly pink in the thickest portion). Remove pork from the oven. While pork is cooking, bring unused glaze in saucepot to a gentle simmer over medium-low heat. Reduce heat to low. Add a little more of the glaze to top of the pork and broil on high for approximately 2 to 3 minutes, or until glaze starts to caramelize. Gently transfer pork and juices from the pan onto a plate. Cover very loosely with foil and allow to rest for 5 minutes to seal in juices.

For the asparagus: Place asparagus on a foil-lined baking sheet lightly coated with fat-free cooking spray. Drizzle with olive oil, rolling asparagus to coat evenly, and season with salt and pepper. Place in 350-degree oven, and bake for approximately 25 minutes, or until slightly caramelized. Serve your recommended portion size of sliced pork and glaze with asparagus. Enjoy!

- This glaze works great on seafood and poultry, too.
- Use leftover pork in wraps, stir-fries, and salads for the week.

Section 7—Mixing Things Up: The Food-Exchange System

The food-exchange system is a quick "go-to guide" for you to learn what food items can be exchanged for others. This system allows you to efficiently make substitutions in your meal plans. Because all foods are made up of protein, carbohydrates, and fat, or a combination of those three, there are countless items that could be included. To keep it simple, I have provided a condensed list of some of the most common and healthiest food items. Once you become comfortable with exchanging your foods and are ready to diversify your options, please see the "Simplifying Your Meals" section (Section 4). Here you will find suggestions on how to add your own food options and customize your meals.

There are four guidelines to exchanging foods in your meal plans:

1. *Your exchange system has different food categories to ensure that each item is correctly exchanged for another.* Any food can be exchanged for any other food in the same category—for example, one type of fruit for another fruit (banana for an apple, and so on). Simply look at the category that particular food belongs to, view your choices, and switch the food. Then follow the same ounce or gram recommendations. For example, if your meal plan calls for 2 ounces of broccoli, you can evenly exchange that for 2 ounces of asparagus or 2 ounces of any other vegetable.

2. *It is important to remember that your meal plans are more like food templates.* Each meal plan is designed with different combinations of protein, fat, and carbohydrates. When using the exchange system, do your best to exchange nutrients that are similar to the food items in each meal plan. For example, if you want a particular type of bread, exchange the type of bread you want for the specified bread in an existing meal that already contains bread. Exchanging food this way will ensure your that meal plans stay in line with your nutrition parameters.

3. *There are two types of measurements listed in your meal plans: weight and volume.* Weight is measured in ounces and grams. Volume is measured in cups and tablespoons. Here are the measurements used in your meal plans.

WEIGHT MEASUREMENTS	
Ounces	1 ounce = 28 grams
Grams	.75 ounce = 21 grams
	.5 ounce = 14 grams
	.25 ounce = 7 grams

VOLUME MEASUREMENTS	
Cups	1 cup = 8 ounces
Ounces	¾ cup = 6 ounces
Tablespoon	½ cup = 4 ounces
Teaspoon	¼ cup = 2 ounces
	1 tablespoon = 3 teaspoons (15 grams)
	½ tablespoon = 1.5 teaspoons (7.5 grams)
	1 teaspoon = 5 grams

It is easiest if you exchange foods within the same measurement types, though exchanging between measuring types is also possible. For example, let's say you wanted to exchange 4 ounces of a baked potato for brown rice. Brown rice is measured cooked and in cup form. If you look at the measurement charts, you see that 4 ounces equals ½ cup. So you would have ½ cup of brown rice for every 4 ounces of potato.

4. *With every system there are some exceptions to the rule.* There are four exceptions to the exchange system:

- Cottage cheese and Greek yogurt both have too much complete protein to be listed in the dairy section and not enough to be an even exchange for a lean or nonlean protein. When substituting cottage cheese or Greek yogurt, look at the calorie amount of each nutrient you are substituting. For example, 4 ounces of chicken comes to 26 grams of protein; 4 ounces of low-fat cottage cheese to 14 grams of protein. To replace low-fat cottage cheese for chicken you would need 8 ounces of cottage cheese (28 grams of protein), instead of 4 ounces of chicken (26 grams of protein).

- Avocado is the only fat that does not work in the exchange system. You can look at the calories of the fat you would like to exchange in order to figure out how much avocado to insert.

- Bread should be exchanged only for bread (since it is measured in slices), and cereal is very dense, so it should be exchanged only for other cereals.

- Beans and corn are starchy vegetables that are very dense and packed with calories. A quarter cup of corn is 40 calories; a half cup of all other vegetables is approximately 40 calories. Look at the calories of both foods you are exchanging, and make an even exchange based on that measurement.

The key to understanding exchanges is to learn about all the different proteins, fats and carbohydrates. Familiarity with your program and meal plans will teach you how to improvise and make meal adjustments without looking at a list or pulling out a calculator. As you begin the program, you should definitely use the exchange system. As your knowledge about food increases, you will become less dependent on meal plans and become more efficient at making quick meal exchanges without any lists.

IMPORTANT SOFTWARE NOTE

Some clients love exchanging foods manually and others prefer using an automated system. If the latter pertains to you, I would suggest visiting VeniceNutrition.com and experiencing the fully automated food exchange and meal building system of Venice Nutrition Online.

FOOD CATEGORIES OF YOUR EXCHANGE SYSTEM

Protein

Complete Protein—Lean

These items are complete sources of protein (meaning they come from an animal or soy) and are low in fat or fat free. Refer to the "Quality of Food" chart on page 106 to learn more about which protein sources are the highest quality.

Bison

Bison

Dairy

Cottage cheese, nonfat
Cottage cheese, low fat
Greek yogurt, nonfat
Greek yogurt, low fat

Fish and Seafood

Catfish
Clams
Cod
Crab
Halibut
Lobster
Mahimahi
Oysters
Scallops
Sea bass
Sea trout

Shrimp
Snapper
Swordfish
Tilapia
Tuna, ahi
Tuna, albacore (water
  packed)
Tuna steak
Yellowtail

Pork

Ham, Boar's Head brand,
  deli meat, low sodium
Pork tenderloin

Poultry

Chicken breast, boneless/
  skinless
Chicken breast, sandwich
  meat, Boar's Head brand,
  deli meat, low sodium

Egg Beaters
Egg whites
Ground turkey (99% fat
  free)
Turkey breast, boneless/
  skinless
Turkey breast, Boar's Head
  brand, deli meat, low
  sodium

Protein Powder

Egg-white protein powder
Soy protein powder
Whey protein powder

Complete Protein—Nonlean

These items are complete sources of protein (they come from animal or soy) and are high in fat. Refer to the "Quality of Food" chart on page 106 to learn more about which protein sources are the highest quality.

Beef

Filet mignon
Flank steak
Ground beef (extra-lean; 96%–99% fat free)
London broil
Rib eye
Roast beef (chuck trimmed)
Round tip
T-bone
Top round
Top sirloin
Veal

Fish

Orange roughy
Salmon, fresh
Salmon, smoked
Sardines (oil packed, drained)
Tuna (solid, white, in oil)

Lamb

Lamb chop (center cut)

Pork

Baby back ribs
Canadian bacon
Pork bacon
Pork chop, trimmed

Poultry

Chicken thigh
Eggs (whole)
Ground turkey (93% fat free)
Turkey bacon
Turkey thigh (fresh, dark meat)

Complete Protein—Dairy and Soy (Lean and Nonlean)

Why are these dairy and soy items in their *own* category? Well, all dairy and soy items are complete proteins, and, with the exception of cottage cheese and Greek yogurt, most contain less protein per serving than the lean and nonlean proteins presented above. For that reason, lean (low in fat) and nonlean (higher in fat) dairy sources as well as soy are listed here. Always check nutrition labels on these dairy and soy items to learn more about their nutritional breakdown and how to best incorporate them into your meals. The only food item that can be eaten as a meal by itself is edamame. Soy milk can be evenly exchanged for all other milks.

Dairy—Lean

Lactaid (lactose-free milk), skim or 1% fat
Milk, skim, nonfat
Milk, 1% fat

Dairy—Nonlean

Cheese, Brie
Cheese, cheddar, low fat
Cheese, cheddar
Cheese, Colby
Cheese, feta
Cheese, goat

Cheese, Jack
Cheese, mozzarella, low fat
Cheese, mozzarella
Cheese, mozzarella, string
Cheese, Muenster
Cheese, Parmesan
Cheese, provolone

Cheese, ricotta, low fat
Cheese, ricotta, whole
Cheese, Romano
Cheese, Swiss
Milk, reduced fat (2% fat)

Milk, whole
Milk, goat
Yogurt, plain, low fat
Yogurt, plain, whole

Soy

Soy milk
Edamame

Carbohydrates

Fruits and Vegetables

Whole fruits and vegetables are an excellent source of carbohydrates because they contain more fiber and nutrients than juice. Because whole fruits and veggies are natural and not processed, they are better for your health and blood-sugar levels. Fruit juice will typically spike your blood-sugar levels. If possible, you should avoid exchanging fruit juice for the items found in your meal plans. If you love juice, drink it in moderation.

Fruit

Apple
Applesauce
Bananas
Blackberries
Blueberries
Cantaloupe
Cherries

Cranberries
Grape juice
Grapefruit
Grapes
Honeydew melon
Nectarines
Oranges

Peaches
Pears
Pineapple
Raspberries
Strawberries
Watermelon

Low-Calorie Vegetables

These vegetables are very low in calories and carbohydrates. When used in small amounts, they are considered "free foods" (that is, you can add them to any meal at any time without worrying about additional calories). For example, it's fine to add lettuce, tomato, and onion to any sandwich for extra flavor and texture.

Arugula leaves
Cucumber

Lettuce
Onion

Tomato
Peppers, jalapeño

Vegetables

Asparagus
Beans (all)
Beets
Black-eyed peas
Broccoli
Brussels sprouts
Carrots
Cauliflower

Collard greens
Corn
Eggplant
Garden salad (lettuce and vegetables)
Mushrooms
Peas, green
Peppers, green and red

Snow peas
Spinach
Squash (all)
Tomato juice
Tomato sauce
Vegetables, mixed
Zucchini

Grains and Potatoes

When choosing grain products—whether it's bread, pasta, cereal, rice, or crackers—aim for the whole-grain or whole-wheat version with a *minimum of 2 grams of fiber per serving*. Whole grains with plenty of fiber, particularly unprocessed, natural items like brown rice and oats, will help stabilize blood-sugar levels best and keep you satisfied longer. Refer to the "Quality of Food" chart on page 106 to learn more about which grains are the highest quality and will yield you the best results.

Limiting the amount of snacks and crackers while aiming for more higher-quality carbohydrates like fruits and vegetables will help to better stabilize blood-sugar levels and assist in achieving faster results.

Bread / Quick Breads / Wraps

Bagels (all flavors)
Bread (all kinds and flavors)
English muffins (all flavors)
Tortilla wraps

Hot and Cold Cereals

Cold cereal (all flavors)
Cereal, corn grits
Cereal, Cream of Rice
Cereal, Cream of Wheat
Cereal, granola (low fat or fat free)

Cereal, oatmeal (unsweetened)

Rice, Pasta, and Potatoes

Couscous
Pasta
Potatoes, white
Potatoes, red
Potatoes, sweet
Quinoa
Rice, brown
Rice, basmati
Yams

Snacks and Crackers

Chips, baked
Chips, tortilla, baked
Crackers (all)
Popcorn, light
Pretzels
Rice cakes

Miscellaneous Carbohydrates

Because these items are high in sugar and lack nutritional value, they should be eaten sparingly.

Syrup, Jams, Jellies, etc.

BBQ sauce
Honey
Jam (all flavors)
Jelly (all flavors)
Marmalade (all flavors)

Splenda, Brown Sugar Blend
   for Baking
Splenda, Sugar Blend for
   Baking
Sugar

Syrup, regular
Syrup, low sugar

Fats

Fats with Incomplete Proteins

The following fats contain incomplete sources of protein (meaning they contain nonanimal or nonsoy, vegetarian sources of protein). These items should be counted only as fat grams when implementing them into your meal plans. When choosing nuts, aim for unsalted and raw. Natural nut butters are healthier and a better choice than processed nut butters because they do not contain sugar or hydrogenated fat.

Nuts (all kinds; for example, almonds)

Nut butters (all kinds; for example peanut butter)

Sunflower seeds

Fats Without Proteins

The following fats contain little to no sources of protein. These items should be counted only as fat grams when implementing them into your meal plans. Natural fat sources such as olive oil and avocado are better for your heart and health than processed fats like sour cream and butter. Please refer to the "Quality of Food" chart on page 106 to learn more about the highest-quality fat sources.

Avocado
Butter
Cream cheese, low fat (*consider this a fat, not dairy, since it has only 1 gram of protein*)

Cream cheese, whole (*consider this a fat, not dairy, since it has only 1 gram of protein*)
Flaxseed, ground
Guacamole

Margarine
Mayonnaise
Mayonnaise, light
Olives
Sour cream
Salad dressings (all)

Canola oil	Flaxseed oil	Vegetable oil
Coconut oil	Olive oil	
Fish oil gelcaps	Peanut oil	

Meal Replacements

Because there are countless protein bars and shakes available in today's market, the brand of meal replacement you choose is up to you. I recommend that you aim for a protein bar or ready-to-drink shake that closely matches your caloric and nutrient ratio parameters, to help stabilize your blood sugar. Here is a list of some of the more balanced protein bars and shakes available. *Venice Nutrition does not specifically endorse nor is associated with any particular meal-replacement product.*

Protein Bars

When choosing a protein bar, look for one that matches or comes close to matching your personal nutritional parameters and has a good balance of protein, carbohydrates, and fat. Protein bars are an excellent meal replacement when you're too busy for whole food or simply on the go. The following protein bars are what I recommend.

| Cliff Builders Protein Bar (all flavors) | Odyssey Bar (all flavors) | Think Thin Bar (all flavors) |
| Detour Bar (all flavors) | Pure Protein Bar (all flavors) | |

Power Crunch (all flavors) **Note:** This bar is made with hydrolyzed whey protein (section 2, explained in strategy 12). It is higher in fat and lower in carbohydrates. Even though the bar's nutrient ratios will not match your ratios, this bar does digest efficiently and should keep your blood sugar stable. For this reason, you can use this bar in your meals.

Protein Drinks

Whereas some ready-to-drink protein shakes are balanced, others may require that you add a food item on the side to match your nutritional parameters. For example, if a premade protein shake contains only protein and fat, you can add a carbohydrate, such as fruit on the side, to create a balanced meal.

Bio-rhythm, Whole Grains Meal Replacement (any flavor)

Lean Body—Ready to Drink Shake, Regular (any flavor)

Muscle Milk—Regular (any flavor)

Muscle Milk—Ready to Drink—Carb Conscious (any flavor)

Muscle Milk–Light (any flavor)

Myoplex (EAS)—Ready to Drink Shake, low carb (any flavor) **Note:** With this shake, you must add a fat (for example, almonds) and a carbohydrate (for example, an apple) to complete the meal.

Myoplex (EAS)—Ready to Drink, Regular (any flavor)

Proto Whey (BNRG) (any flavor)

Pure Protein Shake (any flavor) **Note:** With this shake, you must add a fat (for example, almonds) and a carbohydrate (for example, an apple) to complete the meal.

Premade Desserts

Low-Calorie Desserts

Any balanced lifestyle includes an occasional indulgence like dessert. The following dessert options are low in calories and should be eaten following a balanced meal. (Just lower the carbohydrates in the meal itself to make room for the calories and carbs in the dessert.)

Angel food cake

Cool Whip topping, sugar free (tablespoon)

Frozen Fruit Bar (all flavors)

Ice cream, light (all flavors)

Jell-O pudding snack (all types and flavors)

Popsicle (all flavors)

Condiments, Seasonings, Spices, Etc.

"Free Foods"

In general, condiments, seasonings, and spices provide little nutritional value or calories and can be considered "free foods." The following is a list of food items that you can use to flavor and season your meals. These "free foods" will keep your food "tasty" and provide an excellent feeling of variety.

Condiments

Butter spray, I Can't Believe It's Not Butter or Pam

Capers

Horseradish

Hot sauce

Ketchup

Lemon juice

Lime juice

Mustard

Relish

Salsa

Soy sauce (regular and low sodium)

Sriracha sauce

Vinegar (all flavors)

Worcestershire sauce

Herbs, Dried or Fresh

Basil

Chives

Cilantro

Dill

Fennel

Mint

Oregano

Parsley

Rosemary

Sage

Tarragon

Thyme

Seasonings, Spices, and Flavorings

Allspice

Almond extract

Cayenne pepper

Chili powder

Cinnamon

Cumin

Garlic powder

Garlic, minced

Ginger

Lemon pepper

Mrs. Dash

Nutmeg

Onion powder

Paprika

Pepper, black

Pepper, white

Red pepper flakes

Salt

Vanilla bean

Vanilla extract

Calorie-Free Sugar Substitutes

Equal

Splenda

Sweet'N Low

Stevia and Truvia—*Recommended*. (Stevia and Truvia are made from a sweet herb that is plant based. Because they are natural, Stevia and Truvia are considered the healthiest sweeteners on the market.)

Section 8—Becoming an Expert on Your Nutrition

Chelsea Handler is one of the kindest, most generous, passionate, and, of course, funniest people I have ever known. She is truly an inspiration to me and is one of my favorite people in this world. She is family to me. As Chelsea shared in the foreword, our friendship began many years ago. I have watched her career and life get busier and busier as each year passes, yet regardless of her full schedule, she has always remained committed to the most important thing in her life: her health. I asked Chelsea to write the foreword to this book because she embodies what the Venice Nutrition program is all about. Chelsea, like all of us, has her great nutritional days and her challenging nutritional days. She is a real person. She falls off her plan, she loves to drink her vodka, and she enjoys food.

When I first started working with Chelsea, the goal was never for her to follow a "program" the rest of her life. The goal was for her to learn, through the Venice Nutrition program, to become an expert on her nutrition and her body. This is the education that will provide the freedom and Body Confidence we all want with our health. It is a powerful feeling to know that no matter what life throws at you, you will always have control over your health and how you choose to take care of yourself. The knowledge that at any moment you possess the tools to dial yourself back in is powerful. This is why Chelsea has become such an inspiration. She values her health as much as every other part of her life, and she has become an expert on her nutrition. Chelsea knows what works for her and how far she can push the limits. She also knows when she needs to "raise her game." If her weight or body fat goes up a bit, she doesn't panic or get frustrated. She understands why it went up and simply makes the proper adjustments to quickly drop back to her desired range. The sense of control about her body that Chelsea now possesses—as well as the other the testimonials in this book—exemplifies the results of becoming an expert on your nutrition.

So How Do You Become an Expert on Your Nutrition?

We are all different. Certain things that work for me or that work for Chelsea may not work for you. Becoming an expert on your nutrition means taking all the information in this chapter and molding it into your world. The program will provide you with the nutrition foundation and structure. You need to take that knowledge, infuse it with your personal food preferences, and work the result into your lifestyle.

As you implement the information in this chapter, it is important to remember that your nutrition creates balance within your body. Dieting uses deprivation to force your body to drop weight. This is the main difference between dieting and blood-sugar stabilization. Your nutrition plan will create the ability for your body to consistently release stored body fat, and will provide the environment for your body to build muscle mass (if that is the goal). The way you get your body to burn that fat and build muscle mass is to follow your exercise plan.

. . .

Let's get moving on to chapter 6 and dial in the final component of your Body Confidence Plan.

6

ACTIVATING YOUR ENGINE

Your nutrition releases your stored fat, and your exercise burns up that fat.

I joined my first health club when I was sixteen years old. I was all fired up, eager to get stronger for soccer. Within the first week I became friends with Jon, the owner. Jon was a walking specimen of health. He was lean, fit, and muscular—what most sixteen-year-old males aspire to look like. He was in his fifties, had worked in and owned many gyms since his late twenties, and came to possess a vast amount of knowledge about nutrition and fitness. I have always been one to ask questions (*imagine that!*), so whenever I saw Jon, I would pull out my list of questions and fire away. Thinking back to those times, I know he had the patience of a saint, since my list was long. Initially my questions for Jon were about how I could continue improving my strength and athletic ability. I was training very hard, and my body was improving more each day.

As I continued to progress, gym members began to ask me what I was doing in my workouts, since they could see the progress I was making. The more members I spoke with, the more I became aware of a strange pattern:

it seemed that practically every member of the gym was stuck. Every day I walked into the club and saw the same people doing the same exercises and looking the same. I thought maybe their goals were to maintain. So the next time a member asked me what I was doing, I asked her if her goal was to maintain. Hey, what did I know? I was sixteen. Looking daggers at me, she replied, "Of course not! I work out six days a week, and for what? My body just stays the same." She was quite frustrated. It puzzled me that I was getting great results and no one else in the club seemed to be making any kind of progress. The next time I saw Jon, I chased him down to find the answer.

I told Jon what I had observed. Why did everyone seem to, at the very best, maintain their physiques? Jon looked at me with a big smile and said, "Good question. I wish more people would ask it. The answer is fairly simple. Besides eating healthy [this was 1988, when a low-fat diet was all the rage and very few people taught blood-sugar stabilization], there are three things people need to do to maximize their results with exercise. They need to work out smart, challenge themselves, and enjoy their exercise." I thought to myself that this seemed pretty easy.

Jon continued: "Most people are creatures of habit and resist change. They find a routine and want to stick to it, never really pushing themselves beyond their initial routine. What they do not understand is that their body quickly adapts to that routine. Shaking it up is the only way to progress. This is why people need to work out smarter, learn how to mix up their exercise, and challenge themselves while they are working out." As he spoke, it all began to make sense. All the members who struggled to progress appeared to just go through the motions with their workouts, never diversifying or challenging themselves.

Jon continued with his last point: "People enjoy their exercise because it is new and fresh, but we both know that the same exercises every single day can become monotonous. This monotony takes the fun out of exercise, and when the fun is removed, exercise burnout follows close behind. This type of thinking is exactly why most people's health results progress initially, then shift to maintenance [better known as a plateau], leading to burnout and then, unfortunately, regression. This cycle eventually repeats itself." Within about five minutes, Jon taught me the three most important points I would ever need to know about exercise.

Fast-forward to the present, and Jon's three simple points are as true now as they were then. I have been a member of many gyms since I was sixteen, and every gym reminds me of my first. The majority of the members do not achieve the results they want. They seem to just be going through the motions. I see the same thing with non–gym members. Many people do just enough exercise to feel like they are doing something. I think the main reason that people go through the motions with their exercise is that we are subjected to continual false promotions about exercise. Almost every time I turn on the TV or read a magazine, there seems to be an advertisement about some amazing piece of exercise equipment or some new training method that will give you the body you have always dreamed of. Ad after ad proclaims that it will take only minutes each day to get you abs of steel. Many times, this advertising hype succeeds because people don't know any better. People just do not know enough about exercise to sift through the "hype" and discover the truth. It's time to learn about exercise, solidify your exercise plan, and activate your engine—the final component of your Body Confidence Plan.

Over the years, I have taken Jon's three simple points and developed an exercise system that activates the majority of the body's muscle fibers (your engine). This is the key with exercise. Since fat is primarily burned in muscle, the more muscle you activate during exercise, the more fat you burn (as long as your blood sugar is stable). In addition, if your goal is to increase muscle mass, by performing movements that activate the majority of your muscle fiber you will build the maximum amount of muscle.

Now think about your current exercise routine (if you have one), and ask yourself these three questions:

- Am I working out smart?

- Am I challenging myself?

- Am I passionate about my exercise?

Maybe you feel you are doing great with your exercise. Maybe you are just getting by. Maybe your exercise is nonexistent. Whatever your answers to these questions are, they are not important right now. What is important is that you are asking the right questions. My purpose in writing this chapter is to help you design your exercise plan and, most important, to provide you with enough knowledge to accurately answer yes to the three questions I just posed. These three questions will forever be your litmus test to verify whether you are optimizing your workouts. Whether your Goal Type is 1 or 2, this exercise information applies to you. The only difference between Goal Types will be the prescribed workouts presented later in this chapter.

Now, let's get you working out smarter!

In a nutshell, working out smarter means exercising in a correct and efficient manner. As you have learned, your goal is to optimize each system in your body. To optimize the main systems in your body that are positively impacted through exercise (your muscular, cardiovascular [circulatory], respiratory, endocrine, nervous, and digestive systems), you must first understand the different categories of exercise and the purpose of each.

There are two categories of exercise:

Category 1—Cardiovascular exercise

Category 2—Strength training

Both of these categories have core principles (just as your nutrition has core principles), and once you understand and implement these core principles, you will immediately be working out smarter. In addition, with solid core principles at hand, you will have limitless options for different exercises within each type (similar to limitless food options).

ONE IMPORTANT NOTE PERTAINING TO YOUR EXERCISE PLAN

As I mentioned, my goal in this section is to provide you with the core principles of exercise so you can work out smarter. There are thousands of qualified health professionals, classes, and videos that do a fantastic job of teaching technique and exercise diversity. It is impossible to provide the type of detail in a book format that a one-on-one session, class, or video would provide. In addition, each of our bodies is physically stronger as well as physically weaker in particular areas. The more hands-on learning you get from a qualified health professional about correct exercise technique and preferences, the better. For these reasons, I will focus on teaching you to optimize your exercise, and defer to my fellow health professionals to help maximize your exercise technique and preferences.

Exercise Category 1—Cardio

Cardio is the category of exercise that, by far, burns the highest amount of body fat. *Cardio* is short for *cardiovascular* and is defined as any movement that increases your heart rate and improves your overall cardiovascular system (blood flow and oxygen uptake). Cardio is the most commonly performed exercise and, unfortunately, the least optimized. People do put time aside for their cardio; yet most of the time, they are just performing it at only 30 percent efficiency. Performing inefficient cardio is one of the biggest reasons people seem not to progress very often when they work out. Many times, we think that if we are putting the time into doing cardio, that should be enough to get results. This is just not the case. Results are obtained from working out smarter. The good news is that performing cardio correctly does not require more time; it just allows you to use that time to become better. Cardio can be broken down into five core principles. Once you know and implement these principles, you will perform your cardio more effectively than ever before.

IMPORTANT NOTE

Before we dive into the five principles of cardio I would like to introduce you to the most effective injury prevention technique . . . stretching. A key to helping you stay injury free is increasing your flexibility through stretching. I recommend that you do a full-body stretch five days a week between 10 to 20 minutes per session, preferably before exercise and after a little warmup (muscles stretch better when they are warm). If you are new to stretching I recommend taking a yoga or stretching class, or perhaps purchasing a video. Classes and videos are great ways to learn a solid stretching routine. Stretching consistently each week will ensure your body stays flexible and prepared for all activity.

The five core principles of cardio are these:

1. Implement the two types of cardio.

2. Cardio selection affects how much fat you burn.

3. Cardio intensity and duration matter.

4. Your oxygen line (heart rate) determines everything.

5. Cardio technique is extremely important.

The Two Types of Cardio

Think of a world-class marathon runner's body—very lean, with a small frame. A marathon runner's body is designed to run miles upon miles. Now think about the body of a world-class sprinter—lean, muscular, and with a larger frame. A sprinter's body is designed to explosively exert its muscles over short distances. A marathon runner and a sprinter are extreme examples of the two different types of skeletal muscle we have in our bodies. Skeletal muscle is the muscle you control and use on a daily basis, whether you are walking across the hall, picking up a pen, or scratching your head. It is also the muscle you use when you exercise.

There are two types of skeletal muscle: red and white. On average, most of us have 50 percent red muscle and 50 percent white muscle. Red muscle is called "red" because it is full of blood vessels. As long as oxygen is present (meaning when you are not out of breath), it is the muscle we use. White muscle is exactly that—white. Your white muscle is not designed for long activity; it is the muscle you use when you need to dodge a speeding car or sprint across a room. Your white muscle fibers are the ones designed for explosive movement. Your red muscle fibers are the ones used for slow-paced and methodical movement.

Think back to the example of the marathon runner and sprinter, and it makes sense why each is great at their particular sport. A marathon runner's body typically has more red muscle than white muscle, and a sprinter's body typically has more white muscle than red. This is why each athlete is so gifted at their particular sport. Their dominant muscle allows them to excel at a world-class level.

As I mentioned, each of us has a fifty–fifty ratio of red and white muscle on average. This is really important to understand, since your fat is burned in muscle. If you are doing exercise that recruits only one type of muscle (red or white) and not the other, you are activating only 50 percent of your muscle to burn fat. This means the other 50 percent is not being utilized! This is exactly why people hit plateaus they cannot break through. Their workouts are usually recruiting only one type of muscle: red.

You Must Work Both Your Red and White Muscle

It is pretty easy to determine which type of muscle you are using, because there is only one factor that determines this: the availability of oxygen.

Simply put, if you have a steady flow of oxygen (not huffing and puffing), you are using your red muscle. If you are out of breath, you are primarily using your white muscle. There are two types of cardio that specifically work your red and white muscle. One is *fat burning,* which has consistent oxygen and works your red muscle (fat-burning cardio is also called *aerobic,* which means with oxygen); the other is *high intensity* (also called *interval training*), which lacks consistent oxygen and works your white muscle (also called *anaerobic,* meaning without oxygen). Another way to tell what type of muscle you are using is to notice when your muscle begins to experience a burning sensation or reaches total exhaustion. Think of a time when you ran as fast as you could and within seconds began to feel a burning sensation in your legs. Then, with every additional step, the burn became more intense until eventually you reached exhaustion, stopping your sprint and gasping for air. That burning feeling was caused by not getting enough oxygen to your muscles. Lactic acid was the culprit. Lactic acid is created by your body at times of insufficient oxygen levels and is how your body can temporarily continue providing energy to your muscles so they can keep working. Eventually, if you continue at the same intensity level, your muscles will produce too much lactic acid and reach total exhaustion. This is why when you were sprinting you had to stop eventually. Your legs simply reached their lactic acid threshold.

Also, there are times when your muscles reach total exhaustion and you don't feel an unbearable burning sensation. This occurs when you have not performed cardio for a while and your cardiovascular system (the system that supplies oxygen and blood to your muscles) is out of shape. When you are out of shape and sprinting, you may reach exhaustion before you feel an intense burning sensation in your legs. This is caused by your cardiovascular system's inability to absorb enough oxygen to allow a continued sprint. In this case, your entire cardiovascular system fell victim to fatigue before your leg muscles. With exercise, your conditioning system will eventually improve, and with it your body's ability to efficiently deliver oxygen and blood to working muscles. Whether you reach exhaustion by reaching your lactic acid threshold or by a fatigued and out-of-shape cardiovascular system, when you are out of breath you are working your white muscle.

If you do not encounter a burning sensation (lactic acid) or reach total exhaustion, you are working your red muscle.

There are two myths about lactic acid. The first is that lactic acid is bad for your muscles. This is the furthest thing from the truth. Lactic acid is what your body makes at times of insufficient oxygen levels to provide energy to your muscles. This is a good thing. The second myth is that lactic acid causes muscle soreness. This also has no validity. Lactic acid is quickly removed from your muscle by your bloodstream. Muscle soreness is actually the result of minor tears in your muscle fibers. Whenever your muscles are overloaded or pushed beyond their comfort zone, they become damaged. Your body's response to this damage is to increase the size of that muscle, strengthening it so that the next time it gets overloaded or pushed beyond its limits, it will better be able to handle the challenge. The soreness you feel is the damage in your muscle. It leaves once your muscle is repaired. The good news is that your muscle is now bigger and stronger than it was before, which increases your metabolism. Muscle soreness is necessary if you want to increase your lean body mass.

Examples of Fat-Burning and High-Intensity Cardio Exercises

Since any exercise that has consistent oxygen is fat-burning cardio and any exercise that does not have consistent oxygen is high-intensity cardio, many of the same exercises can be of either type. The intensity level (out of breath or not out of breath) at which you perform your exercise determines which type of cardio you are performing. Here are some examples of each type of cardio. (These exercises are examples of some of your cardio options.)

> **Fat burning**—Walking, hiking, jogging, stair climbing, cycling, jumping rope, swimming, rowing, using an elliptical trainer. (Each of these movements is fat burning as long as a steady supply of oxygen is available.)

> **High intensity**—Sprinting, spinning, running up stairs, any of the movements listed under "Fat burning" performed with bursts of speed. (Each of these movements is high intensity as long as each has a sixty-second "moment of explosion." This means you need to exercise when you are out of breath [completely winded] for sixty seconds, fol-

lowed by a recovery period of one to two minutes when you can catch your breath. Then, you repeat.)

IMPORTANT NOTE

If your goal is to gain weight (Goal Type 2), you will not be performing high-intensity cardio in your exercise plan. The high-intensity level of the cardio works against gaining weight because it triggers your body to shed excess weight due to the intervals of high heart rates. For this reason, you will be performing only fat-burning cardio. This strategy is presented in your workout routine at the end of this section.

Cardio Selection

Each of your cardio exercises has a difference in quality, similar to the way your foods vary in quality.

There are two factors that determine the quality of a cardio exercise. They are:

1. **The amount of muscle the exercise recruits.** You would think that if you were walking on a treadmill on a 15 percent incline, for the same duration and at the same intensity level as on a stationary bike, you would burn the same amount of energy. Even though it seems to make sense, there is a big difference between walking on a treadmill on an incline and using a stationary bike. Since your fat is primarily burned in muscle, your goal is to choose the exercises that recruit the maximum amount of muscle fibers. A treadmill on a 15 percent incline (while you're not holding the handrails) recruits approximately twice as much muscle as a stationary bike. This means that in the same exercise time, by doing a high-quality exercise, you are actually burning twice the amount of fat!

2. **The level of impact the exercise has on the body.** Your body is designed to react to stressors. For this reason, the level of impact an exercise has on your body affects your results. For example, jogging or sprinting is considered a high-impact exercise due to the force of your foot impacting with the ground. Stair climbing or walking is

considered low impact since your foot still makes contact, just at a much lower force. Swimming or cycling is considered nonimpact since your foot does not make impact with the ground during the exercise. The level of impact you choose depends on the health of your body as well as your goals.

Typically, high-impact movements are the best exercises to perform when attempting to drop weight. They stimulate your nervous system while informing your body to shed weight in order to reduce the overall impact of the exercise. (Less body weight equals less overall impact during cardio.) High-impact exercises can wear your body down, so I do not recommend that they be your only form of cardio. Nonimpact exercises are beneficial, especially for people with joint problems; however, since there is no impact, they do not shed body weight and fat at the same rate as high- and low-impact movements.

Overall, low-impact exercises are your best choice. They provide enough stimulus for your body to drop any extra weight, they strengthen your bones, and the impact is too low to create negative stress on your body (which high-impact exercise can).

Here is a list of high-quality exercises compared with low-quality exercises.

Fat-Burning Cardio Exercises

High-quality fat-burning exercises:

Jogging—Since jogging is a high-impact exercise, you should jog on dirt, grass, sand, a track, a treadmill, or any other soft surface. Be cautious of jogging on asphalt or concrete, since both of these surfaces do not absorb the impact of your foot on the ground. This lack of absorption will force the energy back into your leg. Over time, running on asphalt or concrete will most likely cause an injury to one or both of your legs.

Walking—Walking outside on hills, or on a treadmill with an incline (preferably at a 15 percent incline), recruits more muscle than walking on a flat surface.

Climbing stairs (bleachers or stair-climber machine)

Lower-quality fat-burning exercises (nonimpact; does not recruit maximum muscle fibers):

Elliptical trainer

Swimming*

Rowing*

Road cycling and mountain biking*

Stationary bike

High-Intensity Cardio Exercises

As you can see, these exercises are similar to the ones listed in the fat-burning cardio section. Remember that the only difference between fat-burning and high-intensity cardio is the intensity level (oxygen availability) of each. For this reason, the same exercise can be used to perform each type of cardio.

High-quality high-intensity exercises:

Sprinting—Since sprinting is the highest-impact exercise you can perform, the same suggestions given earlier about exercise surfaces when jogging also apply to sprinting.

Running stairs (bleachers or stair-climber machine)

Lower-quality high-intensity exercises (nonimpact; does not recruit maximum muscle fiber):

Elliptical trainer

Swimming*

Rowing*

Spinning

Road cycling and mountain biking*

Stationary bike

*The only exception is when you are road cycling, mountain biking, rowing, or swimming at a sport level (some form of competition training). In this case, these exercises are high quality due to the increased muscle-fiber recruitment caused by the high level athletes train at. This information also applies to the high-intensity cardio exercises presented next.

Once you review your prescribed workouts (at the end of this section), you will achieve better results and break through all plateaus by performing the high-quality cardio selections.

Cardio Intensity and Duration Matter

Your cardio intensity and duration matter because your red and white muscles both respond to different intensity levels and durations. As I mentioned earlier, the amount of available oxygen during exercise determines what type of muscle you use and what type of cardio you perform. The easiest way to monitor the availability of oxygen is by watching your heart rate. Your heart rate increases (measured in beats per minute, or BPM) during exercise. Your exercise intensity level determines whether your heart rate places you in fat-burning mode (moderate heart rate; between 130 and 145 BPM) or high-intensity mode (high heart rate, out of breath; 150 to 175 BPM).

Your Cardio Target Heart Rate

Standard heart-rate formulas are outdated and suggest too low a heart rate for both types of cardio. Training at this lower rate will cause less muscle to be activated and less fat to be burned during the cardio session.

The best heart-rate ranges for you to maintain are:

- Heart rate for fat-burning cardio: 135 to 145 BPM (do your best to keep it at 140 to 145)

- Heart rate for high-intensity cardio: 150 to 175 BPM (do your best to achieve 165 to 175)

Of course, if you have any type of heart disease, consult your doctor about what your heart rate should be.

Three Ways to Measure Your Heart Rate

There are three easy ways to ensure that you are in the correct heart-rate range for your type of cardio:

1. **Wear a heart-rate monitor.** You can get one online or from any sporting-goods store. It is a valuable tool. It will increase your

268

awareness and guarantee that you are maximizing your cardio. You can purchase a good-quality heart rate monitor for fifty to one hundred dollars. I recommend the Polar brand.

2. **Use your cardio machine.** The cardio machines found at the majority of gyms come with sensors that will monitor your heart rate.

3. **Focus on your perceived exertion.** This is definitely less technical and still works great. Basically this means that if you feel you can work harder at your fat-burning cardio (without getting winded), then work harder. If you feel you can push harder on your high-intensity cardio, then push harder.

Your Cardio Duration

To answer the question of how long your cardio sessions should last, I must first explain another difference between your red and white muscle. Your red muscle, since it is designed to work for long periods of time, utilizes both glucose and fat for energy. On the other hand, your white muscle, since it is meant for quick bursts of energy, utilizes only glucose. This is really important when we are talking about cardio duration. Fat-burning cardio does burn fat. The longer your cardio session, the more fat you burn during the session. High-intensity cardio is the opposite. Any high-intensity cardio that gets performed for too long causes your body to begin converting muscle into energy. Since high-intensity cardio utilizes only glucose, after about thirty-five minutes your body runs out of its energy supply. This triggers the same reaction as low blood-sugar levels. Your body begins consuming muscle and converting it to glucose in an effort to provide your body with fuel.

In addition, whereas fat-burning cardio is performed with a consistent heart rate through the entire session, high-intensity cardio is done in intervals. If you are performing thirty-five minutes of high-intensity cardio, you will perform a sixty-second burst of speed, taking your heart rate up to the 160–175 range, then slow down for one to two minutes, bringing your heart rate down to the 120–130 range (regain your breath), and then repeat your one-minute explosion. You would follow the same pattern for the entire duration of your high-intensity cardio. During your recovery time, it is important that you walk or move as slowly as possible. This will get your breath back fast, so you can perform another sixty-second sprint. So . . . if high-intensity cardio uses only glucose for fuel, how does it burn fat?

High-intensity cardio impacts your body's fat-burning ability in three ways:

1. **It depletes your glucose stores,** which increases your appetite and stimulates your body to burn more fat.

2. **It puts high demands on your cardiovascular system,** which accelerates your metabolism for twenty-four to forty-eight hours.

3. **It vastly improves your entire cardiovascular system.** This increase in your conditioning allows you to burn more body fat in everything you do, twenty-four hours a day.

These facts explain why implementing the correct cardio duration is critical to achieving your Body Confidence goals.

Here are the duration guidelines for each type of cardio:

1. **Fat-Burning Cardio**

    a. **Duration per session—thirty to sixty minutes** (fat-burning cardio should always be done for at least thirty minutes, and depending on goal type can go beyond sixty minutes per session).

2. **High-Intensity Cardio**

    a. **Duration per session—twenty to thirty-five minutes** (thirty to thirty-five minutes is the optimal duration for high-intensity cardio. You should *never* go over thirty-five minutes per session without refueling) as explained in the note below.

    b. **All high-intensity cardio is performed in interval fashion,** meaning sixty seconds of speed burst at 160–175 BPM, followed by one to two minutes of recovery, bringing your heart rate to 120–130 BPM, and then repeating this pattern through the entire duration.

IMPORTANT NOTE

If you train in a high-intensity sport (like basketball, cycling, tennis, soccer . . .) that requires more than thirty-five minutes of high-intensity cardio, it is important that you eat throughout your sport to prevent your blood sugar from crashing. You can eat pieces of a protein bar or sip on a balanced protein shake during your activity. This continual fuel supply will keep your blood sugar stable and provide your body the nutrients it needs.

Your Oxygen Line (Heart Rate) Determines Everything

Whenever I discuss cardio I reference a person's "oxygen line." Your oxygen line is an imaginary line that, when crossed, takes you into high-intensity cardio or back into fat-burning cardio. This is a line that is established once you become familiar with both your fat-burning and high-intensity heart rates. Once you know your oxygen line, you will always be clear on which type of cardio (fat burning or high intensity) and what type of muscle (red or white) you are working. This knowledge will enable you to perform your cardio smarter than before. Here is an illustration that recaps your oxygen line and all the points covered so far in this cardio section:

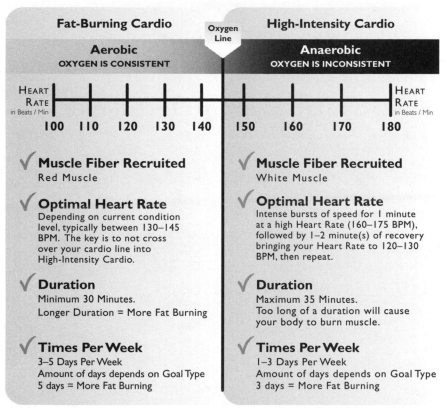

Maximizing Your Cardio

Fat-Burning Cardio	Oxygen Line	High-Intensity Cardio
Aerobic OXYGEN IS CONSISTENT		**Anaerobic** OXYGEN IS INCONSISTENT

HEART RATE in Beats / Min
100 110 120 130 140   150 160 170 180
HEART RATE in Beats / Min

✓ **Muscle Fiber Recruited**
Red Muscle

✓ **Optimal Heart Rate**
Depending on current condition level, typically between 130–145 BPM. The key is to not cross over your cardio line into High-Intensity Cardio.

✓ **Duration**
Minimum 30 Minutes.
Longer Duration = More Fat Burning

✓ **Times Per Week**
3–5 Days Per Week
Amount of days depends on Goal Type
5 days = More Fat Burning

✓ **Muscle Fiber Recruited**
White Muscle

✓ **Optimal Heart Rate**
Intense bursts of speed for 1 minute at a high Heart Rate (160–175 BPM), followed by 1–2 minute(s) of recovery bringing your Heart Rate to 120–130 BPM, then repeat.

✓ **Duration**
Maximum 35 Minutes.
Too long of a duration will cause your body to burn muscle.

✓ **Times Per Week**
1–3 Days Per Week
Amount of days depends on Goal Type
3 days = More Fat Burning

Cardio Technique Is Extremely Important

Next time you are in a gym, look around at the rest of the people doing cardio. Then look at their technique. You will see that most of them are either holding the hand rails as if their life depended on it or are bending over the machine, making you wonder what exercise they are performing in the first place. This goes back to the earlier point I made—that a lot of people exercise just so they can feel they are doing something or they do not know the correct exercise technique. I say, if you are going to spend the time doing it, why not get the most out of it by doing it right? Since cardio is so important to burning body fat, I think it's necessary to cover how to perform it correctly. Proper cardio technique will maximize the activation of your muscle (your engine) and assist in preventing injuries.

This illustration is an example of walking and sprinting. These guidelines of correct cardio technique apply to both fat-burning and high-intensity cardio

Cardiovascular Exercise Technique

This is an example of correct cardio technique while walking or running. Please apply this technique to every instance of cardio you perform. This will ensure optimal muscle fiber recruitment.

1 Keep body upright and head up.

2 Maintain a slight arch in lower back.

3 Tighten entire abdomen region.

4 Keep shoulders back and chest slightly pressed outward.

5 Contract gluteal muscles.

6 Keep knee in line with heel, never leaning over toes!

7 Shift weight to ball of foot, while keeping body upright and knee in line with heel.

8 Heel strike - *the majority of initial weight should be placed on the heel and gluteus (butt).*

9 Push off ball of foot while continue to contract all working muscle fibers.

Please also observe the following guidelines:
- BODY IN BALANCE STATE
- NO HOLDING HANDRAILS OF MACHINE
- BREATHE IN RHYTHM
  example: When walking, inhale every 3–4 steps, then exhale, and repeat that cadence.

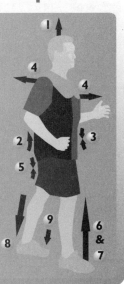

> **IMPORTANT NOTE**
>
> Keeping your joints protected is very important. Healthy joints are necessary to stay consistent with your cardio. For this reason, it is important that you have proper footwear. If your shoes are getting worn out, you should get new, high-quality shoes as soon as possible. Good shoes are great shock absorbers and do wonders protecting your joints.

Category 2—Strength Training

Stretching keeps you flexible, cardio increases your endurance and burns fat, and strength training improves your strength and muscle tone (and muscle size if that is your goal). Strength training is defined as any type of exercise designed to improve the overall strength of your body. There are two core principles, also known as types of strength training: *core training* and *weight training*. Both types of training are extremely beneficial. Choose the type of training you perform based on your Body Confidence goals.

Core Training Strengthens Your Entire Body

Have you ever seen someone you thought was big and strong, and then when they attempted to lift something heavy they were actually pretty weak? This is the classic sign of someone with a weak core. In the most general terms, your core can be defined as your body minus your legs and arms. These muscles are involved in every movement you make, and to truly be strong, you must have a strong core. I was fortunate to be introduced to core training when I was fifteen years old (back in 1987) while recovering from shoulder surgery. During my physical therapy, all of my rehab was based on core training. During each session I would do ten core-specific exercises on a mat, then work on a reformer (used in Pilates) and finish up abdominal work on a Swiss ball (an inflatable exercise ball).

 Being introduced to core training was life changing for me (especially since no one really talked about core training in 1987). I felt, as most fifteen-year-olds do, that I was strong. Man, was I wrong. There are so many tiny muscles in your body. No matter how strong you think your big muscle groups are, you are only as strong as your weakest link. Core training activates and strengthens all of your smaller muscle groups as well as your big muscle groups. The physical therapy I underwent opened my eyes to the importance of activating all of my muscle and ignited a passion for core training. Since then, every time I work out I incorporate core training.

Everyone Should Initially Do Core Training

Core training is primarily designed for people who want to increase flexibility, improve strength, lengthen their body, and develop muscle tone and definition *without* gaining muscle size. Initially, everyone should do core training, regardless of gender or goal type. Then, once you learn how to activate your core, you can move on to the second type of strength training: weights (as long as your goal is to increase the size of your muscles). Typically, about 70 percent of my female clients do *only* core training, because their primary focus is to tighten and tone their muscle.

There Are Three Ways to Learn How to Activate Your Core

Learning how to train your core requires the ability to connect your mind and body. This requires concentration, though with the correct coaching and practice you will master it.

These are three ways to best activate your core:

Pilates—Pilates is core training that focuses more on your strength.

Yoga—Yoga is core training that focuses more on your flexibility.

Core specialists—There are many health professionals who specifically focus on core training.

Pilates, yoga, or working with a core specialist can be done through one-on-one instruction or group classes at a gym or studio. You can also purchase videos of each method.

What matters most is that you learn how to activate your core. With a strong core, your cardio *and* your daily activities will become more efficient. In addition, since fat is burned in muscle, the more muscle (even your small ones) you learn to activate, the more fat you burn.

Weight Training Increases Muscle Size

Once I understood how to activate my core, I took that knowledge and began weight training. Weight training is strength training that focuses on lifting weights to increase muscle size. In the cardio section, I shared what causes muscle soreness (tiny tears in your muscle) and how your body increases the size of the damaged muscle as it attempts to make it strong enough to prevent the muscle from becoming damaged again. In weight training, you continually increase the amount of weight you lift over a period of time to keep damaging the muscle, therefore increasing its size each time.

Here are five important guidelines to follow when weight training:

1. **Choose fundamental movements.** Every year, gyms buy new pieces of weight-training equipment, thinking they will provide their members with a better workout. The reality is that the simpler and more basic the movement is (like pushups, pull-ups, or squats), the better the type of weight-training exercise. Fundamental movements use multiple joints during the exercise, which causes a greater recruitment of muscle fibers and subsequently better stimulates your nervous system. Both of these benefits lead to maximum muscle growth. Here is a list of the six main weight-training movements:

   a. Any movement that takes your body through space, examples being push-ups, dips, pull-ups, squats, and lunges

   b. Any dumbbell movement

   c. Any barbell movement

   d. Any plate-loaded machine (like Hammer Strength)

   e. Free-moving cables

   f. All other machines

   When you weight-train, the majority of all of your workouts should involve fundamental movements from the top three in this list to optimize results. Performing quality weight training will maximize your muscle growth and strength.

2. **Maintain a slow and steady tempo and focus on the eccentric contraction.** Momentum can be a great ally in lifting extra weight. Fast

repetitions will assist in pushing extra poundage, but the problem is that it minimizes your muscle growth. Remember, the goal with exercise is to recruit the largest amount of muscle fibers you can. By lifting weight with an even-paced tempo (slow and steady), you will activate the greatest amount of muscle fibers and rely on your actual strength to lift the weight, not momentum. In addition, the majority of muscle growth is achieved during the eccentric contraction of the exercise. Every weight-training movement has two types of muscle contractions, eccentric and concentric. Eccentric is when the muscle is lengthening, and concentric is when the muscle is shortening. When you curl (*bend*) your arm for a bicep exercise, that is a concentric contraction (*shortening of your bicep muscle*), and when you lower (*straighten*) your arm it is an eccentric contraction (*lengthening of your bicep muscle*). This is important to understand because the majority of muscle fiber damage occurs during the eccentric contraction of an exercise. Remember, muscle grows by tearing your muscle fibers and then grows back stronger with rest and proper fuel. Heavy weights are only positive if you can control the weight and maintain a consistent tempo that focuses on your eccentric contraction. A good rule of thumb is to always do eccentric contractions that last at least two seconds (can be more). This tempo will eliminate momentum from your movements and ensure you are optimizing your eccentric muscle contraction.

3. **Enhance the stretch of each repetition.** Your muscle is covered by a tissue called fascia. Muscle fascia is like plastic wrap. Imagine bread dough wrapped in plastic wrap. That is exactly what your muscles look like when they're covered with fascia. Many times people have a difficult time building muscle (especially "hard gainers," like Don Maclellan from chapter 2) because their muscle fascia is wrapped around their muscle too tight. This is similar to the way that bread dough cannot expand when wrapped in plastic. Think about what happens when you stretch the plastic wrap surrounding the dough. The dough will expand. Your muscle will do the same thing—it will grow faster when your muscle fascia is stretched. Stretching your muscle fascia is accomplished by enhancing the stretch portion during a weight-training exercise. Picture doing a chest dumbbell press.

Lowering the weight toward your chest is the eccentric contraction for your chest (*since your chest muscles are lengthening*) and holding the weight at the bottom of the eccentric contraction is what I suggest you do to stretch your muscle fascia. If you did a set of 8 repetitions, you could have the tempo be 4-4-1: 4 seconds lowering the weight (*eccentric contraction*), 4 seconds holding the weight in the stretch position, and 1 second pushing the weight up (*the concentric contraction*). This type of tempo will ensure that you are enhancing the stretch of the movement and expanding your muscle fascia, leading to maximum muscle growth.

4. **Muscle soreness occurs twenty-four to forty-eight hours *after* your weight training.** If you are not sore after this period of time, you did not create the damage necessary to increase the size of that muscle. *Increase the weight and vary your routine; change exercises, reps, sets, rest, and so on.*

5. **Always wait for the soreness of a muscle to leave before you train that muscle again.** Training sore muscles causes more damage to an already damaged muscle. This prevents it from repairing itself *and* increasing in size.

If your goal is to gain muscle, then you should weight-train. Once you achieve your goal, you can adjust your training by shifting back to core training or lifting lighter weights so you maintain (not gain) muscle mass.

It's Important to Learn How to Weight Train

I am always shocked when I hear people talking about how they have begun weight training without any guidance. For some reason, people think it is a simple act to lift weights correctly. This is definitely a myth. Instead, it's a great way to get injured. Weight training is complicated. It is a skill. Now, once you learn how to weight train correctly, you can do it without guidance.

Initially, if you are going to weight train, I recommend learning from one of these three methods:

Work with a personal trainer—Personal trainers offer one-on-one sessions or group sessions. This is a great way to learn how to weight train correctly.

Take a weight-lifting class—Most gyms and studios offer weight-lifting classes as part of their membership.

Get a video—This is an excellent way to learn weight training in the comfort of your home. The only requirement is that you may need to get some equipment. Many times all you will need (*depending on your goal, of course*) are some dumbbells, an inflated exercise ball, and some bands. Total cost: about sixty dollars.

Your Eight Tips for Exercise Success

Now that we have covered your two categories of exercise and their core principles, I want to share eight tips for exercise success before I present your workout to you. These tips will allow you to make the most out of your exercise plan.

Tip 1—Exercise in the Morning

This obviously depends on your schedule. If working out in the morning is not a possibility, focus on getting your exercise sooner in the day rather than later.

Here are four reasons that exercising in the morning is best:

1. **Since you just slept, your body is rested and has the most amount of energy.** This will allow you to exercise at your highest level.

2. **Activating your muscles (your engine) also activates your metabolism.** This allows your body to burn more fat throughout the day.

3. **Your body releases endorphins** (feel-good hormones). This will help you handle stress and improve your mood for the day.

4. **It creates a sense of accomplishment and relief for the day.** This prevents the internal struggle many of us feel when we have a late workout scheduled and the fatigue is catching up to us in the afternoon. This is when we try to justify missing the workout. Exercising in the morning prevents this struggle and creates a great sense of accomplishment.

Tip 2—Eat Before You Exercise

All the pieces are coming together. You learned that food is your body's source of fuel and that your body is a "refuel as it goes" machine. Due to those two facts, it is a must to eat before you exercise. I know there is a lot of hype suggesting you do cardio on an empty stomach (meaning without eating for hours before exercise). Let's debunk that myth. You know that in order to consistently release stored body fat, your blood sugar needs to be stable. So, how can your blood sugar be stable on an empty stomach? It can't. Without eating, your body needs to tap into its limited stored sugar supplies to create the energy to fuel your muscles during exercise. When you run out of stored sugar, your body begins using amino acids (muscle) to create glucose for energy. In essence, your body begins consuming its muscles to provide energy for your workout. Obviously, this is counterproductive. Eating before exercise ensures that you do not burn muscle (your engine) and will instead burn fat.

Here are two adjustments you may need to make when eating before exercise:

1. We each have a different digestive system, so it is important to experiment with what foods work best for you. You may need to eat a half meal or eat an hour before you exercise. These factors depend on you.

2. If you currently exercise in the morning and do not eat before you exercise, you should start the day with a quarter or half meal. This will allow your body to get accustomed to eating in the morning. As your appetite increases, you can increase the size of your pre-exercise meal.

Tip 3—Always Do High-Intensity Cardio or Strength Training Before Fat-Burning Cardio

Strength training and high-intensity cardio both primarily burn glucose for energy. Fat-burning cardio burns both fat and glucose. If you do your fat-burning cardio first, you will deplete your glucose stores before you do your strength training or high-intensity cardio workout. This will affect the quality of those workouts. In addition, it takes about twenty minutes of consistent fat-burning cardio before you really start burning fat.

By doing your glucose-burning exercise first (either strength training or high-intensity cardio), you will have enough glucose to maximize the workout plus warm up your body for fat-burning cardio. This way you'll immediately start burning more fat, once you begin fat-burning cardio, since your body is already warmed up. This simple adjustment will optimize your body's fuel pathways.

Tip 4—You May Need to Eat Sooner Than Three Hours After Working Out

Your goal is to eat a meal every three to four hours. What if you are hungry before three hours are up? Many times when you have an intense workout (typically after high-intensity cardio), you will be hungry sooner than three hours afterward. This is because you utilized a lot of energy, and your body needs to be refueled. If this happens, simply eat a balanced meal when you feel hungry. A good analogy is automotive once again. Let's say you were driving your car at 110 miles per hour when you typically drive 65 miles per hour. The increase in speed requires more fuel, causing your gas tank to become lower at a faster rate than you are used to. Intense exercise causes the same thing to occur to your body and its food demands.

Tip 5—Disregard All Settings on Cardio Machines

Besides checking your heart rate, all the data that a cardio machine provides you is inaccurate, for two reasons. First, the amount of burned calories that a machine indicates is far from correct. The machine doesn't know your body composition or speed of your metabolism. Its computer is basing the calories you burn solely on your weight, your age, and the intensity of your workout. This number doesn't reflect what actual calories are burned, and whether they were fat calories. Second, you should always choose the machine's manual setting so you can control the incline, level of resistance, and speed. The programs each machine provides will not make your high-intensity cardio intense enough or your fat-burning cardio at the optimal incline/resistance and speed. You want to take the information you've learned in this book's cardio section and apply it to all cardio machines.

Tip 6—Sports Are a Fun Way to Get In Your Cardio

Most sports are a great mixture of fat-burning and high-intensity cardio, and provide an excellent change of pace as well. Some sports that work great for cardio are basketball, singles tennis, soccer, and racquetball. If you choose to play a sport as your cardio, make sure that it keeps you moving around and keeps your heart rate in the correct ranges.

Tip 7—If You Are Short on Time, Always Do Cardio Instead of Strength Training

We all have busy weeks, and sometimes it's just not possible to squeeze in all of your workouts. If this is the case for you, the days you work out should be cardio days. You can skip your strength training that week. Definitely get in at least one high-intensity cardio session as well as one fat-burning cardio session.

This tip does not apply to people who have Goal Type 2. Since their focus is on building strength and muscle, people with Goal Type 2 need to choose strength training over cardio.

Tip 8—Journal Your Exercise to Monitor Your Progress

Temporarily journaling your exercise will allow you to develop baselines for your stretching, cardio, and strength training. It will be easier for you to steadily progress by having a point of reference to continually work from—whether it's how long you held a stretch or the incline you walked on a treadmill or the number of push-ups you did. Each of these examples is easy to remember, which makes it easy to chart your progress by journaling. As with food, once you have reached a point of complete awareness, you no longer need to journal.

A Sample Exercise Journal

Stretching

Type	Duration	Notes

Cardiovascular Exercise

Type	Duration	Heart Rate	Incline	Surface	Notes
High Intensity (consistent HR)					
Fat Burning (consistent HR)					

Core Training

Type	Duration	Notes

Weight Training

Types	Sets	Repetitions	Weight	Rest	Notes

Your Workout Routine

It is time to bring it all together and get you going on your workout routine. You will achieve your goals fastest by performing both categories of exercise during your weekly routine, remembering to stretch, and following your plan as it is presented.

Your weekly routine is based on Goal Type. The prescribed workouts for Goal Type 1 include high-intensity cardio, whereas those for Goal Type 2 do not. You will also notice that the strength-training sessions are longer for Goal Type 2 than they are for Goal Type 1. These differences will provide the right training for you to achieve your goal. Typically, if you want to lose body fat and weight, you do more fat-burning and high-intensity cardio. If you want to gain muscle, you do less cardio and more weights.

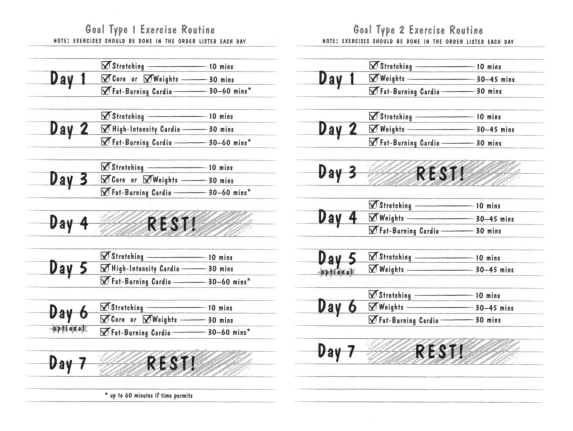

Goal Type 1 Exercise Routine
NOTE: EXERCISES SHOULD BE DONE IN THE ORDER LISTED EACH DAY

Day 1
- ☑ Stretching — 10 mins
- ☑ Core or ☑ Weights — 30 mins
- ☑ Fat-Burning Cardio — 30–60 mins*

Day 2
- ☑ Stretching — 10 mins
- ☑ High-Intensity Cardio — 30 mins
- ☑ Fat-Burning Cardio — 30–60 mins*

Day 3
- ☑ Stretching — 10 mins
- ☑ Core or ☑ Weights — 30 mins
- ☑ Fat-Burning Cardio — 30–60 mins*

Day 4 — REST!

Day 5
- ☑ Stretching — 10 mins
- ☑ High-Intensity Cardio — 30 mins
- ☑ Fat-Burning Cardio — 30–60 mins*

Day 6 (optional)
- ☑ Stretching — 10 mins
- ☑ Core or ☑ Weights — 30 mins
- ☑ Fat-Burning Cardio — 30–60 mins*

Day 7 — REST!

* up to 60 minutes if time permits

Goal Type 2 Exercise Routine
NOTE: EXERCISES SHOULD BE DONE IN THE ORDER LISTED EACH DAY

Day 1
- ☑ Stretching — 10 mins
- ☑ Weights — 30–45 mins
- ☑ Fat-Burning Cardio — 30 mins

Day 2
- ☑ Stretching — 10 mins
- ☑ Weights — 30–45 mins
- ☑ Fat-Burning Cardio — 30 mins

Day 3 — REST!

Day 4
- ☑ Stretching — 10 mins
- ☑ Weights — 30–45 mins
- ☑ Fat-Burning Cardio — 30 mins

Day 5 (optional)
- ☑ Stretching — 10 mins
- ☑ Weights — 30–45 mins

Day 6
- ☑ Stretching — 10 mins
- ☑ Weights — 30–45 mins
- ☑ Fat-Burning Cardio — 30 mins

Day 7 — REST!

Challenge Yourself with Exercise

You now have the tools to work out smarter. Once you implement these tools, your results will come quickly. After a while, though, you will begin to notice your body adapting to your exercise routine, and your fast progress will begin to slow. So how do you keep your progress moving? The answer is simple: challenge yourself. Challenging yourself means raising the level of your exercise and pushing yourself a little harder with each successive workout. Since your body always adapts to new workouts, you always need to stay one step ahead of your body's adaptability.

Here are four things you can do with each workout to ensure that you are challenging yourself:

1. **Change your exercise selections.** Simply switching from walking to jogging, or from jogging to stair climbing, provides a new shock and stimulus to your body. Ideally you should switch your exercise selections for stretching, cardio, and strength training every couple of days. Regarding which cardio exercises to pick, ideally you would want to switch between only the higher-quality exercises.

2. **Adjust your intensity.** The more you work out, the more you will find you can push yourself. Increasing your intensity means walking a little faster, raising the incline or resistance on a cardio machine, holding a Pilates position for five seconds longer than normal, or doing a couple of more reps on the chest press.

3. **Set exercise goals.** Goals are a good way to challenge yourself. If you typically walk two miles a day, pick up the pace and walk two and a quarter miles in the same amount of time. If you have trouble holding a pose in yoga, practice until you can hold that pose. If you sprint for your high-intensity cardio and you can do only eight sprints before you are exhausted, make it a personal goal to achieve ten sprints. This type of goal setting drives you to keep pushing and provides a feeling of victory once you achieve the goal.

4. **Train for a sport.** Remember Eric Standridge's story about how he found his love of running? Well, Eric used running to challenge himself. He started with a 10K run, then a half marathon, and then a full marathon. Eric's running kept him focused on pushing his exercise and continually challenging himself. There are many amateur and recreational sports you can participate in. These might be what fuels you to continue raising the bar on your exercise.

There's no formula for challenging yourself; each of us simply has a feeling when we know we are doing our best or when we are taking it easy. Sometimes we should take it easy during a workout (if you are sick or tired), though the majority of the time, if you want to progress, you need to go for it and raise the bar a little with every workout.

Find Passion in Your Exercise

You are two months into the program, and your results have been fantastic. The food part is easy; you are enjoying the meals and how they work into your day. The only hiccup is that the novelty of your exercise is beginning to wear off. You understand the benefit; it has helped you get great results. And yet you dread going to the gym each day, continually thinking of reasons to skip your workout. Each day you tell yourself, "I'll just get it in tomorrow." You've lost your excitement for exercise, and who can blame you? How exciting is walking on a treadmill or doing strength training at the gym?

The example I just shared is what many of us have gone through or experience each day. I define this lack of excitement as a loss of passion for exercise, and it has been one of my biggest challenges to overcome.

I have always been an athlete, and playing sports or doing outdoor activities is what has inspired me through the years. Unfortunately, as my life got busier, I turned to less varied activities, and it took the joy out of exercise. We begin to go through the motions with our exercise because we know it is what we should do, not what we want to do. This mind-set slowly and steadily begins to drain all of the exercise passion right out of us.

You see, I have lost my passion for exercise many times since I played my final collegiate soccer game. I would become bored with it, feeling like I was living the movie *Groundhog Day* (where the same day repeats over and over again). I dreaded everything about working out. I did feel like I was working toward a destination (a fit and healthy body). The only thing was, I was despising the process.

A few years ago I found myself in one of these ruts, and I missed far too many workouts. I justified these misses by telling myself I didn't have enough time, that my life was just too busy. Even though I knew what I should be doing and I knew the benefits (less stress, more energy, and a leaner body), I was struggling to get out of the rut.

Then one day, an inconvenience turned into a blessing. My car needed to go to the shop for the day, so I decided to walk to the office. (It seemed more fun than a treadmill.) I only live about two miles away, so I put on my walking shoes and hit the pavement. Autumn had just begun, the air was crisp, the leaves were red and orange, and the sky was bright blue. It felt like a perfect day, and gave me the best twenty-five minutes of exercise I'd had in over a year. . . . What dawned on me shortly afterward was that I had lost my passion for exercise. I had let life's circumstances dictate my health pattern rather than creating fun ways to work my exercise into my world.

I had forgotten what I truly get from daily exercise: a quality of life worth living. That evening, on my walk home, I decided I needed to get back to what I loved about exercise and begin enjoying the journey again. It was a simple process: I looked to my past and noted the times when I had passion for exercise. Within five minutes it became clear: Every time I had been passionate about exercise, it was because I was engaged in a sport—soccer, tennis, or cycling. I knew I needed to get back to what I love and at the same time make sure the changes I made could be worked into my schedule. I had about an hour a day to exercise, which immediately put soccer and tennis on the sidelines. Both sports take longer than that to play, including travel, coordinating with other people, and then finally playing the sport. Cycling, however, could be completed in an hour, and I love it. (In the past, I had cycled for six years.) A few weeks later I geared up and began cycling again.

Since that moment, I have looked forward to exercising every day. On the days I miss a bike ride, it feels like a piece of my day was lost . . . a very different story than a few years ago. I now look forward to my weight-training sessions because they help make me stronger for when I ride my bike. My nutrition is more dialed in than ever because the leaner and tighter I am, the faster I ride. I can honestly say that I am now in the best overall shape of my life and have once again found my passion for exercise. I'm making sure that this time it never leaves.

Whether you have been on the program for one month, two months, or six months, if you are not passionate about your exercise, you are one step away from burning out. The reason we love to do new things is that they are new and exciting. The novelty will always wear off—meaning that we must be satisfied with what is left. This is why it is important that you find your passion for exercise now or at least begin the search for that passion. Your passion will keep you consistent, keep you from feeling like you're reliving *Groundhog Day*, and, most important, keep you excited about your workouts.

Ask yourself this: when was I last passionate about exercise? Your answer will fall into two categories:

1. **You will remember a time when you were passionate about exercise.** If this is the case, I suggest finding a way to get some of that exercise you were passionate about back into your routine. . . . Trust me; it will make a huge difference.

2. **You will realize you were never passionate about exercise.** If this is the case, it's time to experiment. Try out many types of activities and see which one fits best. Just keep experimenting until you find the thing that sparks your passion.

Your exercise is a permanent part of your life, and each part needs to be enjoyable. When you are passionate about it, your exercise will never feel like a chore. It will become one of the most exciting parts of your day.

Two excellent examples of how to optimally activate your engine, challenge yourself, and find passion in exercise are the success stories of Brendan Zackey and Tally Sanders. Let's start with Brendan.

rendan and I knew each other well from the gym. He is a tennis pro and loves the game (already had his passion for exercise). I saw him one day after a tennis tournament and asked him how the tournament went. He stood there shaking his head, replying, "Not great. I need to take my game to a higher level." Brendan shared that there were four components of his tennis game that he needed to improve. First, he needed to increase his speed. Brendan was carrying too much weight and body fat, which made him slower on the tennis court. Second, he experienced energy crashes during matches. To counter this, he drank sports drinks (*which are loaded in sugar*) throughout his match, thinking that would increase his energy. Unfortunately, all the drinks did was cause bigger energy crashes (*sugar drinks quickly spike blood-sugar levels, which are followed by blood sugar-crashes*). Third, Brendan wanted more strength. He knew more powerful shots could end points faster, allowing him to conserve more energy in each match. Brendan's final component

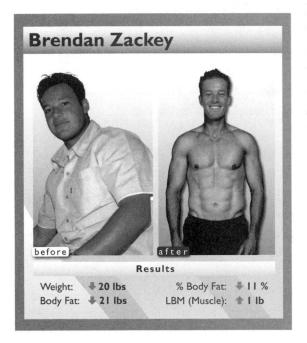

Brendan Zackey

before   after

Results

Weight:	⬇ **20 lbs**	% Body Fat:	⬇ **11 %**
Body Fat:	⬇ **21 lbs**	LBM (Muscle):	⬆ **1 lb**

was to improve his recovery between matches. In many tennis tournaments players have matches in consecutive days. Whenever he played a long match, he would struggle with energy and endurance during the match scheduled on the following day. He felt like his legs could not recover fast enough between matches.

Brendan filled me in on how he ate, revealing that he only had a couple meals each day and they were loaded with carbohydrates and had very little protein. The good news is that his cardio was excellent. He was getting plenty of high-intensity cardio from his tennis training, and on his off days he was jogging forty-five minutes for his fat-burning cardio. I knew all we needed was to get his blood sugar balanced and his body would quickly become lean and tight. Brendan solidified his Body Confidence Plan and his results came fast. Within eight weeks, he dropped twenty pounds and 11 percent body fat. With his extra weight gone, Brendan could now run down any ball on the tennis court. His new quickness became a powerful asset. Brendan's second challenge was his energy crashing during each match. Brendan began eating a high-quality meal one hour before and a piece of a protein bar during each rest period throughout the match. The first time Brendan followed this routine, he was in shock. His energy stayed as strong during the final set as it did the first set. He was now the player who out-hustled his opponent and won crucial points when the match was on the line. Brendan's third challenge was lack of strength and power. He added a solid weight-training routine (four days a week) to his exercise plan, focusing on activating his core and using fundamental weight-training movements to maximize muscle fiber recruitment. Each week, Brendan noticed a higher velocity on his tennis shots. Within eight weeks he achieved the increase in power that he wanted. Brendan's final challenge was his recovery between matches. By eating a solid pre-game meal, snacking on pieces of bars throughout the match, and having a high-quality post-match meal, Brendan recovered within in an hour after his matches. This allowed him to feel fresh for next day's matches.

What was cool about Brendan's progress was that he already had a fantastic skill set for his chosen sport. His challenge was that fatigue always caused him to lose his sharpness on the court. This is what taking your game to the next level is all about, being your best. With a solid Body Confidence Plan at hand, Brendan went from a very good tennis player to a great one.

Tally Sanders also wanted to take her Body Confidence to another level. When I met Tally she was already in good shape. She had qualified for the Ms. Fitness USA competition. Ms. Fitness competitions are demanding, as each athlete is judged on her physique and also her routine. Tally had four things she needed to improve before the national competition: her body composition, endurance, strength, and recovery. As we began working together, Tally was already eating well. The things she needed to improve were her quality of food and nutrient ratios, which required a little balancing to stabilize her blood sugar. With those nutrition adjustments and by adding three days of sprinting to her exercise routine, Tally's physique got much tighter and

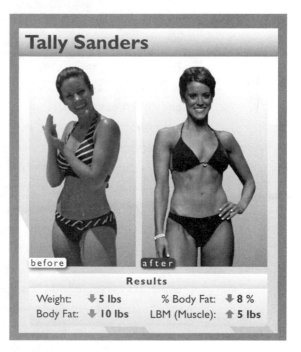

Tally Sanders

before · after

Results

Weight:	⬇ 5 lbs	% Body Fat:	⬇ 8 %
Body Fat:	⬇ 10 lbs	LBM (Muscle):	⬆ 5 lbs

more toned. She focused on eating high-quality meals before her training sessions, drinking a protein shake or eating a bar throughout her practice, and eating a high-quality meal after practice. This meal consistency prevented energy crashes and helped her endurance. Many parts of Tally's routine required strength. What she struggled with most were one-arm pushups, full range (*there's a big difference between partial and full range*). Tally began focusing on core and weight training to improve her overall strength for the parts of her routine that needed it.

Tally's effort was fantastic. In twelve weeks Tally dropped ten pounds of fat, 8 percent body fat, and gained five pounds of lean body mass. All this additional muscle gave her the strength to do a one-arm full-range push-up. Tally's overall weight only dropped five pounds, yet her body completely transformed. Tally did amazingly well in Ms. Fitness USA, and she plans on doing contests just like it for many more years to come. Tally passes her exercise "litmus test" with flying colors . . . she trains smart, challenges herself, and is passionate about her exercise. There is a purpose to Tally's training: each day she strives to take her body to the highest level and be her very best.

YOUR EXERCISE TAKEAWAY

Exercise takes time, period. The cool thing is that now you know how to exercise correctly. We feel the most frustration when we put the time in and do not get the results we want. Many times this happens because we are exercising incorrectly. But this no longer applies to you. You have the answers and the tools to make your workouts efficient and productive.

The next time you hear the latest piece of exercise hype, take a step back and see if it passes your exercise litmus test. You now have the knowledge to tell fact from fiction.

All six components of your Body Confidence Plan are now solidified. Your Body Confidence foundation is complete. The next two chapters are designed to educate you on how to successfully work your program into your world. It is possible to do this, and in so doing you will permanently achieve your goals and take your Body Confidence to the next level.

7

STAYING TRUE TO THE PROCESS

Everything we do in life is a process.

A process is anything we do that combines actions in order to achieve a goal. For this reason, everything we do in life is a process. Each of us has goals we want to accomplish each day, each week, each month, and each year. You may even have goals that reach far into the future—possibly ten, twenty, or thirty years from now. We are continually developing plans and strategies with which we intend to achieve those goals. The execution of these plans and strategies make up the process we go through to reach each goal. Whether the process in question is choosing a house, building a business, strengthening a relationship, raising children, or taking your Body Confidence to the next level, there will be difficult moments. At these moments, you will need to decide if you will abandon the process or stay true to (continue with) the process. This decision may not be as simple as picking black or white. Instead, it might best be described as choosing between different shades of gray. Sometimes, abandoning the process is the right choice. Sometimes, staying true to the process is the wrong choice. Obviously, each process has its own set of circumstances and needs to be evaluated on its own merits. The good news is that the only process we will discuss in this book is the process of learning how to make your health a priority in your life. This is a black-and-white decision. When you experience difficult moments (and you will), your choice is simple: stay true to the process.

Even when we know that we need to stay true to the process, there are still seeds of doubt within all of us—moments when we ask ourselves whether we can achieve our goals. You're reading this book because you want to learn, you want to become an expert on your body, you want to feel your best, and you want to achieve your Body Confidence goals. I know this to be true, because you have already taken the first step; the proof is in your hands! Something similar is true when a new client first walks into my office. There is always a feeling of hesitation while they ask themselves whether they will succeed with their health this time, whether they can actually work their Body Confidence Plan into their day. This is an internal struggle where we try to see how it can be done. Every Venice Nutrition client has felt this; we all feel some anxiety when we know that change is on the horizon. The facts are established. The case has been made. To make your health a priority, you require a "new level of thinking." This means you must change your approach to your health and actually learn how your body works so you can make it work for you.

I am sharing this with you because it is natural right now to be feeling a little overwhelmed. Developing your Body Confidence Plan is an intense moment in your life, and I just presented you with a great deal of information. This is why you and I are a team. We are working together to help you use all your new knowledge as well as the tools you need to apply this knowledge to your world. The tools you will use to accomplish this are the seven concepts of staying true to the process. At your difficult moments, these concepts will provide you with the strength to stay true to the process and permanently remove the thought of ever abandoning your health.

I have always taught the seven concepts of staying true to the process, yet my understanding of what these concepts mean was taken to another level when I became a parent. Hunter has taught me more about life in six years than I learned in my previous thirty-two. He is my greatest teacher. Think of all the amazing processes children go through. They must learn how to walk, talk, write, tie their shoes (this one is tough!), throw a ball, read, and more. The number of processes children must go through is limitless. Kids take on each process with their eyes wide open. Each process brings with it many emotions, like frustration, anger, joy, disappointment, and pride.

Think about what a baby must go through to walk. When Hunter was born, he couldn't even turn his head. Each night Abbi and I lived in fear that he would flip over on his stomach and suffocate. (Infants literally have no control over their bodies.) From the moment we brought him home, every movement he made was part of the process. He had to learn control over his body before he could walk. First he had to gain control of his neck, then learn how to sit up, then crawl, then stand, and eventually walk. I remember how frustrated Hunter would get every time he took three steps only to fall. He would scrunch up his eyes, tighten his lips, and pound the floor in anger. After moping on the floor for a minute, he would grab something close by, pull himself back up, and give it another go. Then he would fall again after three steps. By the third time he fell, his tears would start to flow. Every day his focus was learning how to walk more than three steps.

Then one sunny afternoon, Hunter and I were in our backyard. He was holding the wall and saw me sitting about eight steps away from him. I glanced over and saw a look of determination on his face that I had never seen before. (He had the "eye of the tiger.") He let go of the wall and took one step, then another, then his third, where he began to wobble a bit, struggling to keep his balance. Suddenly he lunged forward with his fourth step, his fifth, then his sixth. He sensed victory, and his face began to lighten up. He took his seventh, then his eighth, and victoriously jumped into my arms. He did it! I picked him up, and we celebrated his amazing accomplishment. He worked every day for fourteen months to walk those eight steps. That is what I call staying true to the process.

I could clearly see that Hunter would eventually accomplish his goal. Abandoning the process he undertook never entered his mind. Hunter, like all kids, has an unbelievable amount of innate determination. Kids believe anything is possible, and they are up for it regardless of the challenge.

I wanted to share this story with you because as I present these seven concepts, I want you to remember everything you have already achieved. We were all kids once, and as kids, we felt that sense of invincibility—that no matter how hard the challenge, we would find a way to win. This is the type of determination everyone is capable of. Every time you reach difficult moments while on the course of achieving Body Confidence, remember Hunter learning to walk, and then push through, staying true to the process.

Let's start with the first concept: pace yourself.

Concept 1—Pace Yourself

Pacing ourselves is typically a big challenge. I know that when I decide I'm going to do something, my initial instinct is to go all in even before I make room in my Quadrant. I've learned the hard way that this "jumping the gun" mind-set will always lead to burnout. Now, the "all in" mind-set is fine if you are ready for it and have made the proper space in your Quadrant. This will maintain balance in your life. The question is, How do you pace yourself?

It typically takes three months to create your Body Confidence foundation and develop the systems in your life that make the plan work for you. Pacing yourself means accepting that doing this is initially a three-month process. Everything you do within these three months is focused on how to make your health a priority. I understand that the natural reaction is to go for the fast results (since this is what we have been taught). No matter what, though—if you correctly implement the program, you will get fast results. The question you want to ask yourself is, What will fast results cost me? Achieving fast results without a proper foundation will always lead to regression. It is important to remember that whatever pace you set for yourself, your Body Confidence goals will be achieved. The real question at that point is, Will those results be temporary or permanent? The answer to this question is determined by the pace you set for working the program into your life. Setting the correct pace provides you with realistic expectations that allow you to stay true to the process.

By following these five strategies, you will set the correct pace.

1. **Understand how to work the four parts of the program.** There are four parts to your three-month (ninety-day) program. Each part is focused on your Body Confidence Plan, and each part's purpose is to lead you through ninety days, from initially implementing your Body Confidence Plan to eventually molding it into your life.

    Here are the objectives for each part:

    Part 1. Implementing Your Jump Start Phase (days 1–10)—Your first ten days are designed to jump-start your metabolism. During this phase it is best for you to follow all the recommendations for your Body Confidence Plan. To accomplish this, it is best to spend a weekend developing a system to prevent unnecessary additional stress. If this means starting the program a week later, so be it.

Getting started under the right circumstances will allow you to feel comfortable and in control.

Part 2. Solidifying Your Body Confidence Plan (days 11–30)— Your next twenty days are designed to expand your meal and exercise preferences. This is the phase where you look at what is working and what is not. Your main focus is to get in rhythm with each component of your plan.

Part 3. Evolving with Your Body Confidence Plan (days 31– 60)—The focus of your next thirty days is on evaluating how your solid plan is working for you on a daily basis. Are your results coming along nicely? Are you missing meals or workouts? Are you struggling with traveling? Have you hit a plateau? Basically, part 3 is when the novelty of the program wears off and you begin to see what is doable for you in the long run and what you want to change. Every day is different, and this part is where you learn how to stay on plan even as your day evolves. While in this part, you should reference the particular chapters that address your challenges. The answers are in this book.

Part 4. Molding Your Body Confidence Plan into Your Life (days 61–90)—Sixty days in, you are now getting close to making your Body Confidence Plan a permanent part of your life. This is the part where life (unforeseen challenges) typically begins to show up: you get sick, go on a big trip, have a family emergency, or go through anything else that is time intensive and forces you to fall "off plan." These challenges allow you to learn what adjustments you need to make to ensure that the same event will not pull you "off plan" again. Once you master this part, you have achieved a permanent Body Confidence foundation.

There are many times that these four parts take more than three months to fully grasp, so it is important to know the direction you are going. This way, you can prepare for each upcoming part and pace yourself based on your own experiences. Your external and internal results will continue to progress throughout each part. As long as you focus on keeping your plan in balance, your Body Confidence goals will be achieved.

2. **Keep it simple.** Many times, people overcomplicate things as they attempt to "do it perfectly." Succeeding with your health is about making your program as simple as possible. Simplifying your meals, exercises, and the other four components of your Body Confidence Plan will help set the proper pace. Look at your program, and start off with what feels the simplest to you. This is a good rule to follow: if it feels like too much, it is too much. If you need to do fewer days of exercise or eat more protein bars, so be it. Once you regain a feeling of comfort, ability, and simplicity, you can begin diversifying once again.

3. **Confirm that you have set realistic time frames for your goals.** After your Jump Start Phase, you will know if your goal time frames have been set correctly. Within your first ten days on the program, you will know what pace is possible. It is important that you make sure that the goals you set match this pace. If not, you need to adjust the time frames of your goals. This adjustment will keep your expectations realistic and prevent unnecessary frustration.

4. **Maintain consistency.** When things are inconsistent, it is difficult to pace yourself. This is why starting out correctly matters: it sets the tone for consistency. Maintaining consistency allows you to correctly pace yourself.

5. **Believe that you will cross the finish line.** It is difficult to set a slower pace if you cannot see the finish line. This is why we typically want to set a faster pace: it gets us across the finish line faster. Whatever pace you set, if you believe you will cross the finish line, speed is irrelevant. You know you will eventually get there.

Concept 2—Accept That You Will Plateau

Plateaus are defined as times when your weight and body-fat percentage remain the same for a period of time. They are the part of the health process that we always know will come, yet we are always surprised when a plateau arrives, hoping that maybe this time we were able to dodge the bullet. You see, plateaus are viewed by many as bullets, since from the surface they are daunting and seem to kill your health progress. You scratch your head, frustrated that you are still doing everything the same and yet your results have halted. The good news is that this plateau mind-set is in your past. When you hit a plateau this time, you have an advantage—your newfound health education and Body Confidence Plan. You know that your health plateau really means you have simply reached your set point. You know that it is impossible for your body to progress at a rapid pace all the time. You understand that your body follows the same pattern as everything else in life: first come moments of progress, followed by moments of recalibration, followed by more moments of progress. This is the natural plateau cycle of life. Your health plateau is just that "moment" that your body takes to recalibrate, to adjust itself and take your improved body composition and all the other positive changes into account. This recalibration period occurs as your body reprograms your metabolism by lowering your set point. Once this reprogramming phase is complete, your body is ready to take another run at progression.

I also want to point out that there is a difference between your body being ready to progress and the actual act of progressing. Once you reach your set point, your body will naturally resist change. This is a protection mechanism that ensures that all the vital parts of your body (like blood volume, amount of essential body fat, water and electrolyte balance) remain stable. Your survival depends on this stability. This is what I mean when I say that your nutrition is used to create balance in your body. Stable blood sugar will get you to your set point and create the proper environment to lower it. The way you lower your set point and break through plateaus is by "raising your game." "Raising your game" means taking your effort to another level. This means fine-tuning each component of your Body Confidence Plan. This means taking action to force your body to progress while lowering your set point in the process.

Think about it: the goal your body strives for is to maintain its set point. Once you reach it (a plateau), why would your body want to progress further? This is the problem: your body doesn't. This is why the initial effort you put in to reach your set point must be increased if your goal is to lower it. I saw a great example of this when a female client of mine went from a Moderate level of health (about 24 percent body fat) to a Fit level of health (19 percent body fat). She was happy with her results (19 percent body fat), though she still wanted to be a little tighter and more toned, to get her body fat to 15 percent. You might think dropping 3 to 4 percent body fat is an easy feat. It is far from easy. Taking your body from a Fit level of health to a Performance level of health requires you to seriously "raise your game"; it is the hardest goal to achieve. My client did not understand this. She thought that she could just keep working her Body Confidence Plan at the same effort that took her body fat to 19 percent. The quality of her plan was already excellent. It needed to be to maintain 19 percent body fat (a great body-fat percentage for women); it was just not strong enough to take her body to 15 percent. This is when she chose to raise her game and apply the six strategies necessary to burst through her plateau and take her body to a Performance level of health (15 percent body fat). Here are the six strategies she applied. They are the same ones you will need to apply if you want to break through your plateaus, regardless of your current level of health:

Strategy 1: Prepare for Your Plateau Now

By accepting a plateau in your future as fact, you will not be shocked or frustrated when your progress slows down. You will then understand why and make the proper adjustments. This knowledge can work in your favor. Instead of implementing these strategies and "raising your game" when you reach your plateau, you can begin steadily working each strategy into your program starting from week 1. This will allow you to improve a little more each week—a comfortable pace. Many times this will prolong the time before you reach your first plateau.

Strategy 2: Choose High-Quality Foods and Meals

Your Jump Start Phase works so well because the majority of your meals are high quality. High-quality foods are optimally digested and metabolized by your body. This optimal digestion stabilizes your blood sugar much more efficiently than medium- and low-quality food. In addition, since high-quality foods are unprocessed, they contain low amounts of sodium. This is why high-quality foods cause less bloating. Focus on meals that contain only high-quality foods, and especially avoid all foods that contain gluten (bread products), dairy, and soy.

In addition, as I shared in chapter 5, for optimal blood-sugar stabilization choose meals that contain both a high-quality simple (fruits and vegetables) and complex (oatmeal, rice, beans, sweet potato) carbohydrate, with of course a high-quality protein and fat. This specific combination of simple and complex carbohydrates (while staying in your recommended nutrition parameters) provides the right balance between a fast (simple) and slow (complex) digested carbohydrate. The more meals you can implement this strategy (with the exception of your meal before bed) the faster you will burst through your plateau.

Strategy 3: Diversify Your Exercise and Increase Your Intensity Levels

As I mentioned in the exercise chapter, you want to continually mix up your exercise and choose a variety of movements. When you raise your game, you take this concept to an entirely new level. To break through a plateau, you want to make the following three adjustments to your exercise. These adjustments will add more time to your workout; however, this is temporary. Once you break through your plateau, you can go back to your normal exercise quantity. No matter what, though, you should still continue choosing the most optimal movements.

Here are your adjustments. (There are differences between goal types.)

1. **For Goal Type 1**

   - Add another day of high-intensity cardio, preferably sprinting. You will get quick results by sprinting three days a week, for thirty minutes each session. If you cannot sprint, do stairs, cycling (spinning), or swimming.

   - Add fifteen to thirty minutes of additional time to each fat-burning cardio session. Do the highest-quality movements.

   - Replace a strength-training session with a high-impact sport or class. Some examples include boxing, kickboxing, singles tennis, racquetball, basketball, or any other high-intensity, high-impact sport. This type of training will activate muscle you have not been using, which will then speed up your metabolism.

2. **For Goal Type 2**

   - Get five days of weight training in each week, between thirty and forty-five minutes per workout.

   - Only perform body-through-space (pushups, dips, pull-ups, squats, etc.), dumbbell, and barbell movements (until you break through your plateau). If possible, add weight to your body-through-space movements (pushups, dips, pull-ups, etc.).

- Focus on lowering your weights at a slower pace and pausing during the stretch position with each repetition of each movement. For example if you are doing a dumbbell chest press, the tempo would be 5–5–1—that is, take five seconds (5) to lower the weight, hold the stretch at the bottom of the movement for five seconds (5), and press the weight up in one second (1). This slower tempo will cause greater muscle damage, and therefore faster muscle growth.

- Keep your repetition range for each set between five and seven reps and make sure you go to muscular failure each set. This rep count and hitting failure will ensure you are lifting heavy enough weights each workout.

Strategy 4: Eat More Frequently

The longer you live the program, the better your body becomes at metabolizing your food. This increased efficiency causes you to become hungry every two and a half to three hours rather than every three to four hours. This is a very good thing. Every meal you eat causes your metabolism to fire up even hotter. More meals equals better results for all goal types. Increase your meals to six or seven per day (eating only when you are hungry, of course).

Strategy 5: Minimize Your Stress

As discussed in chapter 4, stress releases the hormone cortisol. It raises your blood sugar. Too much of this hormone in your blood will cause havoc in your body. If you have high levels of stress, it is almost impossible to break through plateaus. Focus on the five stress-minimizing strategies explained in chapter 4.

Strategy 6: Ask Yourself Whether You Really Want to Raise Your Game

Reaching a Moderate level of health will ensure that your body is working for you. Striving for a Fit or Performance level of health requires a higher level of commitment and discipline. We each have different Body Confidence goals. Before you choose to raise your game, make sure you want to go the extra mile. This is totally your choice. Many of my clients live at a Moderate level, many live at a Fit level, and many live at a Performance level. There is no right or wrong choice; it really just comes down to what you want in your life. The only thing that does matter is that you reach *at least* a Moderate level of health. This will keep your body fat within the proper ranges. As you can tell, breaking through plateaus takes effort. I want you to know that there are no limits to where you can take your body. Bonnie Kieffer is proof of that.

B onnie came to me because she was stuck at a plateau and did not know how to break through it. She had been struggling to lose weight for years, ever since she was pregnant with twins. After her pregnancy she thought she would quickly lose the weight; unfortunately, that was not the case. Her new responsibilities as a mom were exhausting (I hear twins do that), and to make matters worse, she was suffering from hormone imbalances caused by polycystic ovarian syndrome, also known as PCOS. Bonnie's PCOS was affecting the balance of her estrogen and progesterone levels (female hormones) and caused her body to become insulin resistant (her body could not efficiently lower blood sugar). These challenges caused Bonnie to keep all of her pregnancy weight. Within a year, Bonnie had gained even more weight and, to top it off, developed high cholesterol. Her body was in a tailspin, and it seemed to be only getting worse.

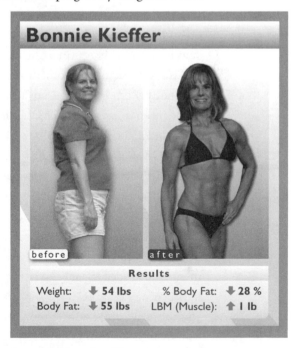

Bonnie Kieffer

before | after

Results

| Weight: | ⬇ 54 lbs | % Body Fat: | ⬇ 28 % |
| Body Fat: | ⬇ 55 lbs | LBM (Muscle): | ⬆ 1 lb |

Later the following year, Bonnie finally reached her "tipping point." She weighed 172 pounds and was at 42 percent body fat. She felt horrible. Before all of her complications, Bonnie lived a healthy lifestyle. She decided to get back to the basics: daily exercise and healthy eating. She was surprised how quickly she dropped twenty pounds. She thought, *This is easy, I'll reach my goals in no time.* (Bonnie wanted to get her weight back to the 120s.) Then a couple of weeks passed, and she made no additional progress. A few more weeks passed and still no progress. Bonnie was confused: she was following the same nutrition and exercise routine that dropped twenty pounds, so why did her progress stop? Another month passed, and Bonnie reached a new level of frustration. She had gotten discouraged, and she thought about quitting her routine altogether. She thought, *What's the point of this? I'm not progressing.* Thankfully, this is the moment I began working with her.

I knew Bonnie's husband, Randy. He told me about what Bonnie was going through. When I first met Bonnie, I could feel her sense of determination and drive. She had lived the last few years with so much frustration. She just wanted to learn how to get back her Body Confidence. Bonnie was already at her set point and felt she had hit a plateau for good. For this reason, we chose to immediately raise her game.

Bonnie shifted from eating healthy to stabilizing her blood sugar with high-quality balanced meals. She went from exercising only her red muscle to adding both categories of exercise into her workout routine, focusing on the highest-quality exercises: sprinting for high-intensity cardio and jogging for fat-burning cardio. Her core strength was weakened by her pregnancy and her years of inactivity. She started working her core twice a week in a core class at her gym. Her effort paid off as she quickly dropped 10 pounds and broke through her first plateau. As her results began to slow again (her body was in the recalibration phase), she raised her game once more by focusing on adding another day of sprinting and fifteen minutes per fat-burning session to her weekly routine. She also began a light weight-training routine to add more strength and some muscle mass (to speed up her metabolism). Additionally, Bonnie focused on increasing the frequency of her meals, getting six or seven in each day. These adjustments propelled Bonnie to drop another 15 pounds, lowered her cholesterol levels to a healthy range, and put her back in the 120s (127 pounds, to be exact).

She was fired up, realizing that she wanted a little more! Summer was around the corner, and Bonnie wanted to do what had been unthinkable to her only a few years before: she wanted to wear a bikini again. She would do it only if her abs looked great. With that goal in mind, Bonnie "raised her game" one more time. She was already so dialed in that the only adjustments she needed to make were to add another fifteen to thirty minutes to her fat-burning cardio sessions (mostly jogging) and lift slightly heavier weights so she would build a little more muscle mass. These final adjustments took Bonnie to her promised land. She finally had abs she was proud of and found her ultimate Body Confidence. Just look how great she fits into a bikini!

Bonnie raised her game three times and took her body from an At Risk level of health to a Performance level of health. Now, that is impressive!

Bonnie has become an inspiration for everyone in her life. Each of them has seen the transformation and still cannot believe what she achieved. There were many inspiring moments for me as well while I worked with Bonnie. The one that means the most to me was when I saw Randy (Bonnie's husband) right after they came back from their summer vacation, where she wore a bikini. Randy and I were talking about how amazing Bonnie's results were, and Randy was telling me how she has become a different person. He spoke about how Bonnie was unhappy and depressed every day when she struggled with her weight. She would never want to go anywhere, ashamed of what she looked like. I listened in disbelief, since I never knew that Bonnie. The Bonnie I knew was happy, confident, and loved life. Randy told me how Bonnie's success not only changed her life, but changed his life and the future of their family. Randy's words reminded me of what making your health a priority and taking your Body Confidence to the next level is all about: living the quality of life you have always wanted.

Concept 3—Acknowledge Your Little Victories

In the goal-setting section (chapter 3) you set short- and long-term Body Confidence goals. As I explained, both types of goals will keep you focused and motivated. Additionally, there is another type of goal that is an important part of staying true to the process. This is your immediate Body Confidence goal. Immediate goals are your "little health victories" each day. An immediate goal could be doing five additional minutes of fat-burning cardio, or remembering to get in your midafternoon meal, or drinking your correct amount of water in a day. They are any actions that take you one step closer to achieving your short- or long-term goal.

We all want to feel like we are winning each day. Acknowledging these little victories provides you with a sense of accomplishment and proves that you are progressing with your health, which in turn inspires you to stay true to the process. Watching Hunter grow and develop makes me extremely aware of this. Every time Hunter does something new, he gets so proud—as he should. We should all feel victorious when we accomplish greatness. Any time you improve your health in some way, regardless of the size of the accomplishment, you should take a moment and acknowledge your little victory.

Just as you determined your short-term and long-term goals, you should write out your immediate goals. Here are three guidelines to follow when setting your immediate Body Confidence goals:

- Choose one healthy action (an immediate goal) each day that will solidify or improve your Body Confidence Plan.

- At the end of the day, acknowledge achieving that immediate goal.

- Each new action becomes a permanent part of your Body Confidence Plan.

This way, you experience "little victories" each day, bringing you closer to achieving your short- and long-term goals.

Concept 4—Create Positive Escapes

I first introduced the concept of creating positive escapes in the stress section of chapter 4. The concept of creating escapes goes beyond stress management. Escapes, positive and negative, are defined as things we do for enjoyment that give our minds a break from the daily grind. These escapes can be anything: reading, watching TV, drinking alcohol, going to the movies, or eating ice cream. They can be anything that provides you a release. When wanting to become healthier, we divide escapes into two categories: *negative* and *positive*.

Negative escapes are any actions that provide a release but work against achieving your Body Confidence goals. (Examples include eating too many "off plan" meals and drinking too much alcohol.) Positive escapes are any actions that provide a release without affecting your progress. (Examples include watching TV, going to the movies, reading, listening to music, and hiking.)

Typically, when people start a health plan, they immediately give up their negative escapes—primarily alcohol, as well as high-fat and carbohydrate foods. Overall, this adjustment is a good idea; the problem is that they do not replace the negative escapes with any positive escapes. This can be problematic, since removing your escapes completely can cause stress and anxiety to build and daily enjoyment to decrease. This is what causes people to abandon their health process.

To prevent this, here are three guidelines:

1. **Make a list of the top ten things you enjoy doing (positive escapes).** This will provide you with enough options.

2. **Limit your negative escapes.** Drinking in moderation and eating a weekly "off plan" meal is fine. Just make sure you stay within those boundaries. Using alcohol or food to relax or de-stress creates unhealthy behaviors and will prevent you from achieving your goals.

3. **Replace all negative escapes with positive escapes.** This will take some practice, and the positives might not initially provide the same release as the negatives. In time, though, your positive escapes will be more enjoyable than your negative escapes. Using positive escapes provides you with the best of both worlds: the release you need, and movement toward your Body Confidence goals.

Concept 5—Evaluate Costs Versus Payoffs

There is a great saying: "Is the juice worth the squeeze?" It means "Is your action worth what you get from it?" This is what the concept of Cost Versus Payoffs is all about. Simply put, everything we do has a cost (negative) and a payoff (positive). Applying this thought process to your health allows you to remove your emotions from the choices you make and instead make your decisions based on facts. For example, let's say you really want to go to dinner and have drinks with your friends, and it has been only three days since your last "off plan" meal. Instead of making an emotional decision and going for it, which most likely will make you feel guilty, just . . . try following this model:

1. **Evaluate the "costs" (the negatives) of eating and drinking with your friends:**

    Your blood sugar will spike.

    You will store a little fat.

    You will be a little bloated.

    You may be hung over the next day.

2. **Evaluate the "payoff" of eating and drinking with your friends (the positives):**

> Your friends are going to your favorite restaurant.
>
> Your friends are going with you, so you get some quality time with them.
>
> You can blow off some steam.

3. **Compare your costs versus your payoffs, and make a choice.**

> If your payoffs are stronger than your costs, then go for it: "the juice is worth the squeeze."
>
> If your costs are stronger than your payoffs, then skip it: "the juice is *not* worth the squeeze."
>
> Here is how I would evaluate the following data: since dinner is at your favorite restaurant, you can blow off some steam, and you get to spend some time with your friends, the payoffs outweigh the costs, and therefore "the juice is worth the squeeze."

This concept really assists you in staying true to the process because it provides you with flexibility. You have a program and a plan to follow, yet you can deal with exceptions should they arise. Knowing that you have this flexibility provides a less rigid mind-set. In addition, it provides you with a gauge that allows you to truly evaluate your actions and see whether they are worth their "costs."

Concept 6—Be Unattached to the Outcome

Being unattached to the outcome means just working the program and not letting the number on the scale or the size of your clothes or your body-fat percentage be the only thing that tells you that you are progressing. You see, I know the importance of setting Body Confidence external goals, and I know that living for those goals can drive you crazy. There is a fine line between working toward achieving a goal and having the goal take you over. Sometimes it is difficult to tell the difference, so . . . think about these four scenarios—clear signs that you are attached to the outcome and the goal is taking you over:

1. You weigh yourself every day and let the number on the scale determine your mood.

2. You get depressed if you "feel" you did not drop enough weight, even though there is no reason you should have dropped that amount of weight.

3. You are *not* enjoying your food or exercise, and you are following the program only to achieve your outcome.

4. You are attempting to be "perfect" on the program so that you can quickly reach your external goal.

In these examples you are basically living for the outcome and forgetting about creating a permanent Body Confidence foundation. If any of these scenarios describe you, it is crucial that you shift your mind-set to become unattached to the outcome. You still set your goals, follow your program, and implement the same strategies. The only adjustment you make is that you no longer focus solely on your "number" goals.

If you simply work the program and make any necessary adjustments, your "number" goals will still be achieved; they will simply become part of the equation instead of the only thing you care about. This shift in mind-set will also play a big part in staying true to the process.

Concept 7—Have Fun

Having fun is rare when you diet, which is why people quit them. As you work the program, remember to have fun. Each day you can look at getting healthier either as a chore or as an experience. Experiences are adventures. This is what your program is all about. Think of all the new foods and fun exercises you will try, as well as the improved energy you will have. As crazy as it sounds, learning how to make your body work for you is fun and liberating.

In order to stay true to the process, you must have fun. Here are three questions you should ask yourself to ensure that you are keeping your program exciting and fun:

1. Am I enjoying my program?

2. What is not fun in my program? (Remove these things and replace them with something more enjoyable.)

3. What can I do to make my program more fun?

By implementing these seven concepts, you will succeed in staying true to the process. A great example of this is the success of my client Sandy Haddock.

*S*andy embodies this mind-set so well. She is a wife and mother, and she consistently struggled with her weight throughout her life. She has always been active; she just chose to eat unhealthy. What can you say? She loves food. As we know, eventually all good things must come to an end, and Sandy's unhealthy eating was beginning to cause large weight gain as she entered into the dreaded territory of menopause. Her metabolism was moving at an all-time low, and her weight was reaching an all-time high. She knew she needed to do something.

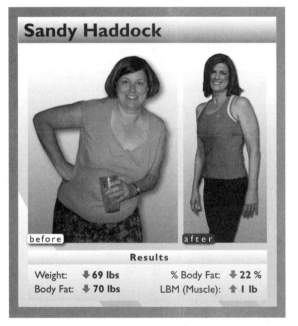

Sandy Haddock

before   after

Results

Weight:	↓ **69 lbs**	% Body Fat:	↓ **22 %**
Body Fat:	↓ **70 lbs**	LBM (Muscle):	↑ **1 lb**

A few of her friends were doing a diet, so she decided to give it try. Sandy's diet was pretty simple: she was told to cut her portion sizes and eat better-quality food. Since she was above her set point, she quickly dropped twenty pounds on the diet. However, as with all diets, Sandy stopped dropping weight the moment she reached her set point. She was eating much healthier—just not stabilizing her blood sugar. Sandy was far from achieving her long-term Body Confidence goal (which was to lose fifty more pounds) and began to regress, so she decided to "abandon the process" of her diet and try a different one that another of her friends was on. Her second diet did more than focus on healthy eating, since this diet had Sandy eating four meals a day. Sandy immediately started losing weight again. She dropped an additional fifteen pounds and then *bam!* She hit another plateau. She still had a good amount of weight (thirty-five pounds) to lose and was frustrated that she would repeatedly drop weight fast and then hit a wall. Sandy chose to "abandon the process" of her second diet once again and chose to start the Venice Nutrition program.

When I met Sandy and talked with her, it made sense that she would drop and then hold: She was eating healthy and fairly frequently, she was just one meal short per day, and her calories and nutrient ratios were off. She was also training only her red muscle and not getting enough omega-3s. Her discipline was strong and she was willing to do the work; she just needed to know what to do. After I designed Sandy's plan, she dived right in and quickly began dropping weight. Every time she would hit a little plateau, she would make the proper adjustments to her program and would then begin progressing again. Within a few months, Sandy achieved her goal weight and body composition. What was more impressive was that Sandy had the courage to "abandon the process" of two diets. The moment she hit a plateau and realized the diet could not do any more for her, she kept searching for a better way. I watched Sandy own the seven concepts of staying true to the process. This was someone who once rarely paid attention to her health. Now Sandy makes her health a priority each day and has permanently achieved her goals. Whenever I see Sandy, it is the highlight of my day as she inspires me with her big smile and the sheer joy she has for her newfound Body Confidence!

CHAPTER TAKEAWAY

Everyone implements these seven concepts a little differently. The key for you is to use each one so you feel your program fits nicely into your world. These concepts are designed to eliminate any feelings of being overwhelmed. Remember that you are the one who sets the pace, so make sure your program makes for an enjoyable experience.

8

WORKING YOUR PROGRAM INTO YOUR WORLD

The key to winning is making the right adjustments to your game plan.

Throughout the book I have mentioned the importance of working the program into your world. So, what exactly does this mean? Think of the game plan for a football game. The coaches design it and the players follow it. The team enters the game with a specific agenda and believes that their plan will lead them to victory. What happens if for some reason the game plan is not working? Maybe the players are struggling, or one of the starters gets hurt, or the opposing team simply has a better plan. At that moment, the team has two choices: they either stick with their original game plan and likely lose, or they adjust their plan and have a better chance at winning. Working the program into your world means making the right adjustments to your game plan so you can win with your health.

Your Body Confidence Plan is the game plan for your health. Right now, you are like the football team before they took the field, prepared with a clear and organized health plan designed to achieve your goals. What happens if you struggle with implementing your game plan like the football team did? For whatever reason, you are having a hard time implementing the strategies we have spoken of. Do you choose to stay the course, hoping things will work themselves out, or do you adjust your plan? When you think about it that way, you already know the answer: you always adjust your plan. You see, right now your Body Confidence Plan is untested within your life. Everyone has different lives. Working the program into your world means adjusting your plan to work for you. Now, of course, you still need to follow all your Body Confidence guidelines; this is a must. What I mean by adjusting is how you will apply these guidelines to your life. There are three actions that will provide you with the knowledge and ability to correctly adjust your plan and successfully work your program into your world.

The three actions are these:

1. Create a Body Confidence System.

2. Know what to do when life shows up.

3. Learn how to include your friends and family.

Action 1—Create a Body Confidence System

We each have a daily routine consisting of the time we awake, the hours we work, when we exercise, how we spend our down time, and eventually when we go to sleep. Within this routine there may be many other little things we do. My point is that each day is fairly structured. Our daily routine provides us with a sense of calmness, consistency, and control. Our daily routine is in essence our daily system, meaning it's composed of many moving parts that work together for a desired outcome: having an efficient and productive day. Just as you have a daily system for the rest of the parts of your life, you also need a daily system for your Body Confidence Plan. Creating a system will help develop consistency and provide you with a sense of daily control with your health. Consistency is how you will achieve your goals.

As you can probably tell by now, I am a systematic and structured person. My wife, Abbi, on the other hand, is a free-flowing spirit and has never been a fan of structure (opposites attract, of course). I am sharing this with you because many times when I mention systems to people, the structured personalities love it and the free spirits hate it. Regardless of your personality type, it is important that you create the Body Confidence System that works for you. Abbi's system works for her, and my system works for me. We are very different, and all that matters is that we both have strong Body Confidence Plans. Our individual health systems help us successfully work the program into our worlds.

Here are the five initial steps to creating a Body Confidence System:

Step 1: Every Sunday, Prepare for Your Upcoming Week

It has happened to all of us: we tried to keep the weekend alive late into Sunday night, leaving us sleep deprived and unprepared come Monday morning. The typical Monday stress seems higher than usual, and it is causing us to scramble just to get our meals in. As each day passes, it feels like we cannot get caught up, and one day dominoes into the next. Finally, the weekend comes once again, we get a moment to breathe, and we realize how important each Sunday night is to prepare for the upcoming week. It seems so minor, yet it is so valuable. By looking at your upcoming week and preparing your plan around your schedule, your adjustments will be proactive rather than reactive.

Here are a few suggestions on how to prepare for your upcoming week:

Determine your approximate mealtimes. If you have a few days that are outside your normal schedule (for example, you have meeting out of the office), get your adjustments in place early so you are prepared.

Prepare for any late nights at work or business dinners. By looking into the future, you can adjust your mealtimes and exercise schedule to accommodate your longer days or business dinners.

Know which days you will be exercising, and plan your workouts. Certain workouts are more intense than others. If you are working twelve hours one day, you may want to do a less intense workout or take the day off on that day, since more intense workouts require more energy.

Schedule your "off plan" meal. This will provide you with something to look forward to and prevent you from falling "off plan" and regretting it afterward.

Your Sunday preparation is centered on your daily routine. Make a checklist that applies to you and sets you up to win each week.

Step 2: Schedule a Weekly Grocery-Shopping Day

The best way to fall "off plan" is by running out of food. It can easily sneak up on you. All of a sudden, you go to the fridge and your favorite foods are just empty containers. When this happens, you are at the mercy of restaurant food and meal replacements (bars and shakes), both of which, when eaten too often, can cause unstable blood sugar because meal replacements are so processed and restaurant food contains extra sodium and fat. You plan on going grocery shopping that night, until something affects your schedule (like working late, your child getting sick, and so on), and now you have to take on the next day unprepared without your food once again. This can all be prevented by scheduling a weekly grocery-shopping day. Which day does not matter. You just need to get enough food to keep your fridge stocked. This is the same principle as preparing for your upcoming week. You always want to be proactive rather than reactive.

Step 3: Pack Your Workout Bag Each Night

Think of a time when you slept through your alarm clock. You woke up, looked at the time, and immediately panicked, realizing you were late. It is at times like these that having your workout bag ready before you wake up feels really good. Mornings are busy enough. The more you prepare each night, the less stressful your morning will be and the more consistent your exercise will become.

Step 4: Have a Cooler, Reusable Ice Packs, and Tupperware

You might be traveling for the day and need to place more items into your MRFK. This is when a cooler is perfect. In addition, having the reusable ice packs will keep your food cold, and Tupperware will keep your food dry and secure. Not to mention that the ice packs and Tupperware can be used over and over again.

I have seen too many melted and gooey protein bars in gym bags. A cooler containing some ice is a great solution.

Step 5: Prepare Your Food in Bulk

Preparing your food in bulk is a great way to eat high-quality food without needing to cook it each day. After a long day, the last thing you probably want to do is cook. Cooking in bulk solves this problem. This is another great reason to have Tupperware.

. . .

These five steps are just the beginning. Systems are a powerful tool because once we are dialed in, everything runs like clockwork. The strange thing is that once we break the pattern, it becomes difficult to regain our rhythm. The Boy Scouts have a motto: Be Prepared. This means "Be ready for anything life throws your way." The way you keep your Body Confidence system running well is to follow the Boy Scout motto yourself. *Be prepared.*

Action 2—Know What to Do When Life Shows Up

You will have weeks without exercise. You will have weeks when you miss meals. You will have weeks when you deprive yourself of sleep. You will also have weeks when your stress levels are out of control. At these times, your life will feel out of balance and chaotic. Your energy will be lower, you will have sugar cravings, and you will want to eat "off plan" meal after meal. All of these circumstances are caused when "life shows up." "Life showing up" is when unforeseen challenges come into your world and create havoc for your Body Confidence Plan and possibly your Quadrant as well. Sometimes, this describes a period of challenges that last only a few days. Sometimes this period will last months. How you respond when life shows up is the key for you to permanently work your program into your world.

These unforeseen challenges may be positive things happening in your life—like getting married, having a baby, buying a new house, or getting a promotion. Each one is a joyous moment that brings more responsibilities and unforeseen challenges along with it. I remember how naive I was when Abbi was pregnant. I played tennis five days a week and thought I could continue that schedule after Hunter was born. Wow, what an awakening! People would always tell me that raising a child is a twenty-four-hour-a-day job. I heard them; I just did not truly understand until Hunter was born. My tennis racket sat in our garage for nine months collecting dust. So much for playing five days a week!

Your unforeseen challenges can also be sad things in your life, like the death of a loved one, a divorce, or loss of employment. Each of these will increase your stress levels and create new obstacles. Your unforeseen challenges may even be little things like a sudden business trip or getting the flu. Basically, life showing up is anything that jeopardizes your consistency.

Since life will show up, the next question is, How do you prevent regression when it does? When life shows up, you go into survival mode. The biggest mistake I see people make when life shows up is that they attempt to keep pushing their program, choosing to ignore their new challenges. This may work for a while. . . . But remember the analogy I used in chapter 4 about the glass of water: if you take a glass of water that is already full and choose to add more water to it, you will spill water everywhere. This is also what happens when you choose to ignore life showing up. You can prevent regression when life shows up; it will take a strong commitment on your part, but it is possible.

There are five elements to adjust in your Body Confidence Plan when life shows up:

1. **Temporarily change your Body Confidence Goal to Maintenance Mode.** It is never easy to change your goals, though you must when life shows up. Sometimes maintenance is a good thing. Think about it. If you maintain your health at times of chaos and progress during times of calm, you will be moving forward with your health overall. There are times to push ahead in life and there are times to survive. When life shows up, your goal is to survive, to maintain.

2. **Make up sleep whenever possible.** Sleep typically gets neglected when life shows up. Since you will be sleep deprived, it's important to do your best to go to sleep as early as you can and take naps when possible. As I mentioned earlier, you want to do your best to follow your sleep schedule. However, rules are made by their exceptions, and when you are struggling to get your sleep in, you need to take it any way and anywhere you can.

3. **Eat any quality of food; just make sure to get five to six balanced meals in.** I have coached many businessmen and businesswomen, and all of them have last-minute business trips. At these times, it is

common for them to eat four bars in a day. Sometimes it is just not possible to get real food into your body. This is why protein bars, protein powder, and ready-to-drink shakes can be lifesavers. What matters most is that you get five to six balanced meals in, even if they are in the form of protein supplements (a low-quality food).

4. **Limit alcohol and "off plan" meals.** Sleep deprivation, low-quality food, and high stress levels can trigger sugar cravings and awaken the feeling of wanting a release. These are the times when alcohol and "off plan" meals are craved the most. When life shows up, your goal is maintenance, and it is hard to maintain when you have too many "off plan" meals or drink too much. These are the times when your discipline needs to kick in and you need to focus on the positive escapes you created in chapter 7. Implement these to give you the release you want.

5. **Minimize high-intensity cardio and heavy weights.** Since your sleep is erratic, your body's battery (adrenal gland) is not fully charged. High-intensity cardio and heavy weight training take a lot of energy, and at times of chaos, they should be limited to a maximum of one time per week. Stretching, fat-burning cardio, and core training are much less intense and should be your primary sources of exercise.

Accepting life showing up as a reality will help prepare you for when it happens. As with creating a system for your Body Confidence Plan, it is always better to be prepared and proactive than reactive.

Action 3—Learn How to Include Your Friends and Family

Growing up, my mom would make two different meals for dinner. One meal was the nondiet meal. This meal was for me, my dad, and my sister Chris. The other meal was the diet meal for my mom and Laurie. The nondiet meal had all the good stuff: a good protein source, mashed potatoes or rice, and some vegetables. The diet meal was usually prepackaged, was very low in calories, and appeared to be a meal for a bird. This was all my mom knew. She thought that in order to lose weight she needed to eat diet foods and that anyone who did not need to lose weight could eat the nondiet foods. My mom had to consistently make two meals for our family. During dinner, you could always feel a sense of separation between the dieters and the nondieters. Laurie and my mom wanted to eat the nondiet meal; they just felt they were not allowed. They felt that something was the matter with them: they were always going to be dieters. Thinking back to those times now frustrates me. It did not have to be like that for my family. Even more troubling is that what occurred in my household back then is even more prevalent in households across the country today.

Taking your Body Confidence to the next level should never create separation between you and your family and friends. You do not need to make two different meals and do double the work. You do not need to be labeled a dieter and feel that you can eat only so-called diet foods. Since the Venice Nutrition Program works for everyone, everyone in your life can eat the same way you do. There is no such thing as dieting on the Venice Nutrition Program. You simply learn how to make food work for you so you can make the foods you love work into your world.

Achieving the Body Confidence you desire is possible only if your program includes your friends and family. You have to feel you can do your program with them at dinner, at social gatherings, on vacation, and when you are out on the town. There are three ways to best include your friends and family in your program:

1. **Lead by example.** The question I always get after a client is on the program for a few weeks is what they should do to inspire a family member or friend to start the program. Since they are feeling so good and getting great results, they want their loved ones to have the same experience. My response is to lead by example. People are always watching. If they see your commitment, their interest is peaked. If they see a realistic and attainable approach, they get excited. If they see you achieve fantastic internal and external results, they are all in. I think everyone should do the Venice Nutrition program, because I think everyone needs to learn how their body works. There's an intangible feeling that accompanies a new level of Body Confidence. Words cannot explain it; you have to feel it. Your friends and family will see this, so if your goal is to improve the health of someone you love, save your words. Your actions are how you lead by example.

2. **Utilize your recipes and "free foods."** Society has labeled health food as bland and boring. As many of us know, this is not true. The moment someone thinks you are on a program, they will become scared of the food you are eating, thinking it is somehow diet food. The way you unlock their thinking is to utilize your recipes and your "free foods." Both of these will spice up your meals and be tasty to your friends and family as well. Your double meal preparation days will become a thing of the past, and now everyone can enjoy the same meal, with the bonus of keeping their blood sugar stable with every bite.

3. **Exercise together.** As you are finding your passion for exercise, think about doing it with your friends and family. A nice family walk after dinner creates great quality time and helps with burning fat. A morning run with a couple of friends holds each of you accountable and provides a sense companionship and fun. Taking a group exercise class with your significant other will get you both to the gym and will help you get motivated to work hard in the class. Joining a sports league provides excellent cardio conditioning and allows you to participate in some healthy competition. The examples are countless. Choosing an exercise that you can do with your friends and family is a powerful way to include them in your program.

Your friends and family are permanent parts of your life. They are part of your world. It is important that your program includes them. This will prevent any feeling of separation and actually enhance your relationships, making them stronger and more fun. Two clients of mine who are stellar examples of how to work the program into your world are Joe and Claudette Foster.

Joe came to me because he needed to drop weight and body fat to improve his performance. Joe is a professional race-car driver, and he needed to lose about forty pounds. The extra weight and body fat was affecting the speed of his car (every pound counts when racing cars), his body's ability to cool down (the inside of a race car runs about 150 degrees during a race), and his overall recovery between races. Joe also wanted to increase his shoulder and neck strength for the actual act of driving. Joe shared how he had dropped weight in the past by drastically cutting calories. Back then, even though he lost the weight, his energy and performance suffered. He thought it had to be one or the other. He didn't know that he could achieve his goal and improve his energy levels and performance at the same time.

Joe, as most professional athletes, is very structured. Due to this structure, I knew once I set him up with his meal plans and exercise guidelines (he loves cycling like me), he would dive right in. The only challenge I saw with Joe was his traveling schedule. During his racing season, he goes from race to race while simultaneously running his racing company. The demands on his time are intense. To ensure that he would not regress when traveling, we needed to work together to create systems for his Body Confidence Plan that worked when he was at home and also when life was more chaotic during a trip. Joe took the concept of making his program work into his world to another level. He adjusted his plan to work optimally at home and on the road. His extra pounds of weight and body fat were melting away.

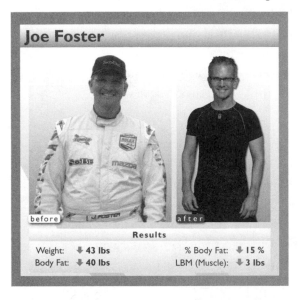

Joe Foster

before   after

Results

| Weight: | ⬇ 43 lbs | % Body Fat: | ⬇ 15 % |
| Body Fat: | ⬇ 40 lbs | LBM (Muscle): | ⬇ 3 lbs |

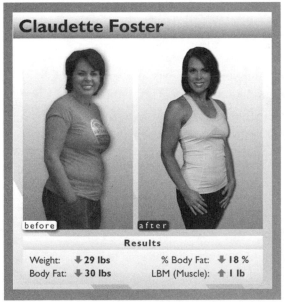

Claudette Foster

before   after

Results

| Weight: | ⬇ 29 lbs | % Body Fat: | ⬇ 18 % |
| Body Fat: | ⬇ 30 lbs | LBM (Muscle): | ⬆ 1 lb |

Joe was quickly down twenty pounds, and this motivated his wife, Claudette, to start the program. (He led by example.) Claudette wanted to drop about thirty pounds and learn how to prepare better meals for their daughters. She saw how Joe was eating real food and thought they should do the program as a family so it could become a way of life for all of them. Claudette and Joe are similar to Abbi and me. Joe is structured, like me, and Claudette is more of a free spirit, like Abbi. She wanted to have more flexibility in her program than Joe. (Joe was eating only high-quality meals.) Claudette also dived right in, focusing on recipes and meals that she could incorporate as a family. She spent time adjusting her Body Confidence Plan and creating a family system

that made it easier for her, Joe, and their girls. Claudette also paced herself with her exercise. She started with fat-burning cardio four days a week. The following week, she added two days of high-intensity cardio. By the third week, she was taking two Pilates classes, and by the fourth week she added a weight-training class. In the end, she was working out five days a week for about an hour a day. Once Claudette achieved her goals, she was getting bored with only doing cardio at the gym. She was looking for a challenge, and what is more challenging than a triathlon (a race where you swim, bike, and run)? She adjusted her gym cardio to train for a triathlon and, in so doing, found her passion for exercise.

It was such a pleasure to watch Joe and Claudette infuse their world with the program. Each day that passes, they continue to evolve and adjust the parts of the program that they want to change and improve. Through consistent effort, the Fosters achieved their Body Confidence goals. Joe lost his forty pounds and is driving better than ever. Claudette dropped thirty pounds and completed her first triathlon. Joe and Claudette created their own systems and made the program a way of life for their family. Their actions have gone way beyond just them. They have both inspired many members of their family, as well as their friends, to take on the program.

What is most motivating to me about Joe and Claudette is their desire to learn. They both wanted to become educated about their bodies. It was as if they knew what was possible and how good they could feel. As you focus on incorporating the three actions that will help work your program into your world, use Joe's and Claudette's success as proof that it is possible. Optimally adjusting your Body Confidence Plan will eventually become second nature, as it has for Joe and Claudette.

You now have the tools. It is time to take action!

9

TAKING ACTION

> There is nothing brilliant or outstanding in my
> record, except perhaps this one thing: I do the things
> that I believe ought to be done. . . . And when
> I make up my mind to do a thing, I act.
>
> **—President Theodore Roosevelt**

I was working late one night and heard a knock on my office door. When I got up from my desk and looked through the window, I saw a man I had never seen before. I opened my door to look closer and saw that he had a look of concern. I introduced myself and asked him how I could help him. He told me his name was Jim Gottschalk and that he had just been diagnosed with type 2 diabetes. Now I understood his look of concern.

Jim is in his sixties, married, the father of two, and a business owner. He had always lived a busy life and never really saw much value in focusing on his health. He smoked for years, ate what he wanted, and rarely exercised. But when he found out he had diabetes, Jim felt like he was in shock. He felt lost, unsure of what to do, and scared (as we would all be under the same circumstances). Jim left his doctor's office after his diagnosis without any nutritional or exercise advice. He was not even given a glucose monitor so he could test his blood sugar. All he got was a prescription for medication to assist in controlling his blood-sugar levels. Jim wanted to do more than just take some pills. Jim also wanted a solid plan. After we spoke for about twenty minutes, I saw the concern on Jim's face begin to dissipate. He went from feeling a sense of hopelessness to understanding that he could influence what happened next.

Jim started his program the following day. We both thought his biggest challenge was going to be changing his poor lifestyle habits. He had lived in a particular way for over sixty years, and changing those habits would involve some big-time reprogramming. But Jim was motivated and wanted to turn his health around after years of neglecting his body. Each week I saw Jim, I was expecting to coach him on methods of making his Body Confidence Plan more consistent, yet that was never necessary. He loved his experience. He got in five meals in each day, exercised five days a week (doing both categories of exercises), and dropped weight and body fat like nobody's business.

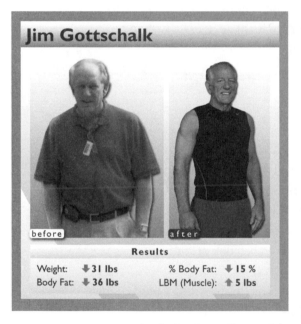

Jim Gottschalk

before   after

Results

Weight:	⬇ 31 lbs	% Body Fat:	⬇ 15 %
Body Fat:	⬇ 36 lbs	LBM (Muscle):	⬆ 5 lbs

Jim implemented each component of his plan like he was born to do it. His weekly consistency and positive results were also helping his blood-sugar levels stabilize and remain that way.

Within six weeks on the program, Jim dropped twenty pounds and took his blood-glucose measurement down to a healthy range for diabetics. Jim now had a new lease on life and felt his best. Jim continued to work his program, each month getting more trim and fit, improving his blood-sugar levels, and achieving Body Confidence. He now has complete control over his diabetes, having lost over thirty pounds and 15 percent body fat. I saw Jim at the store with his wife one day and asked him how he stayed the course with the program after sixty years of bad habits. He replied, "I knew it was time to take action."

Jim's words resonated with me. He was so right! Once you learn what to do, the real success begins when you start to take action. The more I thought about what he said, the more I realized that taking action is an attitude. It is a belief that you are going to make it happen regardless of the task's difficulty or timetable. Knowing the information can get you only so far. . . . You must possess the attitude that will ensure that you will transform knowledge into action.

Three simple traits I think embody the "make it happen" attitude:

1. **Show up**—Woody Allen said, "Eighty percent of success is showing up." I love this quote, because showing up to me is giving everything your full attention and your best effort both mentally and physically. Permanently achieving Body Confidence requires that you consistently show up.

2. **Reach for greatness**—Have you ever met someone who strives to be average? Who wants to feel just OK? In my experience, no one does. Each of us has greatness inside, and each of us wants to find it. Watching Hunter reminds me of this every day: His drive to be his best inspires me to be my best. His passion fuels my passion. Look around, connect with others who are also reaching for greatness, and inspire each other to be your best. When you do this, you can get to places you never thought were possible and reach the level of Body Confidence you have always dreamed of. Jim Gottschalk is living proof.

3. **Choose to be an expert on your body**—While I was growing up, my dad often shared a well-known Chinese proverb to teach me independence: "Give someone a fish and you feed them for a day. Teach them how to fish and you feed them for a lifetime." Diets fail because they never teach you how to "fish for yourself." With each change that you make on your program, you become more of an expert on your body. Each person in a success story featured in this book became an expert on their body as they gained Body Confidence. Be *the* expert on your body.

Megan Hall is another powerful example of taking action. Her story is unique and very special. Megan is an ectomorph (fast metabolism), and she has always been underweight. She ate frequent meals, exercised consistently (both categories), and managed her stress well. Still, keeping her weight stable was a continual struggle. Even though Megan had these challenges, she kept searching (taking action) for a solution, believing there had to be a way she could gain weight. As Megan entered her twenties, things became even more difficult when her hormonal system became unbalanced. Her thyroid was underproducing, her pancreas was struggling to make enough insulin to keep her blood sugar in check, and her low estrogen and progesterone levels caused her to lose her menstrual cycle. This was problematic, since Megan and her husband wanted to have a baby.

When Megan and I first met, I could tell she was wondering if she would ever get better. It was the same look Abbi got when she was injured. I lived in that space with Abbi. It is a tough place to be. Megan felt she was doing everything right and her body just seemed to be getting worse. Her dream was to be a mother. The problem was that without a menstrual cycle, she was definitely not getting pregnant. As I assessed Megan's eating habits, I noticed that her nutrition ratios seemed to be a bit off and that she was a meal short each day. Also, her stress was very high from the uncertainty of her health and the loss of her menstrual cycle. Megan was worried she would never be able to get pregnant. For ectomorphs, high stress triggers weight loss, not gain, because it makes their metabolism even faster.

Megan and I decided to focus on optimizing each part of her Body Confidence Plan, focusing especially on quality of sleep, calories and nutrient ratios, and stress management. Those were the three things that seemed off. Within a couple of weeks on the program, Megan's energy increased and her sugar cravings were gone. Her body seemed to be stabilizing. A few weeks after that, we knew she was stabilizing when she regained her menstrual cycle. When Megan told me that, I could feel the mountain of pressure ease

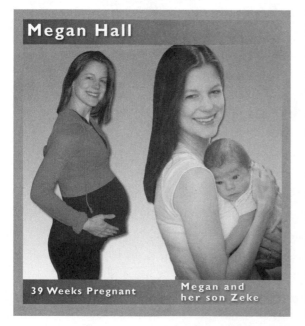

Megan Hall

39 Weeks Pregnant   Megan and her son Zeke

from her shoulders. She began to feel like she was gaining some control over her health. Megan steadily improved, and three months after we started working together, Megan came into my office with a big smile on her face. I said to myself, *She's pregnant!* I was right.

Over the next nine months, Megan experienced many difficulties. She had an underactive thyroid, contracted gestational diabetes (diabetes during pregnancy), and experienced digestive challenges. To say the least, her pregnancy was not easy. Yet throughout her pregnancy Megan worked her plan like a pro. She journaled consistently, made daily adjustments, worked her five stress strategies, and ate high-quality meals. Her effort was the strongest I have ever seen. Megan Hall was the definition of taking action. And of course this story has a happy ending: Megan's dream came true with the birth of her healthy baby boy, Zeke.

I am sharing this story with you because it reinforces everything you have learned so far. Megan did not wave a magic wand; she worked the program into her life and learned how to create balance in her body. By taking action, she became the expert on her body, which helped her conceive.

. . .

My goal during our journey together has been to provide you with the answers you have been seeking and elevate you to a *new level of thinking* about your body. Live with confidence! I ask you, What type of life can you live if you do not have Body Confidence (looking and feeling your best)? With Body Confidence you can live the type of life you want. You can reach your dreams. This realization can forever change your life.

My message to you is that you *can* achieve Body Confidence. It will be scary at times. Change always is. This is why you must be clear on what it will give you (find your "why") so you can stare down your fear and push through to the other side. No matter what challenges you face, you can push through regardless.

As you pursue the path to achieving Body Confidence, know that I believe with every ounce of my being that you can and will succeed. At the moments when self-doubt creeps in, remember that I'm standing up for you, and so is every Venice Nutrition member and coach. You are now part of the Venice Nutrition Community, and each of us believes you can achieve Body Confidence. Everything is possible!

Always remember, there are many things you cannot control in life; the one thing you can *control is how you choose to take care of yourself.*

Now go—reach for the life you want to live. You deserve it!

ACKNOWLEDGMENTS

Writing this book has been one of the most special experiences of my life. Making my dream become a reality was possible only because of teamwork. I would like to acknowledge the team that walked this amazing journey by my side.

My wife, Abbi—You are my foundation, my strength, my forever love. For the past seventeen years, every step I took, you were right there holding my hand. Your love makes me want to be the best man, husband, and father I can be. Thank you for simply being you and always believing in me, especially at the moments when I struggled to believe in myself. I love you. You are the greatest person I have ever known.

My son, Hunter—You are my greatest teacher. Your sheer love for life is intoxicating. Watching you find joy in every moment awakened me to being present and living in the moment with you. Everything about you is golden—your passion, your sense of humor, and most of all your heart. You are my best friend, and I am so proud to be your father. Son, I love you with all of my heart.

Mom and Dad—Your unconditional love provided me with the confidence to follow my dreams. Mom, your positive outlook on life instilled in me the ability to always see the light in things—a priceless gift. Dad, thank you for showing me how to be a father. Your love let me experience the special bond between a father and son. I owe you everything for that lesson; it means the world. Thank you for being the best parents I could have ever asked for. . . . You both gave all of yourselves, and I am forever grateful.

My sisters, Laurie and Chris—Thank you for letting me share our stories. Laurie, you are one of my greatest inspirations. Chris, I believe in you; please remember how special you are. Love you both so much!

Chelsea Handler—Your kindness, generosity, and passion are an inspiration to me. Thank you for creating time to provide me with the guidance and advice I needed. You are simply amazing. I cherish our friendship; we are family. I also want to thank you for believing in me and sharing your story. Your actions show others what is possible with their health and provide them with the motivation to stay the course. Love you, C.J.

Nancy Hancock—Your leadership, patience, and vision made this book come to life. From our first conversation, you just "got" me. My message became our message. My words became our words. We began our journey as author and editor, and we have evolved into partners and friends for life. M.B. was so right . . . you are by far the best editor in the publishing world. Words cannot express my gratitude for all you have done . . . so I will simply say . . . thank you—along with a giant bear hug!

Michael Broussard—M.B., you have been right by my side every step of the process. Your knowledge, expertise, insight, and friendship have meant everything. You kept me calm when I felt the stress coming, you made me laugh when I had a tough day, and you told me the truth when I needed to hear it. I agree with Chelsea 100 percent: you are the best book agent in the business!

Greg Ray and Michelle Lemons-Poscente—Greg and Michelle, what a future we have together. I often think of New York—what an adventure. I knew no matter what happened those three days, the entire ISB team was all in. I will always remember how your and M.B.'s support gave me the strength I needed to be my best. I know this is just the beginning for us, and I look forward to many exciting adventures ahead.

HarperCollins Publishing—From the beginning your team has been magnificent. Thank you for providing me with the opportunity to write the book I have always wanted to write and live a dream. You have my forever appreciation.

Vaughan Risher—You have a special gift in turning my vision into graphics. Being able to share ideas with you and collaborate on concepts helped fine-tune each chapter. Thank you for your consistency, commitment, and creativity. You are one of a kind.

Chef Valerie Cogswell—You possess the rare ability of making healthy food delicious! Thank you for creating such tasty recipes and helping to enhance the meal plans. Your culinary insight is powerful, and your dedication to get things right is what makes you exceptional.

Venice Nutrition Success Stories—Thank you, Shana, Tom, Don, Amy, Eric, Jennifer, Scott, Kati, Dave, Rachel, Paula, Bill, Brendan, Tally, Bonnie, Sandy, Joe, Claudette, Jim, and Megan, for sharing your personal stories with the world. They provide hope for what can be, showing others that they, too, can achieve Body Confidence. You have each touched my heart in a special way. My love to you all.

The Photo Team—Thank you Chris Calhan, Bob Mahoney, Gayle York, and William David Salon for your professionalism, direction, and fantastic quality of work. Your sharpness enabled each photograph to capture the true meaning of Body Confidence. I would also like to thank Matt, Erika, Patti, and the Forum Athletic Club for each of their contributions to the photo shoot and their commitment to Venice Nutrition.

VN Leadership Team—My team—Abbi, Matt, Dave, Donna, Andrea, Vaughan, Valerie, Pam, Joanne, Bryen, Steve, and Nicole: You each know how much you mean to me and that everything we have accomplished is because of our team. Together we have fought the tough battles and won. Through our journey you have each stayed true to the VN message with pure integrity and authenticity. Thank you for always believing.

Venice Nutrition Community: Members, Coaches, and Partners—This book belongs to all of us. Thank you for choosing to lead a new level of thinking in the health industry and for being part of the Venice Nutrition mission.

INDEX

Body Confidence Plan components: sleep, 75–80, 316; stress, 86–93; vitamins, minerals, omega-3 fatty acids, 80–83, 102–3; water, 83–86. *See also* exercise; nutrition

Body Confidence Plan concepts: accept that you will plateau, 296–303; acknowledge your little victories, 303–4; be unattached to the outcomes, 306–7; create positive escapes, 304–5; evaluate Costs Versus Payoffs, 305–6; have fun, 307–9; pace yourself, 294–96. *See also* process

Body Confidence System: every Sunday prepare for upcoming work, 313–14; importance of creating a, 312–13; pack workout bag each night, 314; prepare your food in bulk, 315; schedule weekly grocery-shopping day, 314; traveling with MRFK containers, 314

body fat: body-fat percentage, 46, 47–48, 52; essential, 49; Four Levels of Health, 49–51; methods for measuring, 47; two types of, 46–47

body-fat percentage, 46, 47–48, 52

body-fat scale, 47, 52

body-part measurements, 52

body's fuel: carbohydrates for "brain fuel," 100–101; fat as "fat-burner fuel," 101–3; protein for muscle, 98–100. *See also* meal strategies

body type: ectomorph, 33, 37–40, 326; endomorph, 33, 34, 42–43; mesomorph, 33–34, 40–41; set point relationship to, 33, 36; understanding different, 32–33

Bonnie's story, 301–3

"brain fuel," 100–101

breads, 250

breakfast recipes. *See* recipes

Brendan's story, 288–89

C

caffeine, 115–16, 118

caffeine-free soda, 117

calorie-free sugar substitutes, 254

calories: body's requirement for, 97; "calories in versus calories out"

philosophy on, 3, 15; sauce and salad dressing, 113

calories per meal: blood-sugar stabilization and, 21; female 250-calorie (goal type 1), 138–60; female 300-calorie (goal type 2), 185–207; male 400-calorie (goal type 1), 161–84; male 500-calorie (goal type 2), 208–43

carbohydrates: as "brain fuel," 100–101; broken down into glucose, 20; cravings for, 20, 24–25; food-exchange system on, 249–51; fruits and vegetables, 249–50; grains and potatoes, 250; identify which ones work better for you, 135; meal strategies for eating, 109, 111–12; miscellaneous, 251. *See also* nutrition

cardio duration, 269–70

cardio exercise: description of, 260, 261; fat-burning (or aerobic), 263, 264–65, 266–67, 269–70, 271; five core principles of, 261–73; goal type 2 and, 265; high-intensity (or interval training), 263, 264–65, 267–68, 269–70, 271, 317; maximizing your, 271; proper footwear worn during, 273; protecting your joints, 273; stretching prior to, 261; when to adjust or minimize, 317

cardio exercise principles: cardio selection for fat burning, 261, 265–68; implementing two types of cardio, 261, 262–65; importance of cardio technique, 261, 272; intensity and duration, 261, 268–70; list of five core, 261; oxygen line and heart rate, 261, 268–69, 271

cardio machines, 269, 280

cardio target heart rate, 268–69

cereals, 250

cheat meal, 124–26

chronic stress, 87

Clarke, Steven, 1

Claudette's story, 319–21

climbing stairs, 266

coffee, 116

cold cereals, 250

complete protein: blood-sugar stabilization through, 99–100;

flavorings, 254

flight-or-fight response, 87

food-exchange system: calorie-free sugar substitutes, 254; carbohydrates, 249–51; condiments, 253–54; description of, 137, 244; fats, 251–52; flavorings, 254; four guidelines for using, 244–46; "free foods," 136, 253–54, 319; meal replacements, 252–53; premade desserts, 253; protein, 247–49; seasonings, 253–54; spices, 253–54; VeniceNutrition.com automated, 246; weight and volume measurements for, 245

food pyramid, 3, 18

foods: for breaking through your plateau, 298–99; free foods, 136, 253–54, 319; making adjustments when necessary, 316–17; measure and journal your, 121–22; preparing in bulk, 315; Quality of Food, 104–6, 119; weekly grocery-shopping for, 314. *See also* Jump Start Phase; meal strategies

Foster, Claudette, 319–21

Foster, Joe, 319–21

Four Levels of Health, 49–51

free foods, 136, 253–54, 319

friends and family: Body Confidence process by including, 317–18; exercising together, 319; Joe and Claudette's story on including, 319–21; leading by example, 318; utilizing your recipes/"free foods" with, 319

fruits, 249

fun mind-set: remembering to continue, 307–8; Sandy's story embodying, 308–9

G

gender differences: essential body fat and, 49; female goal type 1, 138–60; menstrual cycle and water retention, 51; nutrition parameters, 128; water requirements, 85. *See also* meal plans

gestational diabetes, 16–17, 326

glucagon hormones, 19–20

glucose: carbohydrates broken down into, 20; low blood-sugar level and need for, 23. *See also* blood-sugar levels

Goal Type 1 (weight loss): Body Confidence goal-setting guidelines for, 59–61; breaking through your plateau exercise strategies, 299; female 250-calorie meal plans, 138–60; goal-setting time frames for, 60–61; Jennifer's story on, 56–58; lose body weight/body fat/tone up as, 53, 56–61; male 400-calorie meal plans, 161–84; Scott's story on, 56, 58–59; setting goal of, 53; workout routine for, 283–84. *See also* Body Confidence goals; health goals; weight

Goal Type 2 (weight gain): breaking through your plateau exercise strategies, 299–300; Dave's story on, 63–64; female 300-calorie meal plans, 185–207; gain weight/increase strength/build muscle mass, 53, 61–67; goal-setting for, 53; goal-setting time frames for, 65–67; guidelines for, 65; Kati's story on, 61–63; male 500-calorie meal plans, 208–43; workout routine for, 283. *See also* Body Confidence goals; health goals; weight

Gottschalk, Jim, 323–24

grocery-shopping, 314

H

Haddock, Sandy, 308–9

Hall, Megan, 325–27

Hall, Zeke, 327

Handler, Chelsea, 255

having fun mind-set, 307–9

HCl (hydrochloric acid), 102

health: balancing your Quadrants, 93–95; blood-sugar stabilization for achieving, 21–23; four levels of, 49–50; knowing your "why" about, 71–74; making a priority of your, 12

health goals: blood-sugar stabilization for achieving your, 21–23; breaking through your plateau by reassuring your, 300–301; your metabolism as starting point to achieve, 31–32. *See also* Goal Type 1 (weight loss); Goal Type 2 (weight gain)

ABOUT THE AUTHOR

Mark Macdonald opened the first Venice Nutrition Consulting Center in Venice Beach, California, in 1999. Since then, the company has grown to include more than 350 centers, 4,000 Nutrition Coaches, and 250,000 clients nationwide. In 2006, eager to bring his successful program to a wider audience, Mark launched Venice Nutrition Online, a fully interactive online version of the program that makes Venice Nutrition available anywhere in the world.

The product of Mark's own lifelong interest in health and fitness, the Venice Nutrition Program is, first and foremost, about empowering every individual to achieve their ideal body. First as a college athlete, and later as a professional fitness model, nutritionist, and personal trainer, Mark grew frustrated by incomplete health "solutions" and restrictive diets. He set out to learn how the human body really works and discovered the power of blood stabilization. After years of study, and extensive work with clients from all walks of life, he designed the powerful three-step system that's now available in *Body Confidence*.

About Venice Nutrition

For over a decade, Venice Nutrition has been educating people on how to realistically work nutrition, fitness, and a healthy lifestyle permanently into their world. We are accomplishing our mission through three tools: the Venice Nutrition Program itself, which focuses on stabilizing an individual's blood-sugar levels with Venice Nutrition's 3-Step System; our Nutrition Coach certification and licensing system, overseen by our Medical Board and available to health professionals and health-related businesses aligned with our mission; and our Workplace Wellness program, designed for companies that want to create a new culture of health throughout their organization. For information about each of these services, or to find a Venice Nutrition Consulting location near you, please visit us at *www.VeniceNutrition.com*.